MAXWELL'S
UNDERSTANDING ENVIRONMENTAL HEALTH

HOW WE LIVE IN THE WORLD

THIRD EDITION

DEBORAH ALMA FALTA, PhD, MPH

Senior Lecturer
Department of Public Health Sciences
Clemson University

JONES & BARTLETT
LEARNING

World Headquarters
Jones & Bartlett Learning
5 Wall Street
Burlington, MA 01803
978-443-5000
info@jblearning.com
www.jblearning.com

Jones & Bartlett Learning books and products are available through most bookstores and online booksellers. To contact Jones & Bartlett Learning directly, call 800-832-0034, fax 978-443-8000, or visit our website, www.jblearning.com.

Substantial discounts on bulk quantities of Jones & Bartlett Learning publications are available to corporations, professional associations, and other qualified organizations. For details and specific discount information, contact the special sales department at Jones & Bartlett Learning via the above contact information or send an email to specialsales@jblearning.com.

34807-1

Production Credits
VP, Product Management: Christine Emerton
Director of Product Management: Laura Pagluica
Product Manager: Sophie Fleck Teague
Content Strategist: Sara Bempkins
Project Specialist: Roberta Sherman
Digital Project Specialist: Rachel DiMaggio
Senior Marketing Manager: Susanne Walker
VP, Manufacturing and Inventory Control: Therese Connell

Composition: Exela Technologies
Project Management: Exela Technologies
Cover Design: Kristin E. Parker
Media Development Editor: Faith Brosnan
Rights Specialist: Rebecca Damon
Cover Image (Title Page, Chapter Opener):
   © Weiming Chen/Getty Images
Printing and Binding: LSC Communications

Library of Congress Cataloging-in-Publication Data
Names: Falta, Deborah Alma, author.
Title: Maxwell's understanding environmental health: how we live in the world / Deborah Alma Falta, MPH, PhD.
Other titles: Understanding environmental health
Description: 3rd edition. | Burlington: Jones & Bartlett Learning, [2022] | Revision of: Understanding environmental health / Nancy Irwin
   Maxwell. 2nd ed. 2014. | Includes bibliographical references and index. | Summary: "Maxwell's Environmental Health takes a unique
   approach to presenting Environmental Health. Rather than organizing topics around the traditional regulatory fields (air and water
   pollution, hazardous wastes, radiation, etc.), this book is structured around the choices we make as individuals and societies that
   result in environmental health hazards. Hence the subtitle: "How We Live in the World"–Provided by publisher.
Identifiers: LCCN 2020042697 | ISBN 9781284207224 (paperback)
Subjects: LCSH: Environmental health.
Classification: LCC RA565 .M383 2022 | DDC 613/.1–dc23
LC record available at https://lccn.loc.gov/2020042697

6048

Printed in the United States of America
25 24 23 22 21   10 9 8 7 6 5 4 3 2 1

Dedicated to

My parents, Dalton and **Kay James**, in appreciation of the ways they demonstrated care for both people and the planet.

—Deborah Alma Falta

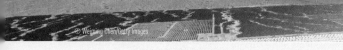
© Weiming Chen/Getty Images

Brief Contents

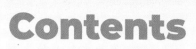
© Weiming Chen/Getty Images

Contents

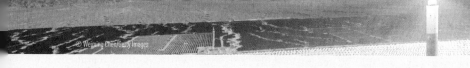
© Weiming Chen/Getty Images

Preface

This third edition updates, and reorganizes, Nancy Maxwell's comprehensive overview of significant concepts in the field of environmental health while ensuring that the information still resounds with her clear, wise, and insightful "voice." A majority of the figures and sidebars are retained from the last edition, but this edition now includes 15 case studies addressing contemporary issues. Another change that readers of the previous edition will notice is that a complete summary table of pertinent federal legislation is now located in the appendix instead of as partial summary tables within each chapter.

The first three chapters of the textbook provide readers with the social, scientific, and technological background for understanding current perspectives about mitigating environmental health risks. Chapter 1 offers several ways to conceptualize the term "environment", stressing ecological, scientific, and social dimensions, then continues on, describing the public health perspective that the field of environmental health focuses on the health risks that humans face from their environment. Economic concepts associated with Hardin's "Tragedy of the Commons" and Environmental Kuznets Curves are introduced to help provide further perspective for understanding why different communities experience different health risks associated with regional and global environmental hazards.

Chapter 2 has been abbreviated to focus primarily on the scientific methods employed to address the question of specific risks associated with environmental exposures. The chapter commences with the characterization of the fate and transport of environmental agents throughout the atmosphere and hydrologic systems. Chapter 2

retains the toxicological, human exposure assessment, and epidemiologic information from the previous edition. Chapter 2 concludes with an overview of the quantitative risk assessment steps involved with specific human health threats from environmental exposures. Several important terms are introduced in Chapter 2 which are highlighted in subsequent chapters with further elaboration of critically associated concepts.

Chapter 3 is new to this edition and specifically addresses the issues related to management of environmental health risks, elaborating on material that had elaborating on material that had been at the end of Chapter 2 in the previous edition. The "cradle-to-grave" life cycle perspective and the story of Love Canal that lead to the passage of CERCLA help to explain the concept of "acceptable risk" as one type of environmental management perspective as compared with other perspectives, such as the Precautionary Principle. Case studies are used to describe the various environmental management perspectives. This chapter also describes the public's willingness to accept any risk from environmental exposures, as influenced by perceptions of personal control, and dread of the outcome demonstrated in recent legal court decisions, such as the recent glyphosate (Roundup) settlement. The chapter concludes with an overview of the various agencies involved with environmental risk protection policies and regulatory strategies.

Chapter 3 in the 2nd edition, titled, "Living with Nature," has now become Chapter 4 and still provides Maxwell's wonderful overview of biological agents of environment concern in the section on infectious diseases. The subsequent material reviewed in this chapter still focuses on those risks from our environment that feel "outside human control," such as electromagnetic radiation and natural disasters.

For the next three chapters, the goal was to provide readers with an understanding of the impact of modern human activities on global resources as well as on human health. The chapters addressing the production of energy and food have been rearranged in this edition from their order in the second edition for two reasons. I have found that my students are particularly interested in, and knowledgeable about, dietary issues, so it helps to engage them and to encourage their confidence to contribute to the course if this material is covered earlier during the semester. Also, the material on food production now follows the material about harmful biological agents (or pests) since modern agricultural practices rely extensively on the use of pesticides. Chapter 5 now includes an introductory discussion of historical concerns as well as contemporary strategies related to sustainably feeding a growing global population. Many of the concepts introduced in Chapter 2 are highlighted in Chapter 5 and explain health concerns associated with modern food production, such as antibiotic resistance and eutrophication of marine environments.

Chapter 6, "Producing Manufactured Goods," addresses the toxicity of organic chemicals and metals, including a case study describing recent health concerns with perfluorinated compounds. An overview of health concerns associated with other occupational exposures is included. Chapter 7 is now the former edition's Chapter 4, addresses "Producing Energy." The material about U.S. fossil fuel resources has been updated to reflect our reduced reliance on imports and incorporates a direct comparison of both the human and environmental impacts associated with energy production (from acquisition to disposal) utilizing various fuel resources. This chapter still provides the information on criteria air pollutants and the Clean Air Act, as well as a comprehensive discussion of climate change associated with the release of greenhouse gases.

The final chapter, "Living in the World We've Made," has the same format as in the previous edition, containing material on liquid and solid waste management with additional information regarding the disposal of plastics and hazardous wastes (including electronics), and medical wastes. The chapter concludes with the emphasis of our modern lifestyle on the ability of our planet to sustain us. Readers are encouraged to continue to learn more and to make informed decisions regarding the risks they are most concerned about and to use their knowledge to advocate for local, national, or global solutions.

Acknowledgments

My passion for the subject of environmental health began as a graduate student in Dr. Dade Moeller's course where he not only shared his knowledge and enthusiasm but also his wise counsel and encouragement. When I began teaching the subject at Clemson University almost 30 years ago, I was so pleased to use Moeller's textbook as a method of sharing his gentle insight. However, I am also indebted to several other authors of environmental health textbooks for their guidance regarding how best to teach this subject. I relied consistently on Dr. Robert Friis' texts to clearly present the basics of environmental health to my primarily undergraduate students, and Dr. Howard Frumkin's comprehensive text to answer specific student queries. I also appreciated the advocacy voiced by Anna Nadakavukaren, as well as that of Nancy Maxwell, throughout their course materials.

I am so grateful to the hundreds of caring and enthusiastic students who demanded that I provide them with a clear, comprehensive, and interesting course. I am also thankful to my Public Health Sciences Department colleagues for allowing me to share the field of environmental health with our students and for supporting our various Earth Day course-related activities for all of these years. I owe a specific debt of gratitude to the members of my doctoral committee (Bob Fjeld, Tim DeVol, Fred Molz, and Bruce Yandle) for their patience and imparted wisdom. Additionally, I offer a broader "thank you" to the entire faculty and staff in the Environmental Engineering and Earth Science Department for their academic support and encouragement.

This project would not have happened without Sophie Teague of Jones & Bartlett Learning, who not only pitched the idea to me but also bolstered my confidence in that I was actually well qualified to attempt this revision effort. Many thanks to Sara Bempkins, as well, for promptly answering my many emailed questions with her positive and upbeat demeanor.

I am grateful to my daughters, Sarah and Lisa, for their enthusiasm and motivation when I felt especially daunted by this undertaking. I appreciate knowing that they believe in me. Finally, I thank my dear husband, Ron Falta, not only for his steady support, encouragement, and clever insights, but for sharing with me his interest in creating a cleaner and healthier environment.

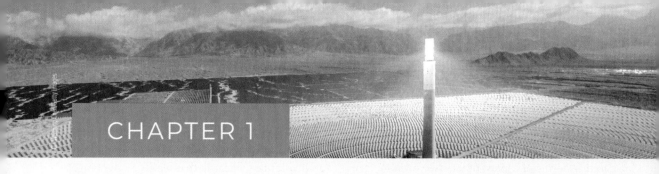

CHAPTER 1

Environmental Hazards to Human Health

LEARNING OBJECTIVES

After studying this chapter, the reader will be able to:

- Define or explain the key terms introduced throughout the chapter
- Provide various conceptual definitions for the term *environment*
- Define and describe the scope of environmental health
- Discuss the social and economic characteristics of environmental health hazards

The title of this chapter is intended to be a warning for those readers who begin this book intent on saving the planet. Although public health practitioners within the environmental health field may care strongly about the ecological health of the world, the discipline's primary concern is centered on the well-being of humans. The goal of environmental health is to promote health for all through a healthy environment and its primary objective to better understand how environmental exposures are hazardous to human health.[1]

1.1 Describing Environmental Health

With this human-centered perspective in mind, one might define the concept of environment as everything within compared to the exterior of the human body.[2] The inner environment consists of a person's various organs and metabolic processes as influenced by unique genetic inheritance compared with the outer environment being all factors outside of the skin. This definition brings up the question of how these external factors influence the interior environment, or to be specific, what are the exposure pathways for external agents to get inside? Ingestion, inhalation, and dermal contact are the obvious exposure routes, but the psychological perception route should not be overlooked.

Another anthropogenic definition of the environment is to describe the indoor versus outside environment. Many environmental health departments partition their specialists into an indoor (or healthy homes) division compared with other groups focused on monitoring and regulating outdoor air or water quality. Despite their focus, all groups must still address the various routes of environmental exposures. For example, secondhand smoke and radon exposure are primary concerns for indoor air specialists compared with outdoor air experts concerned with ozone and particulate matter concentrations.

An environment might also be conceptualized in terms of a person's lifestyle or voluntary exposures, such as smoking or drinking alcohol, compared with involuntary exposures to contaminated air or water in the surrounding environment.[2] These types of involuntary exposures often elicit vocal outrage primarily because they are outside of a person's control, even if the voluntary behaviors are thought to be responsible for causing more human disease. For example, Doll and Hill estimated in the 1980s that less than a quarter of all cancers were attributed to environmental exposures, an estimate that appears to still be fairly accurate.[3]

However, science tells us that the environment is a complex system of living things and natural processes, and that the human species is just one player in this web—albeit a player with a disproportionate impact. All matter exists in either a solid, liquid, or gaseous state that may pose a chemical, biological, or physical exposure. Exposure to chemical hazards includes industrial pollutants, pesticides, lead, and a long list of other agents. Biological hazards encompass the agents of infectious disease, such as the coronavirus, which is responsible for the COVID-19 global pandemic. However, the category is also much broader, ranging from molds that trigger allergic reactions all the way to genetically modified food plants. Physical hazards stem from contact with some form of energy. Radiation, noise, airborne dust particles, mechanical injury hazards, and extremes of heat and cold are all physical hazards.

Compared with the complexities of attempting to define the term *environment*, environmental health may be defined as simply the subfield of public health concerned with the well-being of humans as related to their environment. A more comprehensive description must include the role that humans play in creating an environment that is either healthy or

hazardous.[4] The primary objective of environmental health is concern with assessing and controlling the impact of collective human activities, such as from industrial processes, on the natural resources needed for human survival. Environmental health primarily addresses the involuntary hazards that we face breathing, ingesting, or handling polluted air, water, food, or manufactured goods. For example, addressing the respiratory risks posed to the wait staff in a restaurant associated with secondhand smoke falls within the scope of environmental health whereas promoting smoking cessation campaigns lies outside of the purview of environmental health practice.

1.2 Overview of Chapter Organization

As this text provides an overview of environmental health issues, the focus is fundamentally about how we live in the world. The first few chapters address the social, scientific, and technological characteristics of environmental health. In addition to the concepts introduced in this chapter, Chapter 2, "The Science of Environmental Health," presents readers from different backgrounds with some key toxicologic and human exposure concepts and Chapter 3, "Managing Environmental Health Risks," discusses regulatory principles, and technological mitigation strategies.

Chapter 4, "Living in the Natural World," describes the hazards associated with being grounded in nature and resource competition by other species. Chapter 5, "Producing Food," describes the major approaches used to sustain the ever-growing human population.

In the remaining chapters, the focus shifts to modern Western-style development. By the standards of any earlier era, the residents of today's more developed countries are simply awash in stuff—from appliances and electronic gadgets to household chemicals and plastic objects. The biologist and early environmentalist Barry Commoner once noted that in an ecosystem, nothing ever goes away, [5] and so society's stuff, along with its byproducts, may move around or be transformed in the environment, but will not simply disappear. Thus modern development, wherever it occurs around the world, brings burdens along with its benefits. Chapters 6 through 8 address these questions: Where does stuff come from? Where does stuff go? How do we make, use, and dispose of all of our stuff? And how do all these activities affect human health? For example, when we use oil or uranium as fuel, it doesn't disappear but rather is transformed into energy and waste. Chapter 6, "Producing Manufactured Goods," provides this environmental health context for our durable goods and consumer products as well as addressing water quality concerns associated with modern production practices. Chapter 7, "Producing Energy," describes the environmental health consequences of using fossil and nuclear fuels as well as some alternatives to these energy sources. Chapter 7 also addresses air quality health standards and regulations. When we produce material goods and foods, we transform raw materials into products and waste. The final chapter, "Living in the World We've Made," considers the environmental health concerns of sharing the world we have created. This chapter ranges from local issues— in the communities where people consume food and water, use consumer goods, and produce waste in the form of sewage and trash—to global concerns about sharing the world's resources, present and future.

1.3 Environmental Health Hazards

The specific types of health hazards that humans face from environmental exposures depends greatly upon where they live and their economic status. The majority of acute infections associated with pollution that result in deaths from diarrheal diseases, observed primarily in children, occur in the least developed* and most densely populated homes in the world.[6] Lack of access to safe drinking water, sanitation, and hygiene combined with poor indoor air quality from the use of biomass fuels and inadequate ventilation create homes that pose real risks from biological agents.[7] Homes within the poorest sections of urban communities also lack the space and distancing that traditionally allowed for natural mitigation of airborne or waterborne biohazards when the world was less populated. The environmental engineering adage "dilution is the solution for pollution" is just not feasible in a world of almost 8 billion people where more than half reside in densely populated cities.[8]

As economies develop, these traditional and more biological types of household risks diminish as communities have the resources to provide access to cleaner water and sanitation. However, the urbanization and industrialization associated with improving economies brings about a new set of health hazards associated more with community-level environmental exposures, such as increased traffic and greater concentrations of particulate matter in the air. Exposure to hazardous environmental agents from chemical pollution feature more prominently at the community level. Diseases associated with community-level exposures include more chronic and noninfectious disorders, such as asthma, and concern with diseases involving longer latency periods, such as cancer or developmental disorders.[7]

---

*This text follows the United Nations in using the term *more developed countries* to refer to all European and Northern American countries, plus Japan, Australia, and New Zealand; the term *less developed countries* refers to all of the world's other countries; and the term *least developed countries* refers to a designated subset of the less developed countries (United Nations, Population Division, Department of Economic and Social Affairs, World Population Prospects: The 2010 Revision [table] (POP /DBWPP/Rev.2010/F0-1), 2011. Available at: http://esa .un.org/unpd/wpp/Excel-Data/WPP2010_F01 _LOCATIONS.XLS. Accessed March 2, 2012. Among the less-developed countries, China, India, and Brazil stand out as having large and rapidly growing economies. Although there is no widely agreed-upon definition of "development," the term generally connotes both population health and economic well-being.

From Cholera to Chloroform

The shift in what people worry about in their drinking water demonstrates the evolution from household to community-level pollution concerns. Over the centuries, millions of people have died from infectious diseases spread through contaminated drinking water and waterborne diarrheal diseases still kill far too many children today. One reason John Snow is revered as the *father of epidemiology* (see discussion in the next chapter) is because he recognized the role that domestic sewage played in polluting drinking water supplies during the massive cholera outbreaks in London during the 1850s. The *Vibrio cholerae* bacteria cause excessive diarrhea, if untreated, and potentially fatal dehydration. Modern cholera epidemics still ravage communities, such as the outbreak in Haiti in 2016 after Hurricane Matthew when the water treatment systems were destroyed, and the World Health Organization views cholera as an endemic risk for much of the African continent where there is insufficient infrastructure to treat water.

Implementing sanitation strategies to break this cycle of fecal-oral transmission is considered one of the greatest public health advances of our times.[1] One of the first strategies used, and even suggested by Snow, was the introduction of chlorine into the public water supply to kill the pathogenic agents associated with leading diseases, such as cholera and typhoid fever. Chlorinated drinking water was first introduced in the United States in Jersey City, New Jersey in 1908 and was subsequently adopted in more than 1,000 U.S. cities. Correspondingly, the rates of infectious disease observed in the United States decreased by over an order of magnitude within a decade after public drinking water disinfection was implemented.[1]

By the 1970s, an unintended health hazard associated with chlorinating drinking water emerged associated with its disinfection by-products (DBPs), compounds such as chloroform were formed by the reaction of chlorine with naturally occurring organic matter, such as decaying leaves and other plant material, present in the water sources. Toxicologic and epidemiologic research has implicated DBPs in drinking water with bladder cancer, early-term miscarriage, and birth defects as well as aggravating respiratory conditions such as asthma.[2] Several specific categories of DBPs, such as trihalomethanes, are now regulated in the United States, requiring public drinking water suppliers to ensure that levels of these chemicals do not exceed their health-based Maximum Contaminant Level (MCL) standards. Concern with chlorine-associated DBPs has promoted the use of other disinfectants, such as bromide and ozone, but research continues to implicate these alternatives with their own list of potentially hazardous DBPs. The health concerns associated with DBPs fall into the category of community-level risks associated with chemical exposures and resulting in cancers or diseases with more chronic effects.

1. American Chemistry Council (nd). Chlorine chemistry: chlorine and drinking water. Retrieved May 24, 2020 from https://chlorine.americanchemistry.com/Chlorine/DrinkingWaterFAQ/
2. Richardson SD, Postigo C. Drinking water disinfection by-products. In: Barceló D. ed. *Emerging Organic Contaminants and Human Health. The Handbook of Environmental Chemistry*, Vol 20. Berlin, Heidelberg, Germany: Springer. https://doi-org.libproxy.clemson.edu/10.1007/698_2011_125

Further economic development, as that experienced by most developed economies in the world, presently appeared to counter the degradation of environmental resources with hazardous pollution. Kuznets characterized this phenomenon as an inverted U, now known as the **Environmental Kuznets Curve (EKC)**, where increasing degrees of environmental degradation occur when economies are initially improving, but the impact lessens as the economy obtains adequate affluence to conduct business more cleanly.[9] **Figure 1.1** depicts this relationship between environmental hazards and economic development. The impetus for community stakeholders to advocate for cleaner environmental practices depends on the ecological connections between industrial development and its environmental impacts being clearly observable.

Aquatic biological oxygen demand (BOD) in municipal waterways associated with industrial waste water and atmospheric concentrations of sulfur dioxide from smokestack industries have both demonstrated this type of rise and then falling curve. In both of these examples, the scientific

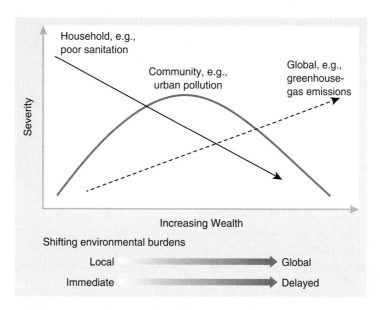

Figure 1.1 Relationship between environmental health severity and increasing wealth as depicted by the environmental kuznets curve.

Reproduced from Smith KR, Ezzati M. How environmental health risks change with development: the epidemiologic and environmental risk transitions revisited. *Annu Rev Environ Resour*, 2005;30:291-333. https://sci-hub.ren /10.1146/annurev.energy.30.050504.144424; https://www.annualreviews.org/doi/pdf/10.1146/annurev.energy.30.050504.144424

and economic connection between the pollution and environmental impact was clearly observable at the community level. Residents who had observed fish kills downstream from industrial discharge pipes could view improvements in water quality when regulations mandated cleaner discharge from such industries at the same time noting that they paid more in taxes to enforce such regulation. The brown smoke associated with SO_2 emissions from burning high-sulfur coal could be observed to become whiter as low-sulfur coal and electrostatic precipitators were substituted, with these higher-priced technologies being incorporated into the cost. Recognition of both the scientific and economic factors connecting anthropogenic activities to environmental degradation appears to be a key influence on whether the EKC trend holds.

A third category of environmental exposures associated with human disease relates to global exposures, such as those from greenhouse gas emissions responsible for climate change.[7] The EKC downward trend has not been observed to occur with global types of pollution because the actual health effects connected to global-level

exposures, such as increases in vector-borne infections, natural disasters, or hunger, are more distally connected than the diseases and their risk factors at the household or community level. The fact that the economies who benefit the most from the anthropogenic release of greenhouse gases, such as fossil fuel combustion for transportation and electricity generation, have not (yet) experienced these associated adverse health impacts has stagnated efforts to mitigate these global hazards.

The economic concept of **externality** further explains this situation. In economic terms, an externality is a cost associated with the use of a resource that is not paid by the user who benefits from its consumption. Hardin explained this concept with his description of a public grazing area ("commons") degraded by its overuse when too many farmers try to feed too much livestock.[9] For each individual user, the benefit of grazing an additional animal vastly outweighs any cost because access to the resource is free. However, the grazing resource has a finite capacity to provide adequate substance and once the number of livestock exceeds its capacity, the resource risks being further depleted with each additional animal. The rational decision to add more livestock at the individual level leads to the ruin of the resource for the group because the cost to maintain the resource is external to individual self-interest.

Before economic development can address human health risks at the global level, the cost of anthropogenic activities external to doing business must be incorporated and the lack of local and community-level perspective about the global ecological connections of all humans trying to survive on the same planet must be addressed. In the 21st century, the underlying reality of environmental health—that our stuff and its byproducts may be transformed or moved around, but does not disappear—is playing out in a changed context. We have begun to see clearly the effects of a general failure to exercise foresight at the societal level: that is, a tendency to make decisions about new products and technologies without much regard for the longer term or the bigger picture. At the same time, globalization is now a fact of life. The natural environment, of course, has always been globally connected, but our appreciation of the global scale of pollution and its impact are more recent. Global trade and travel have become rapid and extensive, with profound implications for environmental health. With this global perspective, it has become clear that Western-style development is not sustainable; that is, the earth simply cannot support the world's entire population in the lifestyle to which the more developed countries have become accustomed. This reality is reflected in the tremendous disparities in environmental health burdens between more-developed and less-developed countries.

Study Question

As you begin your study of environmental health, note any environmental health problems that have been important in your own life or in areas where you have lived.

References

1. Healthy People.gov. Healthy People 2020, Office of Disease Prevention and Health Promotion. (nd) Environmental health. Retrieved April 29, 2020, from https://www.healthypeople.gov/2020/topics-objectives/topic/environmental-health
2. Moeller DW. *Environmental Health* (3rd Ed.). Harvard University Press. 2005.
3. Blot WJ, Tarone RE. Doll and Peto's quantitative estimates of cancer risks: holding generally true for 35 years. *J Nat Cancer Inst.* 2015;107(4):djv044.
4. World Health Organization. Preventing disease through healthy environments: a global assessment of the burden of disease from environmental risks. *WHO.* https://www.who.int/quantifying_ehimpacts/publications/preventing-disease/en/
5. Commoner B. *Making peace with the planet.* Pantheon Press. 1990.
6. Mock CN, Nugent R, Kobusingye O, Smith KR. (2017). *Injury Prevention and Environmental Health* (3rd Ed.). The World Bank.
7. Smith KR, Ezzati M. How environmental health risks change with development: the epidemiologic and environmental risk transitions revisited. *Annu Rev Environ Resour*, 2005;30:291-333.
8. Landrigan PL, Fuller R, Acosta NJR, et al. The *Lancet* Commission on pollution and health. *The Lancet.* 2018;391(10119):462-512.
9. Yandle, B. *Common sense and common law for the environment.* Rowman & Littlefield Publishers, Inc. 1997.

CHAPTER 2

The Science of Environmental Health

LEARNING OBJECTIVES

After studying this chapter, the reader will be able to:

- Define or explain the key terms and concepts introduced throughout the chapter and summarized in **Table 2.1**
- Explain key features of both the atmosphere and hydrologic cycle and explain how these features relate to the distribution of pollutants within the Earth's air and water supply
- Describe how the characteristics of individual chemicals affect their fate and transport in the environment
- Distinguish the key scientific and methodologic domains of environmental health and how they relate to one another
- Present a conceptual model of toxicologic exposure, identifying key events and processes as well as estimates of effects; distinguish between routes and pathways of exposure; and explain the standard units of absorbed dose
- Explain the distinction between descriptive and analytic epidemiologic study designs, compare and contrast the key measures used in surveillance, and discuss criteria for concluding that an association represents a causal connection
- Describe the major steps in a risk assessment for the noncancer and carcinogenic effects of environmental hazards

In this chapter, we describe the science and research methods that enhance our understanding of environmental pollutants and the hazards they pose to people.

- After discussing atmospheric and aqueous characteristics and terms in Section 2.1, we learn about the behavior of contaminants—their chemical or physical transformations, and their movements with or between environmental media, such as air and water. Taken together, these events are commonly

referred to as the **fate and transport** of contaminants in the environment.

- Section 2.2 presents the principles of **toxicology**, the science of the adverse effects of toxic agents—chemicals, including natural toxins, and also physical hazards such as asbestos fibers or radiation—on normal biological structure and function in humans and other living things. In a sense, toxicology continues the story of the fate and transport of environmental contaminants

Table 2.1 Significant Terms and Concepts

Fate and transport	Toxicology	Exposure assessment
Epidemiology	Risk assessment	Limiting factor
Greenhouse effect	Ozone layer	Temperature inversion
Gyre	Thermohaline circulation	Surface water
Aquifer	vadose or unsaturated zone	Saturated zone
Leachate	Lipophilic	Bioconcentration
Bioaccumulation	Xenobiotic	Biomagnification
Persistence	Toxicokinetics	Toxicodynamics
Epigenetics	Teratogenesis	Dose-response
Slope	Threshold	LD_{50}
NOAEL	LOAEL	Biomarkers
Morbidity	Prevalence	Incidence
DALY	Surveillance	Confounding
Rate adjustment	Ecological fallacy	Cross-sectional study
Relative risk, RR	Cohort study	Case-control study
Odds ratio	Bias	Deterministic risk
Stochastic risk	Reference Dose, RfD	Hazard Quotient, HQ
Cancer slope factor, CSF		

into the interior realm, studying their movements, transformations, and ultimate effects in the body.

- The applied science of **exposure assessment** is presented in Section 2.3, providing the methods used to measure or estimate human contact with environmental contaminants. Exposure can be assessed both outside and inside the body, and so exposure assessment not only draws on an understanding of the processes of environmental fate and transport but also on insights from toxicology.
- Section 2.4 describes aspects of **epidemiology** that provide insight into how environmental hazards have directly affected humans. By using specialized quantitative methods and drawing on exposure assessment science, epidemiologic observations

may suggest connections between environmental hazards and health effects before the scientific mechanism is understood.

- The chapter concludes with Section 2.5 describing **risk assessment** as the set of formal procedures for evaluating and integrating scientific information on exposure and toxicity in order to quantify the real-world public health risk of a hazard. Risk assessment is broadly integrative, bringing together information from environmental science, toxicology, exposure assessment, and epidemiology. In environmental health, the formal risk assessment approach is applied mostly to toxicants such as chemicals, particulates, and radiation; however, its influence can also be seen in the evaluation of pathogenic hazards.

2.1 Pollution on Our Planet

The story of human exposure to environmental contaminants begins with the fate and transport of these agents—their transformations and movements—through the atmosphere or an aqueous environment.

The Atmosphere

The Earth's atmosphere, although it may seem formless, has a clear structure and regular patterns of movement.

Layers of the Atmosphere

The innermost layer of the Earth's atmosphere, called the troposphere, extends to an altitude of approximately 8 miles (13 kilometers); within the troposphere, temperature declines with increasing altitude. Most of what we experience as weather takes place in the troposphere.

Air in the troposphere is made up mostly of two colorless, odorless gases: by volume, about 78% nitrogen (N_2) and 21% oxygen (O_2). Human life on this planet is possible because of oxygen, described in ecological terms as a **limiting factor**, a resource required for survival. The concentration of O_2 decreases in the upper regions of the troposphere to levels unsustainable for humans, even at elevation levels for some of our highest mountain peaks. Of the remaining components in the atmosphere, known as trace gases, the most abundant by volume is argon, which is chemically inert; that is, under ordinary conditions, it does not react with other substances. Other trace gases are more important to life on Earth and to public health: In particular, water vapor (H_2O), carbon dioxide (CO_2), methane (CH_4), nitrous oxide (N_2O), and ozone (O_3) all function as greenhouse gases. As the Earth radiates heat energy that it has absorbed from sunlight, greenhouse gases in the troposphere absorb some of that heat and reradiate it back toward the Earth's surface. This return of energy—a natural **greenhouse effect**—keeps the Earth's climate warm enough to support life (see **Figure 2.1**).

Above the troposphere lies the stratosphere, reaching to an altitude of about 30 miles (48 kilometers). Within the stratosphere, temperature rises with increasing altitude. Roughly in the middle of the stratosphere is a layer in which the concentration of ozone is much higher than at other altitudes within the stratosphere. This stratospheric **ozone layer** absorbs much of the incoming ultraviolet radiation from the sun; without this protection, human beings could not live on Earth. (Ozone formed in the troposphere from anthropogenic pollutants, on the other hand, has negative effects on respiratory health, as described later in the context of burning fossil fuels to produce energy.)

Beyond the stratosphere lie the two outer layers of the atmosphere: the mesosphere and the thermosphere. The atmosphere does not have a sharply defined boundary at its outer edge but rather gradually becomes thinner and disappears.

Global and Local Patterns of Air Circulation

On a global scale, prevailing winds at the Earth's surface are easterly in the equatorial region—these are the trade winds, so named because they carried sailing ships on trade routes from Europe to the Americas. In the midlatitudes, both north and south, westerly winds prevail; in the polar regions, easterly winds again prevail. These wind patterns result from the combined effects of two processes—the Earth's rotation and vertical air circulation driven by temperature gradients—and can carry air pollutants over long distances, spreading them both horizontally and vertically.

Regular wind patterns also operate on smaller scales. For example, many coastal locations, where the land heats and cools more rapidly than the adjacent water each day, experience onshore winds during the daytime and nighttime winds that blow out to sea.

More generally, local and regional weather conditions affect the degree of horizontal and vertical mixing of air, and, therefore, the dispersion of pollutants in the air. Such dispersion may actually be visible near a source—for

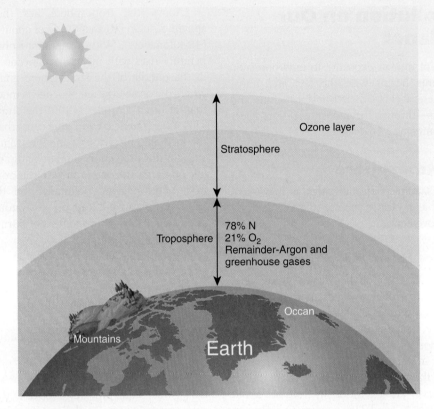

Figure 2.1 The atmosphere.

example, in the form of a plume of smoke trailing from a smokestack, becoming broader and less concentrated with increasing distance from the source.

Sometimes, local weather prevents such dilution of air pollutant concentrations and in extreme cases can turn that pollution into an immediate public health threat. The extreme case of such conditions is a **temperature inversion**, in which a mass of cooler, heavier air becomes trapped at ground level—often in a valley—beneath a layer of warmer, less-dense air. Under this "ceiling," little mixing occurs, and emissions from local sources can accumulate, causing pollutants to reach dangerously high concentrations.

Air pollution comes from either natural or anthropogenic sources. Dust storms, salt evaporation, forest fires, volcanos, mold spores and plant materials, such as pollen, all introduce potentially hazardous pollutants derived from natural sources. Anthropogenic sources are further categorized as either stationary or mobile sources. Emissions from smokestacks, like what is depicted in **Figure 2.2**, are a type of stationary source, and such emissions are part of many industrial processes, such as electricity generation, oil refineries, or incinerators. Mobile anthropogenic sources refer to on- and off-road vehicles, as well as airplanes, ships, and trains, which introduce pollution through combustion engines and their associated "tail-pipe" emissions.

Water in the Ambient Environment

Like the atmosphere, the Earth's water can transport pollutants at global and local scales, in ways both visible and invisible.

The Global Hydrologic Cycle

The Earth's water is connected via a complex web of processes, presented in simplified form in

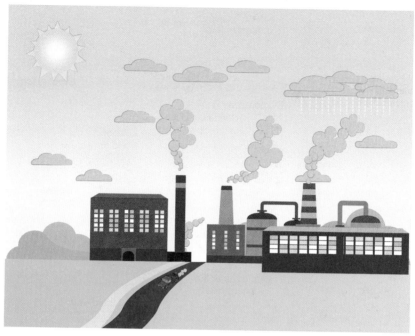

Figure 2.2 Stationary sources of air pollution.

Figure 2.3. Not all aspects of this **hydrologic cycle** are readily apparent: Although oceans, lakes, and rivers are prominent features of the surface environment, both underground water and water vapor are largely invisible.

As shown in Figure 2.3, evaporation and precipitation create a continuous exchange of water between the atmosphere and the Earth's surface. The majority of this exchange occurs between the atmosphere and the ocean. Furthermore, the balance of precipitation and evaporation is different on land and sea: The oceans experience a net loss of water through these processes, while land areas experience a net gain. Most of the excess water from precipitation onto land returns to the oceans via rivers; a much smaller volume returns via groundwater.

Ocean Waters

Ocean currents play an integral role in moderating the Earth's climate, and they also create underwater "climates" supporting populations of fish on which humans depend for food. And, like prevailing winds, ocean currents can carry pollutants for long distances. In January of 1992, a ship en route from Hong Kong to Tacoma, Washington, lost several containers of plastic bath toys overboard during a storm, including 7,200 yellow plastic ducks. The incident occurred near the International Date Line in the Northern Pacific Ocean, south of the Aleutian Islands that extend westward from Alaska. Over the next few years, plastic ducks were recovered at Shemya Island, near the western tip of the Aleutians, at several points along the coast of the Alaska panhandle, and on the Washington and Oregon coasts. In 2003, one well-weathered duck turned up near Kennebunkport, Maine, probably having spun off westward in the Pacific and traveled around the globe.[1]

In oceanology, any large system of circulating ocean currents is termed a **gyre** and there are 11 major gyres described in the world's oceans. The accumulation of marine debris, particularly plastic, has become more of a major concern associated with subtropical gyres than a bunch of floating rubber ducks. Large *garbage patches* form in eddy-like areas within these gyre circulation

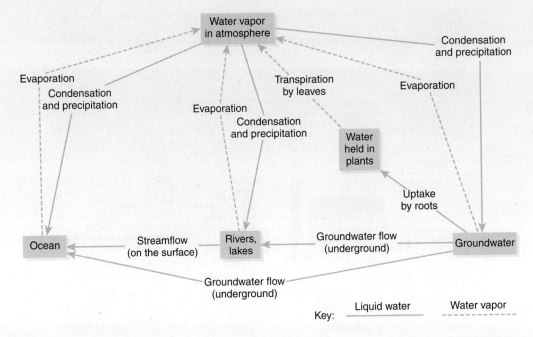

Figure 2.3 Hydrologic cycle.

patterns where debris stalls and creates large masses.[2] Although much of the plastic accumulates, these patches also serve as a source for the release of plastic breakdown products for centuries to come (refer to **Figure 2.4**)

The oceans' major surface currents are driven by friction between air and water and so mimic the global prevailing winds: easterly near the equator and westerly in the midlatitudes. But unlike the winds, these major ocean currents are further deflected by the continents so that they form large rotating cells, flowing clockwise north of the equator and counterclockwise south of the equator. Deeper ocean waters also circulate along predictable paths, moving more slowly than surface waters and looping through all of the world's oceans like a continuous conveyor belt. This process is largely independent of the surface currents, being driven mainly by differences in the density of the water related to temperature and salinity and, therefore, known as the **thermohaline circulation**. The global thermohaline circulation is propelled by events in the North Atlantic. Here, deeper seawater is northbound along the European coast. The northbound water quickly becomes both colder

and saltier (because salt is excluded from ice that is being formed). Both of these changes make the seawater denser, and as a result, it drops suddenly to the ocean floor. This event drives the beginning of a new global circuit by the deep ocean waters influencing how marine pollution is distributed.

Fresh Water

Although the earth's surface is covered largely by water, all but 3% of the planet's water resources are nonpotable ocean water. Humans rely on freshwater for survival, and more than half of all freshwater is unavailable frozen in icecaps and glaciers. Of the remaining freshwater, less than 1% is readily accessible from **surface water** sources, such as lakes and rivers.[3] Typically, a river begins as a set of small streams that converge in stepwise fashion, ultimately uniting as a river. The area drained by a river and the streams that feed it is referred to as the river's drainage basin. Some surface water systems span very large geographic regions; for example, the drainage basin of the Amazon River, with all of its tributaries, extends throughout Brazil.

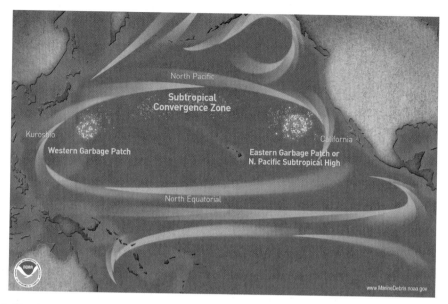

North Pacific

**Subtropical
Convergence Zone**

Kuroshio

Western Garbage Patch

California

**Eastern Garbage Patch or
N. Pacific Subtropical High**

North Equatorial

www.MarineDebris.noaa.gov

Figure 2.4 Plastic garbage patch.

National Oceanic and Atmospheric Administration. https://oceanservice.noaa.gov/facts/garbagepatch.html

Surface water sources of pollution are characterized as either point or nonpoint pollution, an apt description since one may literally *point* to the pollution discharged from industrial or municipal pipes, representing either chemical or biological contamination. Nonpoint sources of water pollution consist of runoff from roads, agricultural activities and construction, sewage overflows, and atmospheric deposition, and can also be chemical or biologic in origin.

Less visible than surface water, and far less familiar to most people, is the water located underground (see the conceptual model in Figure 2.3 and a more comprehensive depiction in **Figure 2.5**). Underground sources of fresh water reside in **aquifers**, geologic material that is porous enough to hold and transmit water through the pore spaces between the geologic material. Aquifers are most often sand or gravel but can be porous rock such as sandstone, or even fractured rock, and they are typically covered by surface soil.

As precipitation soaks into the ground, water moves downward through pore spaces. In the topmost subsurface zone, water may also evaporate or transpire to the atmosphere. Transpiration is a process through which water taken up by the roots of plants is released to the atmosphere through their leaves. Whenever more water enters the topmost zone from precipitation than leaves via evaporation and transpiration, the water moves farther downward.

The area above the water table is called the **vadose** or **unsaturated zone**. In this zone, the pore spaces are partly filled by water. Water that trickles downward through the vadose zone recharges the aquifer—that is, feeds or replenishes it.

Below the vadose zone is the **saturated zone**, in which all pore spaces are filled with water. In the saturated zone, groundwater seeps slowly in response to gradients of elevation and pressure toward a location where water is discharged continuously—for example, via a spring. In most locations, groundwater flows at a rate of only centimeters or inches per day. When speaking of groundwater flow, the term downgradient is used in place of downstream.

The area on the ground surface through which rainfall feeds an aquifer is called the aquifer's recharge area. The lower limit of the aquifer (the floor) is an underlying layer of rock or clay that is impermeable, or nearly so. In a simple geologic

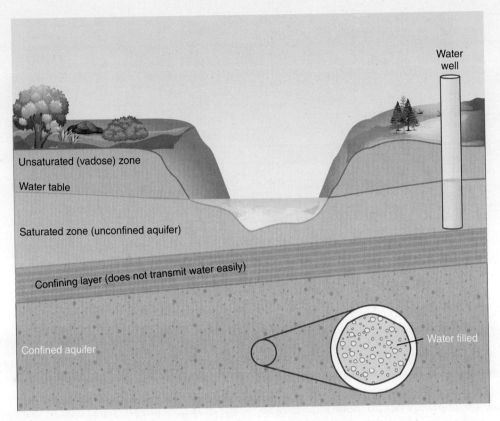

Figure 2.5 Groundwater features.
Special thanks to Ronald W. Falta, Jr.

setting like the one just described, the recharge area is directly above the aquifer, with no intervening impermeable layer. This is called an unconfined aquifer or water table aquifer. The surface of the water table often follows, in muted fashion, the contours of the land surface above. (In fact, contour lines are used to represent the water table surface in maps, much as they are used to represent differences in surface elevation.) If a well is drilled into a water table aquifer—leaving a cylinder made of a fine mesh so that water can flow into the borehole—the water level in the well will be the same as that in the surrounding aquifer.

Wastes or other products placed in the ground or on the Earth's surface within the recharge area of a water table aquifer can contaminate the aquifer. For example, if a chemical such as trichloroethylene is spilled on the ground surface, or dumped into a pit, it can trickle down to the water table. The contamination will then

take the form of a plume as the chemical is carried along slowly with the groundwater, gradually dispersing horizontally and vertically—not unlike an airborne plume of smoke. A well that draws water from within such a plume will produce contaminated water.

Similarly, rainwater percolating downward through wastes placed on the ground surface (or in a pit) can dissolve out or suspend contaminants and carry them along, much as water poured through ground coffee beans dissolves out of the substances that make the water into coffee. Water that has been contaminated by such leaching of contaminants is known as **leachate**.

An aquifer that is sandwiched between layers of impermeable (or nearly impermeable) rock is known as a confined aquifer. Largely isolated from local precipitation, confined aquifers are replenished very slowly and are often considered a finite resource in terms of human lifespans. Today's aquifers were formed long ago and bear the imprint of their geologic histories. In many geologic settings, layers of water-bearing rock alternate with impermeable layers so that aquifers are stacked beneath the Earth's surface. Aquifers vary widely in geographic scale. For example, some 25 aquifers are recognized within Massachusetts; in contrast, the extensive Ogallala Aquifer underlies parts of eight U.S. states from South Dakota to Texas. Once a confined aquifer has been contaminated, from underground storage tanks or purposeful deep-well injection, such as that associated with hazardous waste disposal, it is very difficult and expensive to clean up.

The Fate and Transport of Environmental Contaminants

Environmental contaminants in the ambient environment can be found in air, water, or soil, including soil that is dry and fine enough to become airborne (dust) and soil in bodies of water (sediment). The preceding descriptions of air and water movement in the ambient environment were presented because pollutants are basically passengers along for a ride through the environmental media. However, they are, in a sense, passengers with preferences based on their chemical, biological, or physical properties.

Physical–Chemical Properties of Chemicals

Contaminants have characteristics, known as physical–chemical properties, which affect their behavior in the environment (see **Figure 2.6**). For example, the fate of a liquid chemical spilled on the ground depends partly on its **volatility** (*a*): the tendency to change into gaseous form (to volatilize). In the environment, a highly volatile liquid chemical that is spilled will move rapidly into a gaseous form that cannot easily be cleaned up. Similarly, **aqueous solubility** (*b*) is

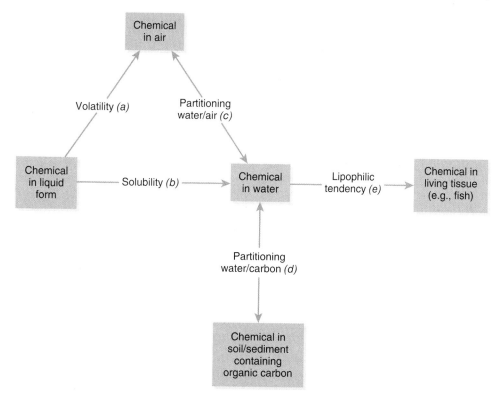

Figure 2.6 Physical-chemical properties of chemicals.

the tendency of a chemical to dissolve in water; a highly water-soluble chemical spilled into a lake is likely to become widely dispersed in the water. (Aqueous solubility is often referred to simply as solubility.)

A third property—a chemical's affinity for water versus air (*c*)—reflects whether the chemical is more soluble than volatile, or vice versa. In conceptual terms, such an affinity represents the division, or partitioning, of the chemical between water and air that would occur if the process reached a state of equilibrium. In practice, the shift toward such an equilibrium state in the environment may be rapid or slow.

Chemicals also show an affinity for soil or sediment—actually, the organic carbon in soil or sediment—versus water (*d*). Chemicals with a high affinity for organic carbon tend to cling to the sediments of a stream, for example, rather than being found in the water. Finally, chemicals vary in their tendency to move from water to an oily medium (*e*). Chemicals having such a tendency are called **lipophilic** (fat-loving) or fat-soluble. Lipophilic chemicals in lakes or streams tend to move into the fatty tissues of aquatic organisms, or bioconcentrate; **bioconcentration** is a biological consequence of these chemicals' lipophilic tendency.*

A chemical that tends to bioconcentrate poses a potential threat to organisms through two further processes. **Bioaccumulation** is the building up of a chemical in an individual organism's tissues over its lifetime as the organism continues to take in more than it excretes. Environmental pollutants that share similar characteristics, such as chemical shape or lipophilic tendencies, to those of human substances are considered **xenobiotics** (*xeno* means foreign), and the location where these foreign chemicals bioaccumulate may be predicted based on the human substance they resemble. For example, a biotransformed chemical product of polychlorinated biphenyls (PCBs) closely resembles the chemical structure

of thyroxine, human growth hormone, and may fool the body into storing it within its fat cells.[4]

Biomagnification is a different process by which a chemical becomes more concentrated in the tissues of organisms at each higher trophic level in a food chain; for example, in big fish that eat smaller fish, and in eagles (or people) that eat the big fish. In contrast to bioconcentration, bioaccumulation and biomagnification are not just properties of individual chemicals but rather processes that take place in organisms and ecosystems.

In practical terms, groups of chemicals with similar properties show similar environmental tendencies. For example, low–molecular-weight solvents such as trichloroethylene and benzene are highly volatile and moderately soluble; they are very likely to become air contaminants but unlikely to cling to soil. At the other extreme, very heavy chemicals such as PCBs and dioxins have very low solubility and volatility; they are unlikely to be air or water contaminants, but rather are found in soil or sediment as well as reside in fat. Chemicals' behavior can also be affected by environmental conditions; for example, a volatile chemical moves from a liquid to a gaseous state more rapidly in warmer weather.

Finally, a chemical in the environment does not persist indefinitely as the same chemical but rather is transformed into other chemicals. A chemical's **persistence** in the environment is often quantified as its half-life in air, water, or soil. The environmental half-life of a chemical in a given medium is the period of time after which one-half of the original quantity is expected to have been chemically or biologically transformed. The term *half-life* is borrowed from radioactive decay; however, unlike radioactive half-life, the environmental half-life of a chemical is only approximate because it is greatly affected by environmental conditions, such as the presence of light or oxygen. The half-life of the pesticide DDT in soil, for example, ranges from about 8 to 15 years. In general, chemicals of higher molecular weight tend to be more persistent. The environmental persistence in soil or sediment of high-molecular-weight, lipophilic contaminants such as DDT or dioxin presents the opportunity for long-term

---

*Some chemicals, including methylmercury, are not highly lipophilic but do concentrate in the muscle tissue of animals.

exposures and thus greater potential for bioaccu-mulation and biomagnification. Even persistent chemicals, however, do not persist indefinitely in the environment, but gradually break down.

2.2 Toxicology: The Science of Poisons

The term *environment* suggests something that merely surrounds us, but we are more permeable than we like to think. People contact—and absorb—environmental contaminants mainly by three major routes of exposure: *inhalation* (mostly through ordinary continuous breathing), *ingestion* (by eating and drinking), and *dermal contact* (via the skin). Toxicology is the study of how the body processes the toxicants to which it is exposed and of the ultimate effects of these toxicants in the body.

In toxicology, the term toxin is reserved for a naturally produced toxic substance, especially one produced by a plant or animal. The term toxicant usually refers to toxic substances that result from human activities, although this definition is stretched to include such naturally occurring agents as toxic metals (e.g., arsenic) or radiation, which are not produced by a plant or animal. In this text, the term *toxicant* is used except when referring specifically to natural plant or animal toxins.

The Disposition of Chemicals in the Body

Whatever the route of exposure, a chemical is absorbed into the body by passing through cell membranes. From the exposure perspective, the linings of the lungs and digestive tract may be thought of as part of the boundary between the external and internal environments—in effect, as extensions of the skin. In fact, absorption via inhalation and ingestion is much more rapid and complete than dermal absorption because the lungs and digestive tract are designed to absorb oxygen and nutrients, whereas the skin is fundamentally a protective barrier.

Exposure to environmental toxicants is often defined as *contact with the human envelope*, and the human envelope is defined in turn as the boundary that separates the interior of the human body from the exterior environment. Exposure is quantified as a **dose**, and **absorbed dose** refers specifically to the amount of some toxicant that passes through the human envelope, entering the body.

After being *absorbed*, chemicals are *distributed* around the body via the bloodstream or the lymph system, and may be *metabolized* (chemically transformed by enzymes) during the course of this journey. Much, though not all, metabolism of chemicals takes place in the liver. The processes of distribution and metabolism interact: A chemical's path through the circulatory system affects how it is metabolized, and how and where it is metabolized determines its chemical form, which in turn affects whether, and how, it is *stored* or *excreted*. These processes are shown in simplified form in **Figure 2.7**. The term metabolite refers to a product of the body's metabolism of a toxicant or toxin.

Lipophilic contaminants, including some pesticides, are stored in fat cells, and lead is deposited in bone (where it substitutes for calcium). However, excretion, by removing some quantity of a toxicant from circulation, can allow some of the same toxicant to be released from storage. Chemicals are not only excreted from the body, mostly in exhaled air, urine, and feces but also in sweat and semen and by deposition in hair and nails, which in this context are seen as being outside of the human envelope. (This is why it doesn't hurt to cut your hair or nails.) Breast milk may also be a route of excretion; from the perspective of the infant, of course, breast milk becomes a source of ingestion exposure.

The combined processes of absorption, distribution, metabolism, storage, and excretion of toxicants are collectively referred to as **toxicokinetics** and determine the disposition of a chemical in the body. The net effect of these processes is reflected in the total burden of the chemical, or of some breakdown product, present in the body at some point in time (the body burden). Of more interest in toxicology, however, is the **biologically effective dose**: The quantity of a toxicant or its breakdown product

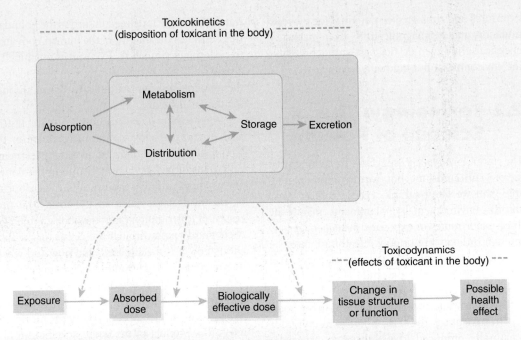

Figure 2.7 Disposition and effects of toxicants in the body.
Special thanks to Wendy Heiger-Bernays and Michael McClean.

that is available to interact with some vulnerable tissue in the body. Such interactions may result in changes in tissue structure or function, which in turn may have an adverse effect on health; the term **toxicodynamics** refers to these latter processes, which constitute the toxicant's actual effects in the body. For example, although there is some speculation that drinking water containing elevated levels of radon may be associated with a small risk of stomach cancer, there is real concern with the lung cancer risk radon gas poses once absorbed from the stomach and carried through the bloodstream to sensitive lung tissue. Together, toxicokinetics and toxicodynamics describe the disposition and effects of toxicants in the body.

The characteristics of the exposure itself—for example, a brief exposure (*acute* exposure) versus a long-lasting and usually lower-level exposure (*chronic* exposure)—may influence the disposition and toxic effects within the body. Exposures to another toxicant may enhance a toxic effect (*synergism*) or interfere with it

(*antagonism*). And finally, many individual characteristics—from age and sex to genetic makeup to health and nutritional status—can affect the fate of a toxicant in the body and make an individual more or less susceptible to its effects. In particular, children's capacity to detoxify chemicals is different from that of adults, and their bodily systems are vulnerable because they are still developing.

Gene–Environment Interaction and Epigenetics

As noted at the beginning of this text, purely genetic hazards do not fall within the scope of environmental health. However, genetic makeup sometimes affects risk through interaction with an environmental exposure, and such gene–environment interactions are currently of great scientific and toxicological interest in environmental health.

There are at least three models of gene–environment interaction. First, a person's genetic makeup (genotype) can increase his or her exposure to an environmental risk factor; for example, a genetic predisposition to nicotine addiction tends to increase exposure to cigarette smoke. Second, genetic makeup can increase a person's susceptibility to an environmental risk factor; for example, different genotypes might result in the production of larger or smaller quantities of enzymes that determine the capacity of cells to repair DNA damage—damage that is the first step on the road to cancer. And finally, genotype and environmental factors can be independent risk factors for a disease, with a combined effect that is additive or more than additive; for example, both a specific genetic trait and cigarette smoking are known to be independent risk factors for Crohn's disease, a chronic inflammatory bowel disease.[5]

An organism's genetic code is found in molecules of **deoxyribonucleic acid (DNA)**, which is present in the nucleus of each cell. This same type of genetic material, with different information encoded, is found in organisms from animals to plants to bacteria and viruses. In higher animals, including humans, chromosomes are matched up in twos: Human genetic material occurs as 46 chromosomes in 23 pairs. The now-familiar double helix structure of the DNA molecule (see the following sidebar titled, "About DNA and the Genetic Code") was first described by British scientists James Watson and Francis Crick in 1953; Crick's working sketch of the molecule appears in **Figure 2.8**.

Mutation is a change to the DNA of a cell. A mutation that causes local damage within a gene—a small part of the DNA molecule gets changed—is called a point mutation. Some point mutations occur spontaneously; others occur when some agent (a *mutagen*) binds chemically to the DNA, causing a change in its structure. Cells have mechanisms to repair DNA damage, but not all damage gets repaired. Mutations that cause broader structural damage to chromosomes—for example, the loss of large sections or reversing parts of a chromosome—are usually fatal to cells. In recent years, environmental scientists

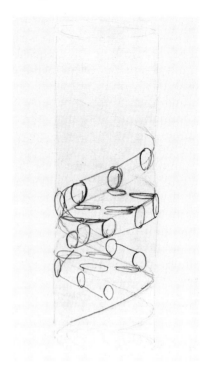

Figure 2.8 Crick's DNA sketch.
Courtesy of Wellcome Library.

About DNA and the Genetic Code

The structure of the DNA molecule is the well-known "double helix," a sort of spiraling ladder in which the long strands are composed of sugars and phosphate groups. Each rung is made up of a pair of bases, and it is the sequence of bases that encodes genetic information. A large molecule of DNA is known as a *chromosome*; sections of chromosomes, each encoding a specific heritable trait, are defined as *genes*, each made up of a set of base pairs. In the rungs of the DNA ladder, the same two bases always pair with one another: adenine with thymine, and guanine with cytosine. When a cell replicates, each chromosome unzips, splitting each of its rungs in two; in this way, each half of the chromosome becomes a template to replicate the other half.

have come to appreciate the importance of *epigenetic effects*—changes in how a gene is *expressed*, without any change to the DNA sequence itself. The term **epigenetics** refers to the concept that some foreign or environmental substance adheres to the genetic surface resulting in either the suppression or expression of different protein enzymes. For example, methyl groups overlaid onto a DNA molecule can change how, or whether, genes are transcribed, the first step toward gene expression. The study of epigenetic effects is a new and rapidly growing area of research. Mutations and epigenetic effects in the cells of the body have varied impacts. As just noted, some mutations are repaired by cellular mechanisms; others have effects so severe that they lead to the death of the cell. Still, other mutations or epigenetic effects become the first step on the path to cancer.

Carcinogenesis

The core scientific endeavor of toxicology is to elucidate how biochemical mechanisms actually lead to toxic effects in the body at the level of molecule, cell, organ, or organ system. This section expands in some detail on one toxic mechanism—carcinogenicity—because it is pertinent to all cancers and because the U.S. regulatory framework handles carcinogenicity differently from all noncancer health effects.

Cancer is a disease of cells. A cancerous cell, dividing without restraint, operates outside of the body's normal controls. A malignant tumor, made up of such cells, first *invades* the tissue where it originated and then *metastasizes* into other tissues, eventually disrupting the functioning of the body. Both genetic and environmental factors can affect an individual's risk of cancer.

Most cancers are believed to result from an accumulation of mutations in genes that direct cell division. Some of these genes (called oncogenes) instruct the cell to divide; others (called tumor suppressor genes) instruct the cell to stop dividing. The mutations that are important for carcinogenesis do one of two things: They either *increase the activity* of genes that instruct the cell to *divide*, or they *inhibit* genes that instruct the cell to *stop dividing*. If enough such mutations accumulate, the result is the runaway proliferation of cells—cancer. Overall, however, the probability of getting enough of the right type of mutations in any given cell is low, making cancer a relatively rare event in the cells of the body.

For some years, the process of *carcinogenesis* has been described as occurring in three stages: initiation, promotion, and progression. Initiation involves a mutation occurring that either enhances instructions to the cell to divide or dampens instructions to stop dividing. This event makes the initiated cell more prone to becoming cancerous. If the mutation is not repaired before the initiated cell divides, the mutation becomes permanent, appearing in all subsequent generations. Promotion describes when an initiated cell can become a population of cells. Such promotion of the initiated cell does not involve further damage to DNA. Instead, through repeated cell division, the initiated cell develops into a large group of identical cells—a benign tumor. Promotion has two effects: It increases the number of initiated cells, and, by making cells divide more often, it narrows the window of opportunity for repair of new mutations. Finally, progression occurs when critical mutations (those that either enhance instructions to the cell to divide or dampen instructions to stop dividing) continue to occur in the initiated cells of the benign tumor. If enough of these mutations accumulate, the result is cascading cell division—a malignant tumor.

Environmental agents can play a role at each of these stages of carcinogenesis: as the cause of the critical mutation that initiates carcinogenesis; as promoters of the initiated cell; and as the cause of the critical mutations that constitute progression, leading to the runaway cell division that is cancer. The term *carcinogen* refers to any agent that increases cancer risk. In more recent thinking, initiation, promotion, and progression are still key elements of carcinogenesis, but the process is no longer conceptualized as a neat time sequence, like a three-act play.

Not all environmental exposures and epigenetic effects cause cancer. A hazardous exposure may cause cell destruction or the resulting tissue or organs to not function correctly, and research into these types of hazards are categorized by the organ systems that they impair. For example, *hepatotoxicity* studies agents that harm the liver, whereas *nephrotoxicity* addresses agents that impact the kidneys and renal function. Some detrimental exposures may result in birth defects. In the language of toxicology, *reproductive toxicity* is the occurrence of an adverse effect on the reproductive system or reproductive capacity of an organism; *developmental toxicity* is the occurrence of an adverse effect on the developing organism, either in utero or during infancy or childhood. **Teratogenesis** refers specifically to the occurrence of a structural defect in the developing organism resulting from an exposure that occurs between conception and birth, and a *teratogen* is a substance that produces such defects.

The Dose–Response Relationship

Whatever the mechanism of toxicity, it is useful to establish the quantitative relationship between dose and a toxic effect (response). Such a **dose–response** relationship is typically summarized in a graph plotting dose on the *x*-axis against response on the *y*-axis. In toxicology, the **slope** of the line in such a graph is typically positive—rising from left to right—reflecting increasing toxicity with increasing dose, as shown schematically in **Figure 2.9a**. A steeper slope indicates a more potent toxic effect—that is, a greater increase in toxic effect for a given increase in dose.

A second important characteristic of a dose–response relationship is the **threshold** (see **Figure 2.9b**). Again, in schematic terms, the threshold dose is the highest dose at which no toxic effect occurs. The practical importance of a threshold (e.g., (*a*) in Figure 2.9b) is that doses

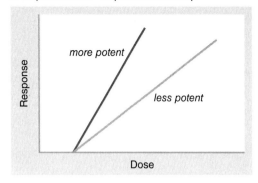

a. Slope of a dose–response relationship

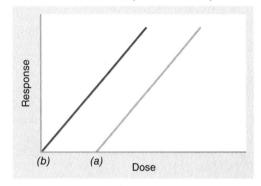

b. Threshold of a dose–response relationship

Figure 2.9 A schematic representation of the basic dose–response relationship.

at or below the threshold dose are without toxic effect. If the threshold dose is zero (*b*), then as a practical matter, there is no threshold and no safe dose.

Now, giving our schematic dose–response relationship a more realistic shape, we show it as a flattened S, referred to as a *dose–response curve* (see **Figure 2.10a**). In such a curve, the flatter slope in the low-dose region (*c*) reflects the body's ability to partially metabolize, detoxify, or excrete a chemical before it causes a response; as these metabolic processes are overwhelmed at higher doses, the slope of the curve becomes steeper in the middle region (*d*). At very high doses, the capacity for a toxic response may be overwhelmed, and this effect

a. Slope

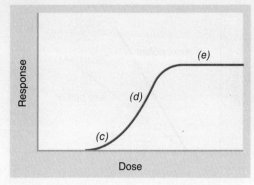

b. Threshold/no threshold

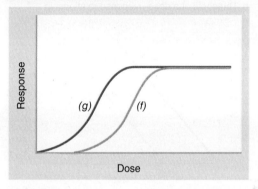

Figure 2.10 The dose-response curve.

appears as a plateau at the top of the dose–response curve (*e*).

Figure 2.10b shows dose–response curves with zero and nonzero thresholds. A wide range of toxicological evidence suggests that nearly all noncancer effects have thresholds; thus, a schematic dose–response curve for noncancer effects has the general form of (*f*). In contrast, the mechanistic model of carcinogenesis as a multi-stage process suggests that any dose, however small, could produce an initiated cell that ultimately results in a malignant tumor; thus, the schematic dose–response curve for cancer has no threshold (i.e., the curve has a threshold of zero), taking the general form of (*g*).

As described later in the context of the toxic effects of chemicals, xenobiotic synthetic organic chemicals mimic or otherwise disrupt the effects of the body's natural hormones. Recent toxicological evidence indicates that at least some of these endocrine-disrupting compounds have dose–response curves with a different shape from those in Figure 2.10.[6] In the classic curves shown in Figure 2.10, the response declines continuously with declining dose (moving from right to left in the graph). But for some endocrine-disrupting compounds, the dose–response curve shows a reversal: an upswing in response in the low-dose region. The result is a curve that is more U-shaped than S-shaped.

Toxicity Testing

Toxicity testing—the practical work of assessing chemicals' toxicity to living things—complements the core scientific work of understanding the biochemical mechanisms of toxicity. This work, done in support of regulatory decision making, is often referred to as regulatory toxicology. In the United States, the National Toxicology Program is the lead entity in conducting regulatory toxicology studies.

In an ideal world, decisions about how to regulate chemicals would be based on studies of health effects in human beings, and in fact, such information is used when it is available. But epidemiologic research is limited by ethical standards that rule out deliberately exposing humans to potentially harmful substances. In contrast, toxicity testing in laboratory animals to serve the interests of human health is generally considered to be ethical. As a result, much of the information used to estimate the toxicity of chemicals in humans comes from toxicity tests in rodents and other laboratory animals. The relatively short lifespan of rodents (about 2 years for mice and rats) also makes such testing practical, because even testing for chronic toxicity can be completed in 2 years.

Preliminary Testing for Toxicity

A 2-year chronic rodent study, which gives information on both cancer and noncancer effects, is a costly undertaking. For this reason, such studies are done only after preliminary screening for toxicity. Toxicity screening is typically conducted in a tiered process, beginning with tests in microorganisms and cell cultures, proceeding to acute and subchronic studies in rodents, and finally to chronic rodent bioassays. Studies in cells or microorganisms are referred to as *in vitro* studies; those in living animals are referred to as *in vivo* studies.

Screening for mutagenic potential in bacteria reflects the current understanding that mutation is integral to carcinogenesis. The mainstay of mutagenicity testing is the Ames test, an assay in which *Salmonella typhimurium* bacteria are exposed to a chemical. The test compares the rate of occurrence of a specific point mutation at different levels of exposure with the test chemical, with and without the addition of rodent liver enzymes (to metabolize the test chemical) and in multiple strains of the bacterium. Most of the organic chemicals that have been clearly identified as human carcinogens have been shown to be genotoxic in laboratory screens such as the Ames test. A separate laboratory assay for larger-scale chromosomal damage in human or animal cell cultures may also be conducted.

In a study of acute oral toxicity, groups of rodents are administered a dose of the test chemical, usually given all at once; several dose levels are used, including some expected to be lethal. Data from such a study are used to calculate the dose that is acutely lethal to 50% of test animals exposed to it; this 50% lethal dose is abbreviated as the **LD$_{50}$**. The LD$_{50}$ is expressed in units of milligrams of toxicant per kilogram of body weight (abbreviated as mg/kg). If exposure is by inhalation, an LC$_{50}$ is calculated; this is the concentration of the chemical in air that is acutely lethal to 50% of test animals in a short time, often 4 hours.

Further preliminary information about a chemical's toxicity in animals is obtained through the subchronic rodent bioassay, a 90-day study. These studies serve at least three purposes. They provide a basis for selecting the doses that will be used in a chronic rodent bioassay. They identify the target organ—in the language of toxicity testing, the organ that is affected first as the dose of a test chemical is increased from zero. And they also identify the need for specialized long-term study of particular effects, such as immunotoxicity, neurotoxicity, or effects on reproduction or fetal development. Although rodent bioassays are a standard approach for assessing the toxicity of chemicals, for some chemicals, testing in rodents has not proved useful in predicting human risk.

The Chronic Rodent Bioassay

The chronic rodent bioassay is about 2 years long, approximately the lifetime of the test animals, and is designed to provide information on both cancer and noncancer effects. Parallel studies are typically conducted in rats and mice; in each study, groups of about 50 animals, male and female, are dosed at three levels; there is also an unexposed control group. Exposure is most commonly by ingestion (in water or food), less often by inhalation.

Very large groups of rodents are needed to study carcinogenicity at the low doses at which people are typically exposed to environmental chemicals. But such enormous rodent studies are impractical in both logistics and cost; instead, rodents are bred to be more genetically susceptible to tumor formation and exposed to very high doses, effectively converting cancer from a rare disease to a common disease and enabling smaller-scale studies. This means that chronic rodent bioassays must be designed to include both a dose high enough to test for cancer without being fatal to the test animals and doses low enough to reveal a no-effect level for noncancer effects, if there is one. The proportion of rodents showing specific effects at each dose is recorded. Specialized testing (e.g., for neurotoxicity, immunotoxicity, or reproductive toxicity) is included.

Results of bioassays in laboratory animals are used to create a dose–response curve for each specific health effect—for example, kidney toxicity. Of course, the results of the assay can document effects only at the doses that were actually administered to the animals in the study, and; therefore, they give a limited view of the true underlying dose–response curve.

Some of the doses used in the study are later given special designations in light of the study's results (see **Figure 2.11a**). For a given effect, the *highest* nonzero dose at which *no* effect was observed in a study is called the **no observed adverse effect level** (**NOAEL**, pronounced "no-ell"), and the *lowest* dose at which an effect *was* observed in a study is called the **lowest observed adverse effect level** (**LOAEL**, pronounced "low-ell"). Neither the NOAEL nor the LOAEL pinpoints the actual threshold of a given effect, such as kidney toxicity, but we can infer that the threshold falls somewhere between the NOAEL and the LOAEL.

However, sometimes *all* of the nonzero doses used in a rodent study show a given noncancer effect; that is, the study does not identify a NOAEL (see **Figure 2.11b**). In this situation, we can infer

only that the threshold is lower than the LOAEL; the study gives no lower bound (other than zero) for the range within which the threshold falls. In this situation, the study does not indicate whether there is, in fact, a nonzero threshold. Furthermore, the study does not indicate the shape of the curve between the LOAEL and zero; in particular, the upswing in effect in the low-dose region that is characteristic of some endocrine-disrupting compounds would not appear in the graph.[6]

For a given toxicant of concern, dose–response curves like these are developed for each cancer and noncancer effect documented in the chronic toxicity study, including the effects documented in specialized studies (e.g., of immunotoxicity, or reproductive or developmental toxicity). These data help toxicologists learn about mechanisms of action and the behavior of toxicants in living systems.

2.3 Exposure Assessment

The preceding sections describe important processes by which chemicals are transported and transformed—in the environment and in the body—and may cause harm. The applied science of exposure assessment is a set of methods to quantify human beings' contact with environmental toxicants. Assessing exposure is quite distinct from assessing toxicity, and both exposure and toxicity are necessary for a health impact to occur.

As described earlier, a conceptual model for toxicology begins with the absorption of a toxicant and ends with its effects in the body (see Figure 2.7). To consider exposure fully, the model in Figure 2.7 needs to be extended backward to begin with the environmental source of a toxicant. This has been done in **Figure 2.12**, while omitting the details of toxicokinetics provided in the earlier diagram. In Figure 2.12, *boxes labeled with capital letters* represent quantifiable estimates or indicators of a toxicant or its effects in the body, and *links labeled with numbers* designate events or processes that connect those estimates.

a. Dose–response curve showing NOAEL and LOAEL

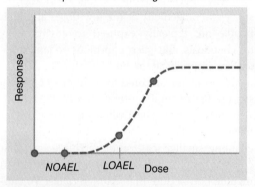

b. Dose–response curve showing only LOAEL

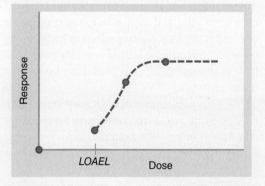

Figure 2.11 NOAEL and LOAEL in a dose–response curve.

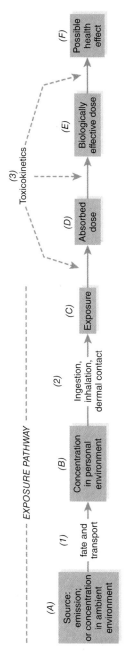

Figure 2.12 Exposure with body disposition.

Special thanks to Wendy Heiger-Bernays and Michael McClean.

Exposure Pathways

Exposure to an environmental contaminant occurs via an exposure pathway that begins with the environmental source of the contaminant (A) and ends with exposure (C), defined as contact between a toxicant and the human envelope. Under certain circumstances, the source (A) is an ongoing emission—for example, the release of lead into the air from the smokestack of a lead smelter. Under other circumstances, the origin of the contamination is harder to pin down in place and time. For example, the lead present in the soil of most U.S. cities today originates from the exhaust of countless moving sources—vehicles using leaded gasoline for decades in the past— and from the lead paint used on millions of houses, some of which are still shedding lead dust into the environment. It isn't really useful to think about these sources of lead as emissions. Rather, it is more useful to think of the source (A) of the lead as its widespread presence in soil, quantified as a concentration.

From either type of source (A in Figure 2.12), chemicals may be transported in air, water, or soil, sometimes being chemically transformed along the way. As a result of the processes of fate and transport, a contaminant may be present at some concentration in a person's immediate surroundings (B).

Exposure Routes

Exposure (C)—contact between a toxicant and the human envelope—occurs by various routes. Most exposures to environmental toxicants occur via three routes: inhalation, ingestion, and dermal contact (2). These are not the only possible routes of exposure to chemicals: Some pharmaceuticals, for example, are delivered by injection into the muscle and others are sprayed into the nostrils to be absorbed through the nasal lining. But exposure to chemicals present in environmental media is usually by inhalation, ingestion, or dermal contact.

People continuously inhale air, of course, and along with it, they inhale dust. At rest, an adult inhales about 360 to 600 liters of air per hour (about 8.6 to 14.4 cubic meters per day).[7] Although children's lung capacity is smaller, they spend more time outdoors than adults do, exercise more, breathe more through the mouth, and tend to entrain a more intense personal dust cloud[8]—a phenomenon sometimes referred to as the "Pigpen effect," after the character in the comic strip *Peanuts*. Skin, too, may come into contact with soil or dust (e.g., while gardening) or water (e.g., while swimming or bathing) or with the toxicant itself, particularly in occupational settings. For young children, even dermal contact with food could be substantial.

People routinely ingest water and food for sustenance. They may also inadvertently swallow small amounts of water (referred to as *incidental* ingestion), perhaps while swimming in a lake or pool. Similarly, if dust is present on the lips, licking the lips leads to incidental ingestion of soil. Touching the lips with the hands conveys soil to the mouth. Both eating and smoking, for example, result in such hand-to-mouth exposures. Under certain circumstances, such incidental ingestion can be substantial—for farmers or construction workers, for example, or for toddlers, who spend a lot of time on the ground (and whose hands spend a lot of time in their mouths).

Contact with an environmental contaminant often occurs through multiple exposure routes. For example, a toddler is exposed to lead in the home mainly by ingestion (incidental ingestion of dust via hand-to-mouth activity) and by inhalation (of airborne dust).

The final elements of Figure 2.12, showing the events following exposure (C), appeared previously in Figure 2.7 and are described in the earlier discussion of toxicology. From the perspective of exposure assessment, the absorbed dose (D) and the biologically effective dose (E), as quantifications of a toxicant in the body, are biological markers, or **biomarkers** of exposure.

Quantifying Exposure

It is common wisdom that "the dose makes the poison"—an idea that dates back to Paracelsus, a physician of the late Middle Ages. So, to be of practical use, the conceptual model in Figure 2.12 needs to be filled out with quantitative information. The work of exposure assessment is to translate the event of exposure into an estimate of the dose of a toxicant. This can be done by measuring or modeling the dose, or an estimate can be made on the basis of questionnaires, records, or other data sources.

Ideally, exposure is quantified inside the body—as the absorbed dose (D) or the biologically effective dose (E)—but often this is not feasible. Instead, external measurements are often made somewhere "upstream" in the exposure model, and mathematical modeling techniques are then used to estimate "downstream" concentrations or doses.

The most basic proxy for dose is simply the concentration of a toxicant in air, water, or soil (A); measurements of these concentrations are made by environmental monitoring. A somewhat better proxy is the concentration of the toxicant at or near the point of human contact (B). Measurements may be taken where exposure occurs (e.g., the concentration of a toxicant in the soil of a yard or the air of a room) called *area monitoring* or alternatively, the measurement can be made in the immediate vicinity of the body. For example, a study of radon exposure might assess the area concentrations in subjects' homes using radon detectors or have study subjects wear a portable dosimeter device collecting radon samples from as close to their breathing zones as possible, even as they move through different environments. Measurements of this type are referred to as *personal monitoring*.

If it is not possible to take a measurement of the concentration of a toxicant at or near the location of exposure (B), it may be necessary to derive an estimate of this concentration, using information from further back along the exposure pathway. In this case, environmental modeling can be used to estimate the concentration of a contaminant at the location of exposure (B). Such

modeling rests on understanding the processes of environmental fate and transport and uses input measurements of the concentration of the contaminant in the ambient environment (A).

Estimates of exposure rest on two kinds of information: a measurement or estimate of the concentration at the location of exposure; and exposure modeling of contact by ingestion, by inhalation, or via the skin. Such modeling rests on assumptions about, for example, the volume of water a person drinks each day, the volume of air he or she inhales (and then exhales), or the area of the skin that is exposed to a contaminant.

For some toxicants, exposure can be quantified inside the body, using one of the following biomarker indicators:

- The absorbed dose (D), the quantity that passed through the human envelope
- The biologically effective dose (E), the concentration in a specific vulnerable tissue

For example, the concentration of mercury in hair or fingernails, the concentration of lead in the blood (used to screen for childhood lead poisoning), and the concentration of alcohol in exhaled air (the police officer's breathalyzer test for drunk drivers) are all biomarkers offering a window onto an *absorbed dose*. Similarly, environmental chemicals such as pesticides, heavy metals, and nicotine (or their metabolites) have been measured postnatally in meconium, the fecal matter that accumulates in the fetus during gestation, providing a biomarker of the prenatal absorbed dose. DNA adducts, formed when a chemical binds to a DNA molecule in the nucleus of a cell, are biomarkers of exposure, and specifically of the *biologically effective dose*. Biomonitoring techniques are relatively expensive, and all impose some burden on the person whose exposure is being assessed, although providing fingernail clippings, for example, is less invasive than providing a sample of urine or blood. And for many toxicants, no techniques are available to make such measurements in the body.

Biological modeling—specifically, toxicokinetic modeling—is sometimes used to predict the ultimate disposition of a chemical from what is known about its toxicokinetics—the absorption, distribution, metabolism, storage, and excretion of the chemical. Toxicokinetic modeling is used to estimate the absorbed dose, the biologically effective dose, or an effect in the form of a change in tissue structure or function from some upstream measure. The majority of mathematical toxicokinetic models rely on compartmentalizing the human body into three or four simple boxes (perhaps representing the digestive tract, bloodstream, and lungs) and estimating the transfer and breakdown of the compound between these compartments, an approach derived from the field of pharmacokinetics. Because sophisticated toxicological understanding is required to develop toxicokinetic models, these models are available for a relatively small number of environmental toxicants, although the fields of radiation protection and radiotherapy have very complex, advanced, and anatomically accurate human models, called dosimetry phantoms.

Units of Absorbed Dose

Absorbed dose is usually expressed in units of milligrams of toxicant per kilogram of body weight per day, written as mg/(kg × day). These units incorporate two important concepts that are probably familiar even if the terminology is not.

First, the mass of contaminant absorbed into the body is normalized to (averaged over) the body weight of the person exposed; that is, it is divided by the body weight. This adjustment accounts for the fact that, for example, 10 mg of Chemical X is a greater insult to a 75-kg man than it is to a 100-kg man.

Similarly, the mass absorbed into the body is averaged over time—usually, expressed as a daily dose. This adjustment accounts for the fact that, for example, 10 mg of Chemical X absorbed by a 75-kg woman at 5 mg/day over a 2-day period is a different insult from 10 mg of Chemical X absorbed by the same woman at 0.5 mg/day over 20 days.

Thus, to calculate someone's absorbed dose of Chemical X from drinking tap water, these pieces of information are needed:

- The concentration of Chemical X in the water
- The rate at which water is ingested (e.g., liters per day)
- The proportion of the Chemical X in the ingested water that is absorbed into the body
- The body weight of the exposed person

For example, the absorbed dose of trichloroethylene to a 70-kg individual who drinks two liters per day of water contaminated with trichloroethylene at 5 μg per liter, assuming 100% absorption of the chemical, is calculated as follows:

$$\frac{\dfrac{5\,\mu g\ chemical}{liter\ water} \times \dfrac{2\ liters\ water}{day} \times 1.0}{70\ kg\ body\ weight}$$

$$= 0.143\ \mu g/(kg \times day)$$

or, in standard dose units, 0.000143 mg/(kg × day)

Similarly, in calculating inhalation exposures, information is needed on the concentration of the chemical in air, the exposed individual's inhalation rate, and the proportion absorbed via the lungs. Calculation of a dermal dose (e.g., a gardener's exposure to a chemical in soil) rests on information about the concentration in soil, how much skin area is exposed, how much soil clings to a given skin area, and the rate at which the chemical is absorbed through the skin.

Other Sources of Exposure Information

Approaches other than direct measurement and mathematical modeling are also used to estimate human exposures to environmental hazards. For example, information about contact with environmental media can be obtained using a questionnaire, in-person interview, telephone interview, or mail survey. Such surveys offer the possibility of direct answers to questions that can't be assessed in the field. For example, how often does the subject apply pesticides in the home? Or, for an exposure via tap water: How much tap water is consumed on a typical day? Does the subject take showers or baths? How often? How long? How hot? Surveys can also be used to gather information on past exposures, such as a woman's job history or her history of using hair dye.

In a variation on the questionnaire approach, subjects in an exposure assessment may keep personal records over a period of time; for example, they may keep diaries of food consumption or time spent in different activities or locations. Historical exposure information may also come from previously existing documentary sources, such as municipal records of contaminant concentrations in drinking water or military records of soldiers' deployments and activities.

Surrogate measures of occupational exposures, such as a worker's job title or the industry in which he or she is employed, are particularly well developed. This is partly because workplace exposures, which may be high and long-lasting, are of special concern. In addition, the occupational setting, which is more regimented than residential or community settings, lends itself to these approaches.

For example, the classification system used in the U.S. Census Bureau's Economic Census defines thousands of industrial sectors ranging from synthetic rubber manufacturing to silver ore mining to shellfish farming. Similarly, job title might be used as a surrogate for potential exposure to latex gloves in a medical setting, distinguishing among nurses, midwives, physicians, medical technologists, and medical assistants. This approach can be taken a step further by developing a job-exposure matrix—a table that provides an estimate of exposure for each combination of job title (in rows) and hazard (in columns). For example, each job title's exposure to each hazard could be rated on a scale of none–low–medium–high based on measurements or even expert judgment.

In recent years, the Geographic Information System (GIS) mapping program has matured into a useful tool for integrating and assessing exposure data. A GIS is a computerized system that combines a database of spatially linked information with application software for spatial analyses and mapping. For example, a GIS might include information on locations where pesticides have been sprayed for mosquito control, or locations of plumes of solvent contamination in groundwater

at different time points, or traffic volumes associated with each quarter-mile segment of a county's roads (representing the concentration of air pollutants produced by vehicles). In essence, such GIS assessments use location as a surrogate for exposure (see **Figure 2.13**).

Epidemiologic researchers can use geographic information systems to link subjects' addresses with environmental data. For example, in a study of the risk of cancer (a disease with a long latency) associated with contamination of private well water, researchers could link each subject's current home address, as well as past addresses, to environmental data on groundwater contamination for the appropriate time periods. This information can be used to estimate exposures at a series of addresses.

2.4 Epidemiology: Human Research Studies

Epidemiology is one of the major sources of information about human health risks from environmental hazards. Epidemiology is the scientific study of the distribution and determinants of health-related states and the application of this study to protect public health.[9] In environmental health, epidemiology provides methods to quantify human health risks observed from exposure to chemicals and other toxicants, as well as risks from noise, injuries, infectious disease, and social factors. Since the major objective of environmental health is to identify hazards and it is unethical to knowingly expose human subjects to such risks, environmental epidemiology primarily relies on observational data where people have either been accidently exposed or exposed at higher occupational levels than those associated with the ambient environment. Rates of disease or other health outcomes are compared between groups known to be exposed at varying levels and/or not exposed at all. Biomarkers of exposure and disease are particularly useful in environmental epidemiology, because these measures allow for possible identification of either exposure or

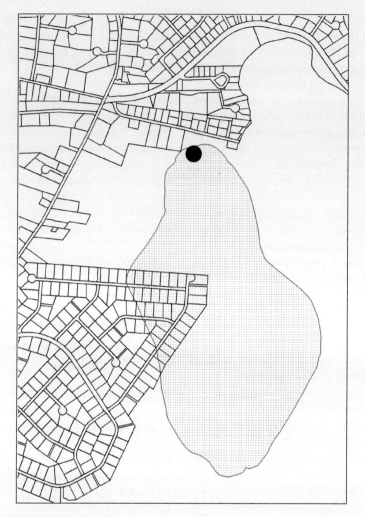

Figure 2.13 This GIS map of a chemical plume in groundwater shows that private wells on nearby properties located upgradient of the source are unaffected by the contamination, whereas wells on more distant properties located downgradient are at risk.

Courtesy of Verónica Vieira.

disease in earlier, preliminary stages that may not be as detrimental to a person's well-being.

Comparing the Sick to the Healthy

The major objective in epidemiology is the comparison of the occurrence of disease among population groups with varying levels of exposure. Historical studies by Jenner and Pott utilized this approach of comparing the sick to healthy among different occupational groups. Jenner helped develop one of the first vaccines after observing that milkmaids developed an alternative, and less virulent disease of cowpox, which seemed to protect them from smallpox. Pott deduced that the excess occurrence of scrotal cancers among chimney sweeps compared with other London workers was most likely due to cancer-causing substances in soot, and Pott's recommendation that sweeps bathe weekly may be one of the very first preventive occupational recommendations.[10]

Comparing the occurrence of disease between population groups requires that records of disease events are kept. Graunt is considered one of the first vital statisticians with his published observations of mortality patterns in the 1600s in England. Graunt's recordkeeping was primarily motivated by concerns with the British maritime industry and the causes of mortality associated with sailors and in the ports where their ships arrived. Graunt created categories for various causes of death, such as from bubonic plague versus childbed fever, a practice further refined by William Farr, the Registrar-General, in London during the mid-1800s. Farr's careful characterization of diseases based on their symptoms and disease characteristics established the basis for the current International Classification of Diseases (ICD) diagnostic codes.[10]

Farr's meticulous and accessible records of cholera deaths in London enabled perhaps the most famous epidemiologic study in the history of public health, conducted by physician John Snow. Hypothesizing that the illness was caused by contaminated drinking water, Snow compared the death rates from cholera according to the water company that supplied individual houses. He documented a more than eightfold increased mortality among people living in houses served by the Southwark and Vauxhall Company, which drew its water from a heavily polluted region of the Thames River, compared with those served by the Lambeth Company, which drew its water from a part of the Thames not contaminated by London's sewage.[11] The design of Snow's study is fundamentally similar to those in use today.

Measures of Disease Frequency

Although keeping good records of deaths from various diseases is still a very significant task for government agencies, mortality data have certain limitations from a research perspective. In addition to exposure to the etiologic trigger or causal agent, death from a particular disease can be affected by various factors that influence survival and access to treatment. In contrast to mortality, the term **morbidity** refers to a diseased (morbid) state and nonfatal rates of disease may be quantified using either prevalence or incidence measures. **Prevalence** quantifies *existing cases* of a disease, specifically, the proportion of a population that has a disease *at a given point in time*. However, the prevalence of a disease in a population still reflects factors associated with survival in addition to possible determinants for the disease. **Incidence** is the occurrence of *new (incident) cases* of a disease in a given population *during a given period of time*. Because only newly diagnosed cases are counted, incidence measures are the preferred measure used to characterize risks in epidemiologic studies trying to identify the etiologic trigger for a disease.

In addition to the number of new cases (incidence) that develop in a population, the prevalence of disease also depends upon the duration of time spent sick by each case. Diseases such as the common cold typically have a duration of only a few days before the patient begins to feel healthy again. However, chronic disease, such as diabetes, may cause a permanent morbid state. Mortality from either acute or chronic disease also obviously affects its duration. The prevalence of HIV/AIDS in Massachusetts on January 1, 2012, for example, not only reflects factors that affect the onset of the illness but also factors that affect how long people survive with the illness, such as treatment options and the availability of medical care. For this reason, although prevalence figures may be useful, for example, in planning for health services, they are not generally useful in assessing potential risk factors for disease, including environmental risk factors.

Another measure for morbidity, called the **Disability Adjusted Life Year (DALY)** characterizes not only the association between environmental risk factors and disease frequency but also the impact those factors have upon the quality of one's life. One DALY is equivalent to the loss of one year of productive life lived due to poor health, so fractions of a DALY can indicate how much disability was experienced during that year, even if a death did not occur. For example, an individual with well-controlled diabetes might enjoy excellent health during a year and barely contribute even a fraction of one DALY, whereas a diabetic with poorly controlled blood sugars may experience the amputation of a limb, equivalent to a full DALY. The summarized value of DALYs for different communities are often compared in environmental research, such as the DALYs associated with air quality (DALYs might be measured in terms of number of days experiencing attacks of asthma) or contaminated drinking water supplies (DALYs determined by the rate of diarrheal diseases among children).

Descriptive Epidemiology

Epidemiologic efforts are often divided into descriptive compared with analytic activities, and **descriptive epidemiology**'s primary task is to characterize the distribution of disease occurrence in populations by person, place, or temporal patterns. Gender, age, and ethnicity are often assessed for any demographic clue regarding who experiences more or less disease. Rural compared with urban residence is commonly used in air pollution studies for assessing where people live and who has more or less disease. Infectious disease outbreaks typically have a rapid peak in cases over a few days or weeks compared with the decrease in stroke-related mortality observed during the past three to four decades. Careful assessment of *who*, *where*, and *when* disease occurs hopefully suggests possible reasons *why*, which is one of the main objectives for descriptive epidemiology—the formulation of plausible hypotheses associating an environmental exposure with a specific health outcome of interest. Descriptive epidemiologic methods, particularly disease surveillance, are the primary activities of environmental health practitioners in city, county, and state health departments. For this reason, this text puts greater emphasis on these descriptive approaches than on the research study designs that are the focus of most textbooks and courses in epidemiology.

Surveillance

To conduct environmental health **surveillance** is to survey the landscape of illness. Surveillance is fundamentally a comparative exercise. The objective of surveillance is to track and compare disease rates in populations across places, across diseases, or over time. In environmental health, surveillance data often highlight unusual patterns that may provide clues to an environmental risk factor for disease. In public health, more broadly, surveillance data are used for policy and planning purposes.

In the United States, state departments of public health typically gather and report disease data. Most of the 50 states have a cancer registry—an agency that receives a report of each cancer diagnosis in the state (including the residential address of the patient) and uses this information to track the incidence of various types of cancer and document geographic patterns. The U.S. Centers for Disease Control and Prevention (CDC) gathers data from all of these agencies. A separate program under the auspices of the National Cancer Institute (Surveillance Epidemiology and End Results, or SEER), gathers cancer data for selected locations around the country, including states with no central cancer registry. Between them, these two programs collect cancer data for the entire U.S. population.[12] Other health outcomes, from HIV/AIDS to birth defects to gunshot injuries, may also be tracked by state or federal agencies. At the federal level, the CDC conducts surveillance, including infectious disease surveillance (see **Figure 2.14**). In addition, the CDC helps states develop their surveillance capacities.

The concept of surveillance can be extended to include biomonitoring at the population level. Such *surveillance biomonitoring* often documents exposure rather than illness—for example, monitoring of blood lead concentrations in young children. The concept of surveillance can be further

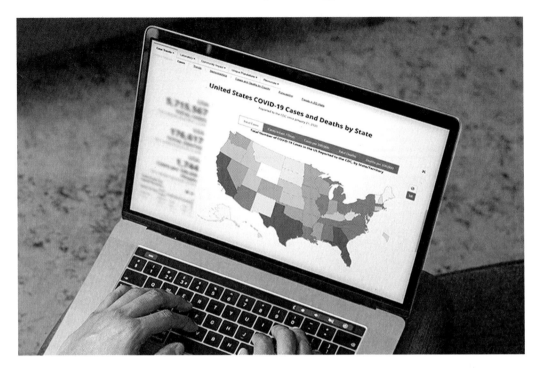

Figure 2.14 CDC workers assess the national distribution of an outbreak.
CDC.

extended to include tracking of health hazards, such as the release of toxic chemicals.

Crude, Specific, and Adjusted Rates

Mortality or morbidity measures that use the actual, observed numbers for disease are considered *crude* rates and are most commonly used in disease surveillance tied to a given population and time period. These actual rates are typically reported per some standard unit multiplier, such as 1,000 live-births or 100,000 people to allow for rates to be compared among populations of different total sizes. For example, in 2016, there were 245,299 new cases of Female Breast Cancer reported in the United States, 16,057 new cases in New York State compared with only 1,304 in New Hampshire. However, New York has a much larger total population of women than New Hampshire. Once the number of incident

cases is divided by the state population of women, New York's incidence rate of 129.1 per 100,000 women is lower than the rate of 145.6 per 100,000 in New Hampshire.[13]

The frequency of many diseases is different in males and females; similarly, disease occurrence often varies by age group. Therefore, if the crude disease frequency for a disease, such as lung cancer, is different in two towns, the difference may be caused partly or entirely by differences in the age and gender makeup of the towns' populations. Similarly, if the crude rates for lung cancer are equivalent in two towns, this statistic may obscure a genuine difference in risk. In the example shown in **Table 2.2**, the annual incidence of female breast cancer is 60% higher in Location A than it is in Location B. However, the table also shows that the female population of Location A is somewhat older than that of Location B. Because it is well known that

Table 2.2 Annual Incidence of Female Breast Cancer and Age Distribution of the Female Population in Two Locations for a Given Time Period

Location	Crude Annual Incidence	Proportion of Population in Each Age Group		
		Premenopausal	Perimenopausal	Postmenopausal
Location A	0.0021	0.55	0.09	0.36
Location B	0.0013	0.65	0.10	0.25

breast cancer is more common in older women, the age makeup in Location A may explain, or partly explain, the higher incidence there. The concern with age distorting this comparison of the rates between these two locations is that age **confounds** the relationship, a concept that will be explained subsequently.

Given that comparing rates across location and time periods is a fundamental task of surveillance; issues like this one create a concern with making an unfair and inaccurate comparison and must be addressed. The effects of gender on disease rates are usually resolved by reporting rates separately for males and females, or as *specific rates*. The effects of age, on the other hand, are usually handled through reporting methods that statistically adjust for differences in age distribution using either a direct or indirect standardization method.

Any method of **rate adjustment** must take account of the separate effects of two factors:

- A population's age distribution (the proportion of the population that falls into each age category)
- The age-specific rate of disease in each age category

Both approaches often use a third population as a reference—a sort of intermediary for comparison. The majority of descriptive epidemiologic data at the national or international level is reported as age-adjusted rates, employing a direct method of standardization. The indirect method is required typically for more regional comparisons where disease rates are suppressed to protect the privacy of cases.

The Ecological Study

Age-adjusted rates are often used in a type of descriptive epidemiologic study conducted using only group-level data called the ecological study. The adjusted mortality or morbidity rates for a specific disease between different populations are compared to aggregated rates representing some type of environmental exposure. For example, across all of the towns of a state, is the mortality rate associated with the volume of toxic industrial releases? With lower average educational attainment? Is the incidence of childhood lead poisoning associated with the presence of an older housing stock? With the percentage of the population in poverty? By providing a rich portrait of the public's health, analyses such as these can enhance our understanding of bare surveillance figures.

The ecologic comparison may also be quantified if these exposure and disease rate values for each group are plotted on an X and Y graph, resulting in a scatter plot then assessed for a linear correlation or trend. The correlational coefficient associated with the trend helps quantify the degree of association between exposure and disease. For example, a hypothetical ecologic study of air pollution and respiratory distress in different regions might depict regional air pollution as the number of days each region experiences hazardous air quality during the year as monitored and reported by the United States Environmental Protection Agency's Air Quality Index. Each region's respiratory distress could be measured as the number of emergency room visits for acute asthma attacks documented that same year.

The drawback of these correlational types of comparisons is that whatever trend is observed from group-level data may not be true at the individual level. In epidemiologic terms, the **ecological fallacy** is that those represented by the exposure measure may not be the same individuals represented by the disease rates. In the previous example, there is no way to know when using aggregated group statistics that those who went to the ER with asthma actually breathed the outdoor air on those hazardous days. Using only data at the population level, it is impossible to know. The ecologic study design is considered useful to *generate* a hypothesis about an association but not to *test* such a hypothesis.

The Case Series

A case report or case series does direct focus at the individual level of those experiencing the disease of concern and assessment for any noteworthy characteristic that such cases might have in common. Taken together, the cases might simply be a medical mystery, or they might be seen as an early clue to a risk factor for an illness. For example, a case series of a rare cancer in homosexual men, published in 1982, first flagged the condition that eventually came to be known as AIDS.[14] Similarly, a series of cases of a rare vaginal cancer in young women provided an early clue to the effects of prenatal exposure to the synthetic hormone diethylstilbestrol (DES),[15] prescribed for more than 20 years in the mid-20th century with the belief that it would prevent miscarriage. However, since such analyses do not include an assessment of the amount of exposure for disease-free individuals, this type of descriptive study also cannot quantify or prove any definitive association.

Analytic Epidemiology

In contrast to descriptive epidemiology, **analytic epidemiology** refers to studies designed to specifically test a hypothesized association between exposure and outcome. In an observational study, as the name suggests, the investigator does not manipulate exposures but merely observes and gathers information on exposures and outcomes. In contrast, in an experimental study, the investigator assigns study subjects to different exposure or treatment groups, and then gathers information on outcomes, a process familiar from clinical drug trials. Due to ethical concerns, the vast majority of environmental epidemiologic studies conducted are observational ones, except for a few exceptions, such as the community-level fluoridation experiments that demonstrated a benefit in reducing cavities to those towns receiving the extra fluoride in their drinking water. Most epidemiologic studies involve assembling groups of specific individuals. The three major types of individual-level observational studies used in analytic research are cross-sectional studies, cohort studies, and case-control studies.

In any such study, in which individuals are enrolled and information is gathered from them, research standards require that participants give their *informed consent* to participate after having been given information about the potential risks and benefits of taking part in a study. Without informed consent, research subjects may be exposed to risks that are not apparent to them; historically, members of disenfranchised groups have been particularly at risk of such treatment. In one infamous episode, U.S. Public Health Service researchers at the Tuskegee Institute in Alabama studied the progression of syphilis in African American men for four decades beginning in 1932, without offering them treatment with penicillin after it became the accepted treatment for syphilis in the mid-1940s.[16] These events led to reforms at the U.S. Public Health Service and ultimately to current requirements for the informed consent of participants in research.

Observational, Analytic Study Designs

Surveying the prevalence of exposures and disease among a group of sampled individuals is the simplest type of study design, called the **cross-sectional study**. In this study design, the subjects (e.g., a group of workers at a particular facility or in a given industry) are classified on a specific exposure (e.g., exposed or not exposed to a chemical in the workplace) and their current health status for a variety of health outcomes (e.g., a specific neurological deficit or a diagnosis of diabetes). Because cross-sectional exposure and health data are typically collected at the same point in time, a key limitation of the cross-sectional design is that it may not be possible to determine if the exposure preceded the outcome. The results of a cross-sectional study investigating a hypothesized association may be summarized by dividing the prevalence of disease among an exposed group by the amount of disease observed among nonexposed study subjects or background baseline prevalence rates for that community. This ratio comparison of disease prevalence between groups is called a **Relative Risk (RR)** and quantifies the strength of the association between exposure and disease. A RR of 2 indicates that the prevalence of disease is twice as high among the exposed group as the nonexposed group, whereas a RR equal to 0.5 depicts a beneficial association where there is half as much disease observed for the exposed population compared with the background (or assumed lesser exposed) groups.

In a **cohort study** (e.g., a study of smoking as a risk factor for lung cancer), subjects are selected according to their exposure status (smoker, nonsmoker) and are then compared on disease status (lung cancer, no lung cancer). The key question in a cohort study is: Other things being equal, are the smokers more likely than the nonsmokers to be diagnosed with lung cancer? Cohort studies can be done either prospectively or retrospectively. That is, the subject can be enrolled in a current cohort study *before* the health outcome of concern has occurred (a prospective design), and the investigator goes forward in time to follow up on which health outcomes occur. Alternatively, the subjects can be enrolled using historical exposure data such as past employment records in a current cohort study *after* the health outcome of concern has also already occurred. In both cases, the subjects are selected based on exposure status and the activity of the study is to assess the incidence of disease among subjects free of disease at the time of their exposure.

A RR comparing disease incidence for exposed and unexposed groups provides a quantitative summary result for the hypothesized exposure. In addition, high-quality cohort studies may also provide an assessment of the absolute benefit or risk associated with exposure by subtracting the incidence rate among the unexposed from the exposed group's incidence rate. The resulting value indicates how much disease may be directly attributed to exposure.

In a **case-control study**, subjects are selected according to their disease status (e.g., lung cancer [cases], no lung cancer [controls]), and their past exposures are then compared (e.g., smoker, nonsmoker). The key question in a case-control study is: Other things being equal, are the lung cancer cases more likely than the controls to have smoked? The case-control design is often used to study rare diseases, such as cancer, because it is impractical to select and follow a cohort of the size needed to generate enough cases for a statistically robust analysis. A limitation of the case-control approach is that it neither provides accurate prevalence nor incidence information. The amount of disease in a case-control study depends upon how many cases and controls (subjects free of the disease under study) the investigators choose to include. However, the **Odds Ratio**, indicative of the probability of exposure for cases compared to controls, is an accepted approximation for the RR derived in other analytic studies.

In any epidemiologic study, careful assessment of both the risk factor of concern and the health outcome of interest is essential. If subjects are misclassified on either risk factor or outcome, this misclassification will cloud any association that might actually exist, making it difficult or even impossible to discern. The assessment of exposure to environmental risk factors poses unique challenges and uses a distinct set of methods, as described earlier. Long latency periods, exposure to multiple mixtures of hazards, and modest relative risks for specific exposures pose methodological challenges in environmental epidemiology.

Evaluating Epidemiologic Associations

In evaluating the results of an individual-level epidemiologic study, the researcher must first assess the statistical significance of the association—that is, assess whether the finding might simply be due to chance. To be considered *statistically significant*, the probability that a finding is simply due to chance must be acceptably low. Often, a less than 5% probability (expressed as $p = 0.05$) is considered acceptable.

In addition, for a study finding to be considered valid, it must not be attributable to bias or confounding. **Bias** is a systematic error in the way that subjects were selected or information was gathered. **Confounding** (from the Latin, to pour together), mentioned earlier with regard to the need to adjust rates, occurs when a factor that is associated with the risk factor of interest is itself a risk factor for the health outcome of concern. For example, in a study of body mass index (BMI) and risk of heart attack, if people with a higher BMI are also likely to be older (and if older age is itself a risk factor for heart attack), part of the apparent effect of higher BMI is actually a result of older age. To see beyond this "pouring together" of the two effects and avoid mistakenly attributing the effect of age to BMI, information on age must be collected and the separate effects of the two risk factors must be teased out by statistical analysis.

The term *effect modification* is used in epidemiology when the joint effect of two risk factors is either greater than or less than the effect expected to result from adding their individual effects. Effect modification is analogous to the toxicologic concepts of synergism (the enhancement of a toxic effect) and antagonism (interference with a toxic effect), discussed earlier in the context of toxicology. For example, epidemiologic studies of the lung cancer risk of asbestos exposure have shown that cigarette smoking multiplies the risk of asbestos exposure—a synergistic effect. Unlike bias and confounding, which are nuisance effects to be controlled, effect modification is of substantive interest.

Finally, in judging whether a causal connection has been shown, as opposed to merely a valid and statistically significant association, researchers generally consider several factors, including these put forward by British epidemiologist Sir Austin Bradford Hill in a seminal 1965 article:[17]

- The strength of the association documented (e.g., a finding of a fivefold risk is more convincing than a finding of a 1.5-fold risk)
- The consistency of findings across epidemiologic studies
- An appropriate temporal relationship—that is, exposure to the putative risk factor precedes the development of the disease
- The finding of a dose–response relationship—that is, risk increases with increasing exposure
- The biological plausibility of the finding in light of current scientific understanding

2.5 Environmental Risk Assessment

Research in epidemiology and toxicology tells us a great deal about the health effects of pollutants in humans and laboratory animals. However, such scientific knowledge accumulates slowly, and questions about a particular compound, or gaps in theoretical understanding, may be pending for years or even decades. Meanwhile, government agencies are charged with regulating hazards, such as setting a limit for the concentration of a chemical in drinking water or deciding how to deal with leachate runoff from a hazardous waste site. In deciding what action to take, regulators do not have the luxury of waiting for scientific certainty to make their decisions easier. In effect, regulators need working answers for scientific questions that scientists have not yet answered.

The process used to bridge this gap is known as *environmental risk assessment*, a methodology for integrating and interpreting scientific data using default procedures for bridging gaps in scientific knowledge in a manner that is both consistent and health-protective. Risk assessments focus on the actual or potential release of contaminants to the environment and attempt to quantitatively describe the impact of this release upon human health. The basic risk assessment framework—estimating health risk on the basis of exposure and toxicity—can be applied to more than individual chemicals or hazardous waste sites. For example, it can be used to estimate the health risk to workers from an industrial process or population risks from air pollutants in automobile exhaust. Formal risk assessment guidelines and protocols have been established that are industry-specific, such as those for the Nuclear Regulatory Commission, or created in response to a federal law, such as the Risk Assessment Guidance for Superfund to be discussed in the next chapter. Rather than adhere to any specific guidance or its inherent terminology, the process of environmental risk assessment is presented here in general terms involving the basic steps suggested earlier in the conceptual model depicted in Figure 2.12, those of analyzing the release, transport, exposure, and health effects associated with environmental hazards.

Risk Assessment Steps

Release Analysis

The first step of many risk assessments requires the identification of the type of contaminant being released, such as an organic compound or pathogenic agent, and the rate at which this contaminant is emitted. The initial source characterized in this step may occur because of an accidental spill, derive from naturally occurring source, or be projected based on process knowledge for a proposed new industrial procedure. Although human exposure could occur at the point where the contaminant is first released to the environment, as in the case of a gas explosion enveloping those in its vicinity, release analyses typically provide the emission rate from a source, such as a smokestack, some distance away from human exposure (refer to A in Figure 2.12).

Transport Analysis

The next step in risk assessment is to determine the contaminant concentration at the point of human exposure based on the source emission rate and the contaminant's fate and transport through environmental pathways (refer to B in Figure 2.12). If possible, samples of water, soil, sediments, and/or air are collected and analyzed and the concentrations at which individual chemicals are found, in different environmental media at different locations, are reported. If the risk assessment is being performed to characterize a proposed hazard, these environmental media concentrations must be predicted using previous scientific knowledge and environmental modeling. Many environmental engineers and scientists spend their careers trying to understand the movement of specific categories of contamination through specific pathways, such as air or water. For example, given the measured concentration of a fairly insoluble chemical in groundwater at an industrial site, what is the expected concentration in water from a private well located 10 miles downgradient of the site?

Exposure Analysis

The objective for this step in risk assessment is to identify the plausible scenarios by which humans might experience an exposure from the contaminant concentrations characterized in the previous step and to determine the dose received from contact with the contamination in their air, water, or food. Identifying populations exposed to the chemical of concern, including susceptible or highly exposed subgroups, should consider all important sources of exposure, with their associated pathways and routes of exposure, taking account of the physical–the chemistry of the chemical.

The risk assessor constructs plausible scenarios for exposure, identifying groups of people who might be exposed to contaminated environmental media on the site (or from the site) and the activities that could bring them into contact with these media. Assumptions made about exposure are intended to include the great majority of the

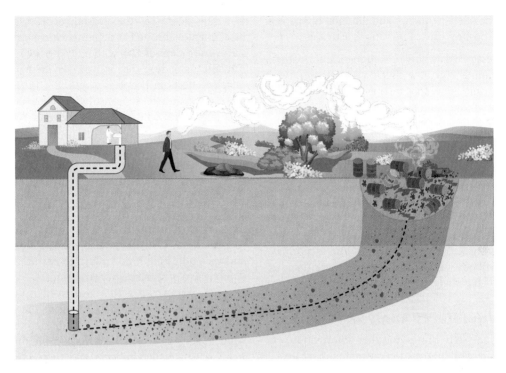

Figure 2.15 Exposure scenarios.

population that is exposed to the site. The exposure scenarios often cover not only current uses of the site but also reasonably foreseeable future uses (refer to examples provided in **Figure 2.15**).

In defining exposure scenarios, the risk assessor identifies likely exposure pathways leading to ingestion, inhalation, or dermal exposures to contaminants in various environmental media. For example, the exposure assessment component of a risk assessment for an industrial site abutting a residential neighborhood might include some of these potential exposure pathways for nearby residents:

- Ingestion, inhalation, and dermal exposures to contaminated well water used as tap water
- Dermal and incidental ingestion exposures to contaminated surface water and dermal contact with sediment in a neighborhood pond used for swimming
- Exposures to dust carried from the site by air movements
- Incidental ingestion of soil, dermal contact with soil, or inhalation of vapors on the site

itself (e.g., by children cutting through the site on their way to and from school)
- Consumption of homegrown produce or of fish caught in contaminated waters
- Ingestion of breast milk by infants

The second major task is to translate each relevant pathway into a concrete dose estimate. Such calculations require a number of inputs, which can be measured, estimated or modeled, or assumed. For example, the risk assessor must quantify the following factors:

- Concentrations of chemicals in various media on the site
- The fate and transport of chemicals or environmental media (e.g., the movement of airborne dust from the site into a residential area or the bioconcentration of a chemical from pond water into fish tissue)
- People's contact with environmental media resulting from various activities (e.g., the quantity of fish ingested)

- The likely frequency and duration of people's exposures caused by various activities

Research data provide some basic information, for example, on how much water people typically drink skin exposure area, as well as typical inhalation rates and skin exposure area—and the United States Environmental Protection Agency (EPA) has established default values for these factors. However, a risk assessment often requires many other assumptions to be made. How often do residents likely eat locally caught fish, and how much do they eat? How often and for how long do children swim in a contaminated pond? Dose estimates are typically quantified using units of mg/(kg × day)—that is, the dose is normalized to body weight and averaged over time, as described earlier.

Health Effects Analysis

The final step brings together information on exposure with information on contaminant toxicity to allow the risk assessor to quantitatively estimate risks to human health, including an estimate of the uncertainties that are built into it. Different approaches are used to assess the health effects associated with the received dose of contaminant depending on whether a deterministic or stochastic risk[18] is associated with the contaminant based on toxicologic and epidemiologic knowledge. **Deterministic risks** are defined as those health effects whose severity increases with increasing dose; noncancer types of health effects are considered deterministic risks. For example, increasing doses of alcohol are associated with an escalation of symptoms from just being buzzed to comatose. Exposures associated with cancer risks are defined as stochastic risks because the *probability* of developing the cancer increases with increasing dose, not the severity of the disease.

Risk Assessment for Noncancer Deterministic Effects. In assessing the noncancer health effects of a chemical, the procedures used are shaped by the assumption that deterministic effects have a threshold. Specifically, the existence of a threshold implies that, in principle, there

is a safe dose. For this reason, dose–response assessment is directed at defining what is called a **reference dose (RfD)**, with units mg/(kg × day). The RfD is a dose that is expected to have no adverse effects in people—specifically, in people who are particularly sensitive to the chemical's effects and who are exposed over a 70-year lifetime.

Unfortunately, the literature on a chemical rarely includes an epidemiologic study of lifelong exposure in a sensitive subpopulation. Indeed, the literature might include no dose–response information at all in humans. Therefore, the RfD for a chemical is usually derived by starting with some other dose that is available in the literature and then adjusting it downward to ensure that it is protective of sensitive human beings.

For example, if a RfD is derived from the NOAEL in a chronic rodent bioassay, the starting value (the rodent NOAEL) is adjusted downward to account for the fact that people may be more sensitive than rodents and then adjusted downward again to account for the fact that some people may be more sensitive than most people. If the starting value is a chronic rodent LOAEL rather than a NOAEL, or if the value comes from a short-term rodent study rather than a chronic rodent study, additional downward adjustments are made in deriving the RfD to account for these limitations in the toxicological knowledge base. A further downward adjustment may be made to account for gaps in the toxicity data for a chemical.

The actual procedure for making these downward adjustments is to divide the starting value (such as a chronic rodent LOAEL) by one or more *uncertainty factors*, each of which is a hedge against the effects of a specific limitation in the available toxicity data. There are two key decisions in this process. The first is the selection of the dose to be used as the starting value (often the dose for the most sensitive effect in the most sensitive species—a health-protective choice). The second is the assignment of values of the specific uncertainty factors by which the starting value is reduced in deriving the reference dose. For example, should the starting value be reduced by a factor of 3 to account for a specific limitation in the available data? Or more conservatively, by a factor of 10? These decisions are made by an expert panel, with the opportunity for review by others.

The development of a RfD is a lengthy process requiring that existing research findings be reviewed and an array of new toxicity studies be undertaken. As a result, the EPA currently publishes reference doses for about 370 chemicals of the many thousands that are produced and used in the United States.

Because the result of a dose–response assessment for noncancer effects is a dose, the risk is characterized by the simple comparison of the actual or estimated dose (from the exposure assessment step) to this RfD:

$$\text{hazard quotient (unitless)} = \frac{\text{actual or estimated dose (mg/[kg} \times \text{day])}}{\text{reference dose (mg/[kg} \times \text{day])}}$$

A **hazard quotient** greater than 1.0 indicates that the actual or estimated dose exceeds the reference dose, pointing to potential harm to people who are exposed at the actual or estimated dose of the substance. In the exposure assessment discussion earlier, the absorbed dose for an individual drinking well water contaminated with trichloroethylene (TCE) estimated an absorbed daily dose of 0.000143 mg of TCE per kg. The oral RfD for TCE is 0.0005 mg/kg/day,[19] resulting in a hazard quotient equal to 0.286, indicating ingestion at levels less than half of the threshold value considered risky. If people are exposed to a set of substances that affect the same organ or organ system (and ideally, by the same toxicologic mechanism), a **hazard index** is calculated as the sum of the hazard quotients for the individual substances.

Risk Assessment for Stochastic Carcinogenic Effects. In a risk assessment for carcinogenicity, the assumption is that the stochastic effects have no threshold. This assumption implies that in principle, any dose, no matter how low, carries some probability of harm. In this context, the concept of a reference dose, or safe dose, is not useful. Rather, the objective is to quantify the probability of developing cancer at the received dose. Evaluation of a chemical's carcinogenicity considers the results of epidemiologic studies as well as chronic animal bioassays, mutagenicity assays, and other short-term tests. The outcome is a designation of the chemical's likely human carcinogenicity, based on expert evaluation of the full body of scientific evidence. Agencies including the EPA and the International Agency for Research on Cancer (IARC, an arm of the World Health Organization) have defined *weight-of-the-evidence categories* for carcinogenicity (see **Table 2.3**).

A stochastic risk assessment relies on a **cancer slope factor (CSF)**: the slope of the dose–response curve, for humans, in the low-dose range wherein human exposures actually occur. The cancer slope factor has units of incremental risk (probability of cancer) per unit increase in dose. The derivation of a CSF poses substantial methodological challenges. Only occasionally

Table 2.3 Weight-of-the-Evidence Categories for Carcinogenicity, as Defined by the International Agency for Research on Cancer and the U.S. Environmental Protection Agency

International Agency for Research on Cancer	U.S. Environmental Protection Agency
Group 1: Carcinogenic to humans	Carcinogenic to humans
Group 2A: Probably carcinogenic to humans	Likely to be carcinogenic to humans
Group 2B: Possibly carcinogenic to humans	Suggestive evidence of carcinogenic potential
Group 3: Not classifiable as to carcinogenicity to humans	Inadequate information to assess carcinogenic potential
Group 4: Probably not carcinogenic to humans	Not likely to be carcinogenic to humans

does the epidemiologic literature provide dose–response information, and; therefore, the CSF is typically derived from a rodent bioassay. And, as described earlier, for practical reasons, rodents in such studies are given very high doses of the test chemical. Thus the carcinogenicity data yielded by a rodent bioassay must be extrapolated in two ways: from rodents to people and from very high experimental doses to much lower real-world exposures.

Sophisticated mathematical models are used to estimate the slope of the human dose–response curve in the low-dose range from rodent data at high doses. Ideally, these models take account of differences in species and differences in dose regimens, while incorporating a health-protective stance. Specifically, assumptions that lead to a steeper slope estimate in the low-dose region are protective of public health. The CSF for a particular chemical is decided by an expert panel, with opportunity for review by others. At present, the EPA publishes a cancer slope factor for approximately 100 chemicals.

Because the result of a dose–response assessment for cancer effects is a slope, with units of risk (probability) per unit dose, the cancer health risk is estimated by multiplying the actual or estimated dose (from the exposure assessment step) by the CSF:

$$\text{dose (mg/[kg} \times \text{day])} \times \text{cancer slope factor (risk per mg/[kg} \times \text{day])} = \text{risk}$$

This estimated risk is the *incremental lifetime cancer risk*—the additional cancer risk, over a 70-year lifetime, which would result from the exposures that were assessed. The absorbed dose of TCE used in the previous hazard quotient calculation may also be used to estimate the stochastic risk of kidney cancer. The CSF for TCE is 0.046 mg/kg/day,[19] resulting in an incremental lifetime cancer risk estimate equal to 6.6 additional kidney cancers per million. The acceptability of a risk at this level will be discussed further in the next chapter, although this range of risk of a few additional cancers out of a million does represent the point where protective regulatory standards are often enacted.

As part of a risk assessment, the core work is to gather the available toxicity values (reference dose, weight-of-the-evidence classification, and cancer slope factor) for the contaminants of concern, and to derive missing toxicity values, if necessary. Depending on circumstances, the dose–response step may be relatively straightforward or may require sophisticated scientific work.

The final product goal of a risk assessment is to quantitatively summarize the cancer risk and noncancer hazards associated with exposure to the contaminants of concern under the exposure scenarios considered. This characterization should include a discussion of the uncertainties embedded in the risk assessment. The risk assessment provides an essential summation of the best (and most protective) estimates that science can provide regarding the possible health hazards associated with an environmental exposure.

Study Questions

1. Describe key aspects of the atmosphere related to human well-being, such as oxygen's role as a limiting factor, the greenhouse effect, and the tropospheric ozone layer.
2. Identify types of stationary and mobile anthropogenic air pollutants.
3. Describe the hydrologic cycle in specific terms, especially related to sources of fresh drinking water. Also, provide examples of point and nonpoint source pollution.
4. Characterize the physical–chemical properties of environmental contaminants related to their behavior in the environment.

5. Assess the advantages and disadvantages of toxicology compared with epidemiology as sources of information about the human health effects of environmental chemicals.

6. Describe the assumptions associated with estimating absorbed and biologically effective doses.

7. Explain why risk assessors use a reference dose to quantify noncarcinogenic toxicity but use a cancer slope factor to quantify carcinogenic toxicity.

8. Review the terms introduced in this chapter and listed in Table 2.1.

References

1. Hohn D. Moby-Duck, or, the synthetic wilderness of childhood. *Harper's Magazine*, 2007;39–62.

2. Eriksen M, Thiel M, Lebreton L. Nature of plastic marine pollution in the subtropical gyres. In: Takada H, Karapanagioti H, ed. *Hazardous Chemicals Associated With Plastics in the Marine Environment. The Handbook of Environmental Chemistry*, vol 78. https://doi.org/10.1007/698_2016_123

3. Bureau of Reclamation California—Great Basin. (2020). Water Facts – Worldwide Water Supply. Retrieved June 7, 2020 from: https://www.usbr.gov/mp/arwec/water-facts-ww-water-sup.html

4. Lans MC, Spiertz C, Brouwer A, Koeman JH. Different competition of thyroxine binding to transthyretin and thyroxine-binding globulin by hydroxy-PCBs, PCDDs and PCDFs. *Eur J Pharmacol Envir Toxicol Pharmacol.* 1994;270(2-3):129-136.

5. Lewis CM, Whitwell S, Forbes A, Sanderson J, Mathew CG, Marteau TM. Estimating risks of common complex diseases across genetic and environmental factors: the example of Crohn disease. *J Med Genet.* 2007;44(11):689-694.

6. Vandenberg LN, Colborn T, Hayes TB, et al. Hormones and endocrine-disrupting chemicals: low-dose effects and nonmonotonic dose responses. *Endocr Rev*, 2012;33(3):378-455.

7. Witschi HR, Last JA. Toxic responses of the respiratory system. In: Klaassen CD, ed. *Casarett & Doull's Toxicology: The Basic Science of Poisons* (5th Ed.). McGraw-Hill.

8. Trasande L, Thurston GD. The role of air pollution in asthma and other pediatric morbidities. *Journal of Allergy and Clinical Immunology*, 2005;115(4):689-699.

9. Last JM, Spasoff RA, Harris SS. 2000. *A Dictionary of Epidemiology.* 4th ed. Oxford University Press.

10. Merrill R. History of epidemiology. *Introduction to Epidemiology.* Jones & Bartlett Learning. 2010.

11. Snow J. *On the Mode of Communication of Cholera*, 2nd ed. *London, England: Churchill, 1855. Reprinted as Snow on Cholera.* Hafner Publishing Company.

12. Centers for Disease Control and Prevention. (n.d.). National Program of Cancer Registries (NPCR). Available at https://www.cdc.gov/cancer/npcr/index.htm

13. Centers for Disease Control and Prevention. (n.d.) United States Cancer Statistics: Data Visualizations. Retrieved June 3, 2020 from https://gis.cdc.gov/Cancer/USCS/DataViz.html

14. Centers for Disease Control and Prevention. A cluster of Kaposi's sarcoma and Pneumocystis carinii pneumonia among homosexual male residents of Los Angeles and Orange Counties, California. *Morb Mortal Wkly Rep.* 1982;31(23):305-307.

15. Herbst A, Ulfelder H, Poskanzer DC. Adenocarcinoma of the vagina: association of maternal stilbestrol therapy with tumor appearance in young women. *N Engl J Med.* 1971;284:878-881.

16. Centers for Disease Control and Prevention. The Tuskegee timeline. Retrieved June 25, 2012 from www.cdc.gov/tuskegee/timeline.htm

17. Hill AB. The environment and disease: association or causation? *Proceedings of the Royal Society of Medicine*, 1965;58:295-300.

18. Fjeld RA, Eisenberg NA, Compton KL. *Quantitative Environmental Risk Analysis for Human Health.* John Wiley & Sons, Inc. 2007.

19. National Center for Environmental Assessment, United States Environmental Protection Agency. Integrated risk information system chemical assessment summary - trichloroethylene; CASRN 79-01-6. Retrieved June 14, 2020 from18 https://cfpub.epa.gov/ncea/iris/iris_documents/documents/subst/0199_summary.pdf#nameddest=rfd

CHAPTER 3

Managing Environmental Health Risks

LEARNING OBJECTIVES

After studying this chapter, the reader will be able to:

- Define or explain the key terms introduced throughout the chapter
- Define risk management and characterize its societal, economic, and regulatory components
- Discuss the factors that influence the acceptability of an environmental risk
- Describe aspects of environmental justice
- Articulate how the principle of having the polluter pay has been incorporated into federal hazardous waste legislation
- Identify leading local, federal, and international environmental risk protection organizations
- Describe how health-based standards are developed and enforced
- Explain how sustainability may be incorporated into the environmental risk management, decision-making process

In addition to considering the best scientific estimates of harm associated with an environmental agent, management of environmental health risks must also balance the benefits and costs associated with taking action and also consider the social context of such actions. This chapter begins by describing, in Section 3.1, the societal factors that influence the *acceptability* of risk from environmental exposures either with or without risk mitigation efforts. Careful *risk communication* between experts and the public regarding how the risk is conceptualized is a complex and significant part of this process. Deciding who should pay for any environmental risk protective action is an issue closely related to its societal acceptability and Section 3.2 discusses various *economic perspectives*. The current *regulatory structure* for addressing environmental health hazards in the United States is briefly described in Section 3.3 with the significant federal agencies summarized in Table 3.1. Section 3.4 provides an overview of the policies and tools available for risk mitigation and the chapter concludes with Section 3.5 addressing how global-level environmental health risks will require more flexible and *sustainable approaches* toward protective policies. **Figure 3.1** depicts the key factors that contribute to the risk management decision-making process.

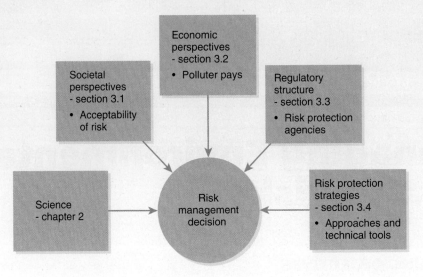

Figure 3.1 Components of Environmental Risk Management Decisions.

3.1 Identifying Acceptable Risk

Risk management encompasses the very broad range of actions taken to control or mitigate environmental health hazards. Risk management decisions are often informed by the results of a formal risk assessment, the process described in the last chapter producing the *best scientific* estimate of the hazard associated with environmental exposure. In addition to considering whatever scientific insight is available, risk management also includes several other dimensions, such as any associated legal and regulatory framework, the range of technical options available for controlling the hazard at hand, economic costs and benefits of various mitigation actions, and the often diametrically opposed perspectives of various stakeholders regarding the acceptability of any risk. This is not a simple matter.

Historically, *acceptable risk* has been defined at different times and in different contexts as a specific numeric risk, the lowest risk that is reasonably achievable, the lowest risk that can be achieved using the best available technology, a negligible risk (too small to be of concern), or a risk that is comparable to similar existing risks and

does not warrant any corrective action. The U.S. federal cutoff to require action to reduce the level of a contaminant in drinking water occurs when a cancer risk assessment indicates a lifetime excess cancer risk of one additional cancer in 10,000.[1] For comparison, the current U.S. lifetime risk of experiencing any type of cancer is approximately 40% based on data from 2014 through 2016[2], or four additional cancers out of 10. This U.S. lifetime cancer risk must combine the risks for both smokers and nonsmokers since data on smoking are not typically indicated in cancer rates, although it is well known that smoking contributes greatly to one's risk of developing cancer. Of course, aspects of the voluntary or involuntary nature of exposure and control of the risk affect how acceptable a risk may be, and the majority of environmental risks reflect involuntary exposures. If the risk level ultimately established by the **environmental risk management** process is deemed *unacceptable*, legal action is often threatened.

Risk Communication

Whatever the hazard, sharing information about its specific risk is an important part of the risk management process. Such activities are referred to as

risk communication. Clearly, communication between substantive experts and members of the public about environmental health concerns is important. Informed consent by participants in research studies, as well as community-based focus groups between community members and governmental agents tasked with *"doing something,"* are examples of such communication. However, the term *risk communication* is more often used narrowly to refer to the exchange or transmission of information about an environmental health hazard between experts and those affected by the hazard. The affected group might be people living near a hazardous waste site, for example, or parents whose children's school is located near a proposed new industrial development.

Communication about environmental health hazards between members of the public and scientists or other experts is often complicated by differences in the way these groups perceive risks. Technical experts tend to think of risks in strictly quantitative terms, whereas the public's perception of risks is more affected by other factors. Indeed, the public perception of risk has been formulated as "hazard plus outrage"[3]—that is, the quantitative estimate of risk can be ramped up by a sense of outrage, which is elicited by certain characteristics of the risk.

Research has identified a number of characteristics of hazards that tend to contribute to public outrage. Research by technical experts sought to understand the public's tendency to under- or overestimate risks relative to scientific estimates, while research by psychologists sought to uncover how nonexperts conceptualize risk. Taken together, these two lines of research identified features of hazards that, for members of the public, tend to make the associated risk seem numerically higher and also somehow less bearable.[4-8] That is, these features of hazards tend to generate outrage:

- The consequences of the hazard are serious or irreversible (e.g., death or permanent disability).
- The hazard kills large numbers of people at once (e.g., the risk of a single plane crash that

causes 300 deaths, as opposed to the risk of 200 car accidents that cause 300 deaths).
- The hazard simply evokes a gut dread in most people (e.g., radiation).
- The hazard is new or unfamiliar, or its consequences are unknown (e.g., genetic engineering as opposed to car accidents).
- The hazard was not appreciated as such before an unexpected event (e.g., the flood of molasses that killed 21 people after the rupture of a large storage tank in Boston in 1919).
- The consequences of the hazard are delayed (e.g., cancer, with its long latency period) rather than immediate.
- The hazard is perceived as not being within an individual's personal control (e.g., a commercial aviation accident as opposed to a car accident while driving).
- The hazard is taken on involuntarily or without knowledge of the risk (e.g., the risk of exposure to secondhand smoke as opposed to the risk of smoking).
- The hazard is not natural, but rather man-made (e.g., toxic synthetic chemicals).
- The hazard is seen as avoidable or unnecessary, as opposed to, for example, occupational hazards or chemotherapy to treat cancer.
- The victims are nearby (although faraway victims can be brought close by media coverage, especially coverage of identifiable individuals, such as miners trapped by a cave-in).

Many environmental health hazards have one or more of these outrage-generating characteristics. In addition, risks that affect people in their homes, such as chemical contamination of drinking water, elicit a powerful emotional response because they strike at the heart of family, security, and even personal identity.[9] Furthermore, the public's outrage tends to be magnified if there are no benefits clearly associated with a risk, if the risk receives a lot of media attention, if the risk results from unethical activities or an unfair process, or if the risk was created by people or institutions they do not trust.[10] Outrage may also be particularly acute in those with past experience of injustice, including residents of lower-income neighborhoods or members of historically disadvantaged racial or ethnic groups. The recent exposure of almost 5% of children in Flint, Michigan, to unsafe levels of lead in their drinking water when the city opted to save money by switching its drinking water supply is a recent outrageous example, with a state civil rights review committee calling it the "result of systematic racism."[11]

Professionals who communicate about environmental health risks must understand and acknowledge the roots of outrage in a given situation, and they must be committed to genuine two-way communication with diverse **stakeholders**—those who are affected by the problem at hand and who will be affected by the chosen solution. As a general rule, effective risk communication about environmental health issues requires careful planning; genuine collaboration with stakeholders; careful listening and clear speaking; acknowledgment of outrage, honesty, and compassion; and skill in working with the media.[10]

Stakeholders and Environmental Justice

The term stakeholder refers to any person or group with a vested interest in the decided outcome, including property owners and community residents, industries and/or their employees, municipal entities and political representatives, corporate and environmental lobbyists, and often legal or special guardian representatives of vulnerable members of a population. Many environmental laws mandate the formal consideration of various stakeholder perspectives during the decision-making process, including addressing aspects of **environmental justice**, which the Environmental Protection Agency (EPA) defines as "the fair treatment and meaningful involvement of all people regardless of race, color, national origin, or income with respect to the development, implementation, and enforcement of environmental laws, regulations, and

policies."[12] In 2005, the agency named several areas in which it has made environmental justice a priority, including reducing the incidence of elevated blood lead levels and asthma attacks, reducing exposure to toxic air pollutants, ensuring that water is safe to drink and that fish and shellfish are safe to eat, and the cleanup and redevelopment of contaminated industrial sites (sometimes called *brownfields*).[13] The concept of environmental justice also includes equitable access within a community to factors such as clean water or safe air to breathe.

In addition to the federal requirement that the EPA include stakeholders at several points during the formal risk management decision-making process, other laws exist that also adhere to environmental justice principles. Employees, for example, have the right to know what types of exposures they might receive on the job. Occupational laws mandate that Material Safety Data Sheets (MSDS) be available to workers near their point of potential exposure with detailed information about the physical and chemical properties of any potentially hazardous substances. Preliminary training must be provided to help familiarize workers with the location of the MSDS as well as any protective equipment in their workspace, such as fume hoods or eye wash sinks.

The Emergency Planning and Community Right-to-Know Act (EPCRA) calls for information about industrial releases to be made publicly available for citizens residing near these industries. The idea was that such openness would lead to more responsible behavior by manufacturers simply by changing the norms for corporate disclosure and public awareness. Passage of the law was motivated partly by a 1984 industrial accident at a Union Carbide plant in Bhopal, India, in which thousands of people living near the plant were killed or horribly injured by the release of a cloud of highly toxic gas, methyl isocyanate. This event sparked public outrage against Union Carbide both in the United States and internationally, increasing awareness of industrial pollution and of the social disparities in its impacts.

The EPCRA called for the establishment of state and local emergency response commissions to plan for, and respond to, industrial accidents. The law also set up ongoing reporting requirements for manufacturing facilities. Each year, facilities must report the quantities (in pounds) of a long list of chemicals that they have released to air or water, or placed on land, or transferred offsite. This database, called the Toxics Release Inventory (TRI), is publicly available online in a format that allows the user to generate custom reports, such as the quantities of specific chemicals released by specific facilities. EPCRA also requires manufacturers to submit MSDS (which, as described earlier, must be made available to workers) to the local emergency response commission. The requirement that manufacturers be transparent about the makeup and toxicity of their waste streams to the surrounding community addresses aspects of both environmental justice and risk communication.

When environmental hazards are deemed to unfairly expose someone to an unacceptable level of risk, the risk management process may be perceived as having *failed,* resulting in the initiation of legal action. Specifically, the aggrieved party may sue and place the risk management decision in the hands of a jury of their peers. The courtroom setting often demonstrates how public perceptions of control, trust, and fear of the unknown diminish scientific insight into the true magnitude of harm associated with an environmental agent. Recent multimillion-dollar settlements have been awarded by juries even when the available science is ambiguous regarding the degree of harm associated with an exposure, but the lawyers were able to sway public perception. In the case of glyphosate, an herbicide manufactured by Monsanto under the tradename Roundup, industry lawyers have also been able to call the credibility of the international agency, IARC into question (refer to the **Case Study**, *Science in the Court*). In recent settlements against Johnson & Johnson, the predominant maker of talc-based baby powder, the possible contamination of talc with asbestos has swayed juries to award damages, even when industry testing has failed to find

asbestos in their products. In this case, the well-known risks of asbestos seemed to set a precedent for the potential of harm from baby powder and the company is settling claims and discontinuing the sale of talcum products to "buy peace," although arguing that they did no harm.[14]

Precautionary Principle

In the United States today, attitudes about the level of acceptable risk relate to the fact that most risk management decisions come once the public is exposed—after an industrial process has been put into use, after a toxicant has been released into the environment, after the opportunity to prevent or minimize a hazard has been lost. Historically, the tendency in the United States has been to introduce new chemicals or processes freely and only later consider their ramifications. Concerns about pesticide residues lingering on fruit, for example, or the controversy over Bisphenol-A exposures in plastics are both situations where public concern about the hazards emerged before there was much available science to assess the risk.

At the other end of the spectrum, a strict preventive approach would require full knowledge of all potential impacts before introducing any new chemical or process—an almost impossible prerequisite. The **precautionary principle** of risk management parallels our commonsense notions about taking precautions (e.g., "look before you leap," "better safe than sorry"). If a significant potential for serious harm exists, but conclusive evidence of harm is lacking, protective action should be taken in advance as a precaution against the harm. Rather than demonstrating harm as grounds to regulate a chemical or process after it is in use, we should take steps to prevent or minimize harm from the outset. The precautionary principle embodies the long-standing preference in public health for primary prevention over secondary prevention whenever possible. Essentially, decisions made in the spirit of precaution avoid the worst possible outcome of a decision made under conditions of uncertainty.

The precautionary principle specifies that the burden of proof should rest with the party

Science in the Court

In California, a jury recently awarded $289 million to a school custodian that claimed his non-Hodgkin's lymphoma was caused by spraying Roundup every summer to keep down weeds in the playground. There are currently 125,000 cancer lawsuits involving Roundup pending in the US.[1]

Roundup was introduced by the Monsanto Chemical Company in 1974. Glyphosate functions to inhibit an enzyme in plants responsible for the synthesis of essential amino acids needed to build proteins[2] and because animals lack this biosynthetic pathway, glyphosate was considered nontoxic to humans. The use of Roundup increased tremendously when Monsanto introduced genetically modified "Roundup ready" seeds that allowed for crops to be sprayed while growing that would resist the herbicide's effects while weeds withered around them. Although large agricultural businesses are responsible for 90% of the usage of these Roundup products, nonagribusiness usage, such as that in private homes and gardens, is still a lot and grew by over 300-fold from 1974 to 2014.[2] The success of its Roundup products made Monsanto quite profitable and the German-based Bayer AG chemical company paid $63 billion to acquire Monsanto in 2018.[1]

Bayer also inherited responsibility for growing liability concerns associated with glyphosate. One might ask why, if glyphosate was originally thought to be nontoxic, are so many people successfully suing over their glyphosate exposures? The courtroom setting means that the attitudes and beliefs of the jurors will influence their judgment and a large agrichemical business involved in controversial technologies, such as genetic modification, is likely to be viewed with distrust and is also viewed as having *deep pockets*.

Unfortunately, science has also muddied the waters by contributing conflicting information. The U.S. EPA asserted that glyphosate *was not likely to be carcinogenic* to humans in its most recent review of available toxicologic and epidemiologic evidence, whereas the International Agency for Research on Cancer (IARC) classified it as Group 2A, *probably carcinogenic to humans*.[3] There are technical reasons why these two agencies who are supposed to render unbiased, impartial scientific judgments arrived at opposite conclusions. The EPA focused its research on the health effects data when glyphosate was used *as directed by labeling*, typically in large agricultural settings, whereas IARC considered study data from *all likely types of exposure*, including studies of "shorts and flip-flop wearing" household users of Roundup[3] (the most common type of plaintiff in these lawsuits). The EPA also reviewed more unpublished data that included many more studies indicating negative results than the IARC reviewers who relied on peer-reviewed published resources. The lack of transparency regarding who did the research (*or at least funded it*) for these unpublished resources has harmed the credibility of the EPA's conclusions. However, the credibility and transparency of the IARC's review has also been called into question over last-minute edits omitting evidence from negative studies without any explanation. Outrage over the IARC assessment's seeming lack of disclosure and selective use of data has even resulted in the chair of the U.S. Congressional Committee on Science, Space, and Technology to recommend withholding governmental funding for IARC work in the future.[2]

1. Feeley J, Loh T, Bloomberg. Bayer reaches verbal deal to settle up to 85,000 Roundup cancer lawsuits. *Fortune.* Retrieved June 19, 2020 from https://fortune.com/2020/05/25/bayer-roundup-cancer-lawsuit-settle/

2. Richmond ME. Glyphosate: a review of its global use, environmental impact, and potential health effects on humans and other species. *J Envir Stud Sci.* 2018;8:416-434.

3. Benbrook CM. How did the US EPA and IARC reach diametrically opposed conclusions on the genotoxicity of glyphosate-based herbicides? *Envir Sci Europe*, 2019;31:2.

initiating a new activity, that a wide range of alternatives for action should be considered, and that the decision-making process should be broadly inclusive.[15] Thus the precautionary approach is tied to societal goals, asking whether an activity is needed, to what degree its negative impacts can be prevented while still meeting the societal goals, and whether there are other ways to meet the goals with less risk.[16] The list of lost opportunities for precaution is a long one and includes depletion of global fisheries, broad use of asbestos and various synthetic organic chemicals, and the practices that led to the outbreak of "mad cow disease" and human illness in the 1980s and 1990s.[17]

In fact, some U.S. policy initiatives and some international agreements do reflect a precautionary approach. For example, the U.S. Toxic Substances Control Act is precautionary in spirit, as was the Delaney clause, a now-repealed food safety measure that tried to prevent the use of any food additive if it had been demonstrated to cause cancer in any species. Two major international agreements that directly affect public health—the Kyoto Protocol on global climate change and the Montreal Protocol on Substances that Deplete the Ozone Layer—reflect a precautionary approach to problems that are global in scale and respond only slowly to control measures. Furthermore, the European Union has established a program for the **R**egistration, **E**valuation, **A**uthorisation and Restriction of **Ch**emicals (REACH), under which new chemicals can be authorized only after toxicity testing (with more testing required for higher-volume chemicals) and a weighing of their potential risks against their potential socioeconomic benefits.[18]

3.2 Costs Associated with Environmental Hazards

Stakeholder perspective regarding the acceptability of a risk also includes consideration of the economic benefits and costs associated with any risk mitigation action. Simply put, *it matters who pays.* Will the costs to cleanup be paid by those who made the mess in the first place? Or will risk mitigation expenses be borne by taxpayers? Perhaps the consumer of a product will pay more for having it manufactured more safely? Then there are environmental laws, such as the Endangered Species Act, where the beneficiary is not even human but the costs to protect the endangered habitat may be too prohibitive to allow for a proposed development that would benefit people. The costs associated with many environmental laws relate to the philosophical principle upon which the law was established,

such as species protection or environmental justice. However, two major federal statutes in the United States are founded on the economic principle that the *polluter pays*.

The Resource Conservation and Recovery Act (RCRA) was enacted in response to growing concerns during the 1960s about ever-increasing amounts of municipal and industrial solid waste. The national law, subsequently amended to include hazardous waste, instituted a manifest system where waste generation and disposal is clearly documented from *cradle-to-grave*. As depicted in **Figure 3.2**, any materials involved with the manufacturing process needed to be documented from their point of origin through their manufacturing usage to their final disposal arrangements. The goal of RCRA is that the cost of any resource degradation be incorporated into the industry's business expenses.[19]

Attempting to ensure that polluters pay for the messes they make is even more fundamentally engrained in the United States Comprehensive Environmental Response, Compensation and Liability Act (CERCLA). Also known as the Superfund Act, CERCLA was enacted in response to several shocking discoveries during the 1960s and 1970s of abandoned areas with large amounts of hazardous waste.[20] The story of the Love Canal exemplifies what led to CERCLA.

The political fallout associated with the Love Canal (refer to **Figure 3.3**) led directly to the passage of CERCLA and the creation of a federal *Superfund*. Although the EPA is required to attempt to identify private parties responsible for cleaning up, CERCLA also created mechanisms to accrue federal monies associated with cleanup for hazardous waste sites when legal liability could not be assigned to a private previous or current landowner. The Agency for Toxic Substances and Disease Registry (ATSDR, see Table 3.1) was established to help with the evaluation of discovered hazardous waste sites and the ranking of the sites for placement on the National Priority List, a listing that allows for the use of these federal funds for cleanup. Although a detailed overview of the complete CERCLA process is not appropriate here, it is worth mentioning a few more of its risk

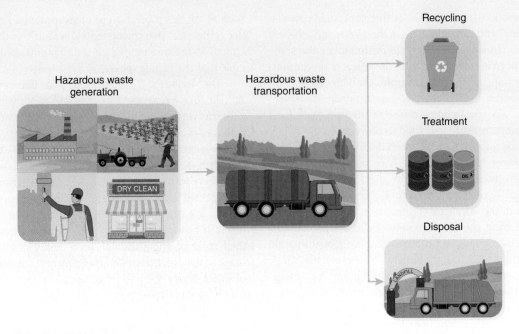

Figure 3.2 RCRA cradle-to-grave System.

U.S. Environmental Protection Agency. Cradle to Grave System. Retrieved from: https://www.epa.gov/sites/production/files/2016-02/cradletogravegraphicgreen.jpg

Love Lost

In 1978, President Carter declared a federal health emergency for the Love Canal neighborhood in Niagara Falls, New York, and encouraged the evacuation of hundreds of residents. Putrid odors and chemical slime in a myriad of colors had been discovered in the basements of many of these recently built homes, oozing in from the surrounding soil. Outside of the homes, children were warned away from strangely smelling puddles in their backyards. The source of contamination was a mixture of chemical waste disposed of by the Hooker Chemical and Plastics Corporation in the remnant of the Love Canal.[1]

William Love had been a developer in the late 1890s with hopes of building a utopian community powered by a six milelong canal between the upper and lower portions of Niagara Falls. However, Love ran out of money and abandoned his plans after excavating only one mile. The city of Niagara Falls initially used it for municipal construction waste, then sold it to Hooker Company, which used it for chemical waste disposal for over 20 years. By 1953, over 22,000 tons of waste had been dumped in and the pit was full and the wastes sealed under dirt and a clay liner.[1]

Subsequently, the local school district purchased the land from Hooker for construction of a new school for the growing community. At this time, about a decade before Rachel Carson published Silent Spring, the hazards associated with chemical wastes were not a salient concern. Of note, however, the Hooker Corporation did include a carefully-worded disclaimer with the sale of the property, disclaiming responsibility for any side-effects from future chemical exposure.[1] Over the next 20 years, the neighborhood grew around the school with occasional complaints to local officials about strange odors or children experiencing skin rashes and burns after playing outside. However, it wasn't until heavy rains in 1976 caused the chemical wastes to overflow the canal and contaminate the entire neighborhood that local residents demanded that something be done. By this time, the environmental movement was in full swing and with the formation of the EPA a few years earlier, residents were motivated to act and had a regulatory avenue for voicing their concerns.

1. Brook M. *The tragedy of Love Canal*. Retrieved June 22, 2020 from https://www.damninteresting.com /the-tragedy-of-the-love-canal/. 2006.

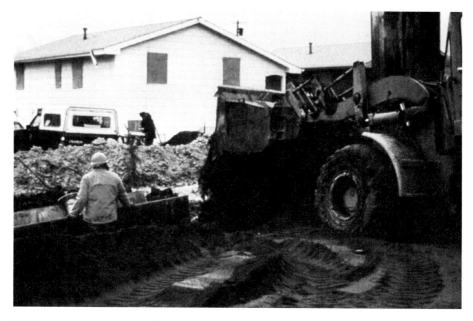

Figure 3.3 The Love Canal neighborhood, built over a chemical waste dump, became the scene of bulldozers and boarded-up houses.

Courtesy of CDC Public Health Image Library. ID# 5534. Content providers CDC. Available at: http://phil.cdc.gov/phil/home.asp. Accessed October 3, 2012.

management details (refer to **Figure 3.4**). One of the initial actions required by CERCLA when assessing a site is to conduct a *baseline risk assessment*, to help determine the risk associated with taking "no- action" to remediate the site. If this risk is deemed unacceptable, based on mandated stakeholder input as well as current regulatory statutes, alternative remedial actions must be fully described, including costs, time frame, and degree of risk reduction achieved. The CERCLA process requires that these remedial actions be shared and the final decision documented and recorded with follow-up through the final delisting for a site, once clean.[20]

3.3 The Regulatory Structure for Managing Environmental Health Risks

The preceding discussions about how hazardous waste is federally managed suggests just how complicated the U.S. regulatory infrastructure is for addressing environmental health. Several federal agencies and organizations (refer to **Table 3.1**) exist to manage the process stipulated by laws enacted by Congress. The majority of federal environmental statutes date back to the early 1970s when the environmental degradation associated with the chemical industrial revolution's prosperity could no longer be ignored by the public. Prior to discoveries such as the Love Canal, city skies were already being darkened by heavy concentrations of particulate matter in the air and urban rivers often contained water with unnatural hues, such as bright orange from discharged textile dyes. In 1969, the oil-slick contaminated surface of the Cuyahoga River in Cleveland, Ohio, actually caught *on fire*, a shocking event that further catalyzed the public demand that the government *do* something to protect the environment (refer to **Figure 3.5**).

One of the first environmental laws in the United States was enacted the same year as the Cuyahoga river fire, the National Environmental Policy Act (NEPA), requiring that all branches of government give proper consideration to the

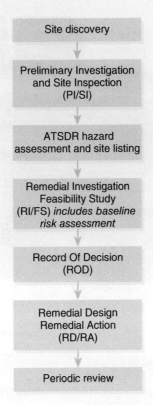

Figure 3.4 Overview of the CERCLA Process.

Data from United States Environmental Protection Agency. https://www.epa.gov/risk/risk-assessment
-guidance-superfund-rags-part

environmental impacts of any proposed major federal action. The EPA was established the next year to oversee the implementation of NEPA mandates and the development of regulations that ensure that Americans have clean air, land, and water.

Much of the work done to manage environmental health risks actually involves state and local health departments. Many city and town governments are responsible for providing water supply, sewer service, and trash removal. Local governments inspect and regulate food service establishments, manage episodes of foodborne illness, and respond to other infectious disease outbreaks. Local health departments also work to manage various environmental hazards related to housing conditions, from controlling rodents to preventing lead poisoning and asthma. Noise is also regulated through local ordinances.

In addition to the U.S. federal, state, and local infrastructure addressing environmental policies, several international agencies also play a role in risk management. The World Health Organization (WHO) coordinates health efforts for the United Nations, including overseeing the previously mentioned IARC. Similar international agencies under the guidance of WHO exist to address other types of environmental health concerns such as those

Table 3.1 U.S. Agencies and Organizations Most Pertinent to Research and Practice in Environmental Health

Agencies Within Departments of the Executive Branch of the U.S. Government

U.S. Department of Health and Human Services
 National Institutes of Health—conducts and supports research and dissemination of information on human health
  National Cancer Institute—conducts and supports research and dissemination of information on the causes, prevention, diagnosis, treatment, and control of cancer
  National Institute for Environmental Health Sciences—works to understand environmental influences on the development and progression of human disease
   National Toxicology Program—evaluates agents of public health concern by developing and applying the methods of toxicology and molecular biology (an interagency program; core agencies are NIEHS, NIOSH, and FDA)
  National Library of Medicine—collects and organizes biomedical science information and makes it available to scientists, health professionals, and the public
 Centers for Disease Control and Prevention—helps individuals and communities protect their health through the promotion of health; prevention of disease, injury, and disability; and preparedness for new threats

National Institute for Occupational Safety and Health—conducts research and provides information and recommendations to help prevent work-related injuries and illnesses

Agency for Toxic Substances and Disease Registry—implements health-related sections of laws that protect the public from hazardous wastes and spills, including waste facilities and Superfund sites, by assessing hazards and preventing exposures and health effects

Food and Drug Administration—works to ensure the safety and efficacy of the food supply, drugs and vaccines, other biological products, supplements, cosmetics, and medical devices

U.S. Department of Labor

Occupational Safety and Health Administration—works to ensure safe and healthful working conditions by setting and enforcing standards, and by providing training, outreach, education, and assistance

Mine Safety and Health Administration—develops and enforces safety and health standards; inspects mines, investigates accidents, provides technical assistance and training

U.S. Department of Energy

Energy Information Administration—collects, analyzes, and disseminates information on energy for policymakers and the public

Office of Civilian Radioactive Waste Management—manages and disposes of high-level radioactive wastes and spent nuclear fuel

U.S. Department of Agriculture

Agricultural Marketing Service—develops quality-grade standards for agricultural commodities and administers programs that regulate marketing

Food Safety and Inspection Service—ensures that the nation's commercial supply of meat, poultry, and egg products is safe, wholesome, and correctly labeled and packaged

Animal and Plant Health Inspection Service—protects and promotes U.S. agricultural health, including animal welfare

National Agricultural Statistics Service—conducts monthly and annual surveys and prepares USDA data and estimates of production, supply, prices, and other information

Economic Research Service—provides economic research and analyses to inform decision making on issues related to agriculture, food, natural resources, and rural America

Independent Agencies of the Executive Branch of the U.S. Government

U.S. Environmental Protection Agency—responsible for protecting human health and the environment

U.S. Nuclear Regulatory Commission—regulates commercial nuclear power plants and other civilian uses of nuclear materials through licensing, inspection, and enforcement

U.S. Consumer Product Safety Commission—responsible for protecting the public from unreasonable risks of injury or death from consumer products

Private, Nonprofit Institutions in the United States

The National Academies—produce reports on matters of science and technology in support of policymaking, public understanding, and scientific advancement

National Academy of Sciences—one of the National Academies; a society of scholars engaged in scientific and engineering research, who provide independent advice to government

Institute of Medicine—one of the National Academies; a society of scholars in health, medicine, and health care, who provide independent advice to government

National Research Council—the operating arm of the National Academies; produces independent expert reports and undertakes other scientific activities to inform policy and actions

Note: Descriptions are derived directly from information on agency websites listed as source

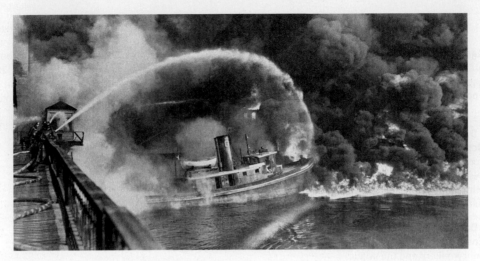

Figure 3.5 The Cuyahoga river on fire.
© Bettmann/Getty Images

related to climate change, radiation exposure, or food safety.

3.4 The Nuts and Bolts of Risk Protection

Establishing Standards

What can risk managers actually *do* to protect humans from environmental hazards? One approach is to establish specific health-based standards. Several of the agencies described in Section 3.3 have the primary task of conducting the research to establish these standards, such as the National Institute for Occupational Safety and Health (NIOSH) or the National Toxicology Program. The EPA standards for concentrations of individual chemicals in drinking water are derived from the results of chemical risk assessments.[21] Thus, if a risk assessment has shown that Chemical X is a carcinogen, any exposure to the chemical is assumed to carry some cancer risk, and the goal for the concentration of Chemical X in drinking water is set at zero. The enforceable standard is then set at a concentration that is considered feasible to achieve. Both policy decisions—the choice of a goal and of a feasible standard—are risk management decisions.

Similarly, if a risk assessment has shown Chemical Z to be noncarcinogenic, and a reference dose has been derived, a drinking water standard can be derived from the reference dose. This is done by back-calculating the concentration in drinking water that corresponds to the reference dose, given certain assumptions about body weight and daily consumption of drinking water. For example, suppose that the reference dose for Chemical Z is 0.000143 μg/(kg × day), or 0.143 μg/(kg × day). Then, a backward calculation would look like this*:

$$\frac{0.143 \text{ μg Chemical Z/(kg} \times \text{day)} \times 70 \text{ kg body weight}}{2 \text{ liters water/day}}$$

$$= \frac{5 \text{ μg Chemical Z}}{\text{liter water}}$$

The enforceable standard for the concentration of Chemical Z in drinking water might then be set at a concentration somewhat lower than 5 μg/L to account for the fact that people will have additional exposures from sources other than drinking water.

---

*The corresponding forward calculation appeared earlier in this chapter as an example of calculating a dose of trichloroethylene in drinking water.

In addition to chemical-specific drinking water standards, risk assessments also contribute to the development of air quality standards for indoor, outdoor, and occupational exposures. The occupational setting also stipulates a variety of other exposure limits (or standards) to protect workers from job-specific risks, such as radiation, noise, or repetitive motion. Standards may be established based on the total cumulative risk associated with a specific environmental pathway, such as well water obtained downgradient from a federal NPL hazardous waste site or the maximum amount of pollutants permitted to be discharged into a lake or other body of water.

Enforcing Standards

In order to enforce compliance with health standards, sampling and monitoring programs exist. In occupational settings, workers may wear personal monitoring devices, such as badge dosimeters, or have the air quality sampled in different regions of the manufacturing facility. Typically, large industries hire industrial hygienists and may have entire departments to assess the types of exposures that their employees receive and to manage the regulatory compliance reporting associated with industry-specific, health-based occupational standards. The Toxic Release Inventory program mentioned previously is another type of reporting required of many industries.

Another regulated approach to monitoring requires that public drinking water suppliers sample their water for a long list of possible contaminants, and report any instances of *violations*, when a sample exceeds the allowed concentration for that pollutant, to the regional EPA and state health authorities. A further interesting aspect related to enforcing drinking water compliance is that these public water suppliers have to also inform their consumers about any water-quality violations by creating and sending out yearly Consumer Confidence Reports. These public documents must provide tabular information about any water-quality violations during the year (refer to **Figure 3.6**) as well as provide information about the source, treatment, and management of the

drinking water so their clients may make educated decisions regarding any potential health risks.[22]

Outdoor air quality standards are assessed by sampling for several specific pollutants using specialized equipment set up in different locations across a designated region. Regional EPA offices must monitor compliance and regions that are identified as exceeding the standards, or *noncompliant*, risk the loss of federal highway safety funding. Another approach to sampling what is already *in* the air actually assesses what is being emitted *into* the air. Industries are often required to prove that they meet specific smokestack emission standards and car manufacturers must report their tailpipe emissions. The laws related to these various types of emission standards often rely on specifically mandated Best Available Technologies (BAT) more than just environmental sampling. Electrostatic precipitators, smokestack scrubbers, and catalytic reactors are all examples of air pollution control technologies that industries may be required to use. Another approach to reducing air pollutant emissions was the requirement for coal-fired power plants to switch from high-sulfur to low-sulfur content coal.

Mandating the use of such specific pollution control approaches, such as BAT, has been criticized as overly proscriptive and termed a *"command and control"* approach to risk management.[23] Although criticized as the most burdensome method for reducing risks, this top-down, command and control approach is embedded at the heart of many federal environmental statutes addressing pollution. The key criticism of the BAT approach is that it addresses *how* a process must function instead of focusing on the desired *outcome* of reducing emissions. Groups wanting to benefit from an environmental risk protection decision are likely to pursue political support for their best interests, even if it is less cost-effective, rather than strive to create better pollution mitigation policies. For example, within the current regulatory structure adhering to the command-and-control approach, there have been instances where stricter standards were required for new industrial polluters to *join* the market compared with the standards required for those already-existing industries that were

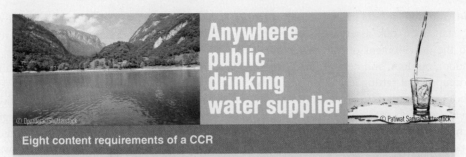

Eight content requirements of a CCR

- *Item 1*: **Water System Information**–Name/phone number of a contact person; information on public participation oppertunities.
- *Item 2*: **Source(s) of water.**
- *Item 3*: Definitions - Maximum contaminant level (MCL); MCL goal (MCLG); Treatment tecnique (TT); Action level (AL); Maximum residual disinfectant level (MRDL); MRDL goal (MRDLG).
- *Item 4*: **Detected contaminants** - A table summarizing reported concentrations and relevant MCLs and MCLGs or MRDLs and MRDLGs; known source of detected contaminants; health effects language.
- *Item 5*: **Information on monitoring for *Cryptosporidium*, Radon, and other contaminats** (if detected).
- *Item 6*: **Compliance with other drinking water regulations** (any violations and ground water rule [GWR] special notices).
- *Item 7*: **Varences and exemptions** (if applicable).
- *Item 8*: **Required education information** - Explanation of contaminants in drinking water and boltled water; information to vulnerable populations about *Cryptospondium*, statements on nitrate, arsenic, and lead.

Optional information

CWSs are not limited to providing only the required information in their CCR. CWSs may want to include:

- An explanation (or include a diagram of) the CWSs treatment processes.
- Source water protection efforts and/or water conservation tips.
- Costs of making the water safe to drink.
- A statement from the mayor or general manager.
- **Information to educate customers about:** Taste and odor issues, affiliations with programs such as the partnership for safe water, opportunities for public partcipation etc.

Contaminants	MCLG	AL	Your Water (90th%)	Sample Date	# of Samples Exceeding the AL	Violation	Typical Sources
Inorganic Contaminant							
Lead-lead at consumers tap (ppb)	0	15	9	2008	1 of 20	No	Corrosion of household plumbing systems; erosion of natural deposits.

Figure 3.6 Components of consumer confidence report.

U.S. Environmental Protection Agency, Office of Water. (August, 2009). Consumer Confidence Report Rule: A Quick Reference Guide. Retrieved from: https://nepis.epa.gov/Exe/ZyNET.exe/P100529A.txt?ZyActionD=ZyDocument&Client =EPA&Index=2006%20Thru%202010&Docs=&Query=&Time=&EndTime=&SearchMethod=1&TocRestrict=n&Toc=&TocEntry=&QField=&QFieldYear=&QFieldMonth=&QFieldDay=&UseQField=&IntQFieldOp=0&ExtQFieldOp=0&XmlQuery =&File=D%3A%5CZYFILES%5CINDEX%20DATA%5C06THRU10%5CTXT%5C00000010%5CP100529A.txt&User=ANONYMOUS&Password=anonymous&SortMethod=h%7C-&MaximumDocuments=1&FuzzyDegree=0&ImageQuality=r75g8 /r75g8/x150y150g16/i425&Display=p%7Cf&DefSeekPage=x&SearchBack=ZyActionL&Back=ZyActionS&BackDesc=Results%20page&MaximumPages=1&ZyEntry=2

grandfathered in.[23] Technology designations such as BAT may actually discourage competition and prevent the implementation of newer, cleaner, or more cost-effective methods. The political maneuvers done to influence regulatory decisions also create unlikely alliances between groups truly advocating for a protective policy and those who desire to benefit from the decision, akin to temperance groups arguing to limit Sunday sales of alcohol and the bootleggers happy to see competition eliminated.*

3.5 Managing Global Health Risks Going Forward

On the whole, the risk assessment/risk management paradigm that is dominant in U.S. regulation calls for existing health hazards to be quantified and then managed, one by one. This approach is by nature slow and cumbersome and more fundamentally, the absence of foresight that it embodies has led to numerous missed opportunities for primary prevention of human health impacts from environmental hazards. The current approach also reflects the *community-level* concerns and expectations for access to clean, natural resources and safely manufactured products that emerged beginning in the late 1960s and 1970s. Alternatives to the current technology-based, command and control risk management approach must move away from such an entrenched regulatory infrastructure to allow for more flexibility and diverse approaches to mitigating *global-scale, environmentally hazardous exposures.*

One approach is to adopt more incentive-based standards. To be effective, such standards focus on the greater environment, such as an entire watershed or the air quality across an entire region or even across national borders. For example, all of the counties and their municipalities that rely on the same watershed might be tasked with working together to ensure that the river does not exceed any existing federal water quality health standards, such as the Clean Water Act's Total Maximum Daily Loads (TMDL) standards for a waterway. The various entities that impact the river's quality have to cooperate and work directly with each other and have the flexibility to form creative partnerships to stay within legal compliance. However, this incentive-based approach varies from the current method of enforcing TMDLs that requires governmental regulators to grant discharge permits and monitor pollution for each individual contributor to the river. Several such cooperative river associations exist in Europe and a few within the United States, such as the Carson River Coalition made up of five counties in both California and Nevada and over 20 agencies and organizations within the watershed.[24]

Another example of an incentive-based approach was the Clean Air Act's successful sulfur dioxide (SO_2) cap and trade program to combat SO_2's contribution to acid rain. The law capped total SO_2 emissions for the nation's 3,200 coal-fired power plants and divided these emissions into discrete government-issued allowances to emit SO_2, *permits to pollute* in effect. A market was created where facilities could buy and sell these allowances with each facility choosing their most cost-effective option, whether it be to reduce emissions and sell their shares or pay for more allowances to cover SO_2 emissions. The total amount of allowances and, therefore, SO_2 emitted, however, could not increase. For many facilities, instituting SO_2 reduction through a change in equipment or process was the better option and overall aggregate annual SO_2 emissions actually declined below the program's initial cap.[25] This type of allowance trading structure is also called cap and trade and has been proposed as a possible solution for reducing carbon dioxide emissions associated with climate change.

This chapter has described several environmental risk protection tenets or beliefs that are embedded within existing environmental statutes, such as "make the polluter pay" or "ensure environmental justice." Future risk

---

*For an entertaining depiction of these unlikely alliances, readers are encouraged to watch the YouTube video featuring Dr. Bruce Yandle titled Bootleggers and Baptists Theory of Environmental Regulation, https://www .youtube.com/watch?v=msQ_khFmKtU

management decisions must also encompass the principle of environment sustainability. The United Nations World Commission on Environment and Development defined "sustainability (as) the ability to meet the needs of the present without compromising the ability of future generations to meet their own needs."[26] Efforts to reduce the amount of pollution generated by developing greener technologies as well as greater efforts to encourage recycling represent the ideals of sustainability.

The cradle-to-grave approach described earlier in this chapter as part of RCRA management of hazardous waste (see Figure 3.2) has also been adapted with a more sustainable twist, titled the *cradle-to-cradle* approach.[27] Rather than just focus on the life cycle of a product from its creation until its disposal, the cradle-to-cradle approach encourages adding a feedback loop where the resource may be re-used within the same process or perhaps repurposed for another use. (Refer to **Figure 3.7**, which indicates this additional feedback concept associated with the cradle-to-cradle approach that adds to the cradle-to-grave approach depicted as a one-way process.)

The conceptualization of this approach in Figure 3.7 is often used to analyze every step in the entire life cycle of a manufacturing process or the provision of resources, such as electricity or drinking water. **Life Cycle Analysis** may be used to assess different methods at each step in a process, such as how the basic resource is acquired, perhaps replacing the mining of ore with a process to recycle the resource postindustrial usage. The environmental costs and benefits of building the recycling system on site could be compared with the issues associated with transporting raw material from where it is mined. Often, the life cycle approach is used to determine alternatives within the production stage, such as substituting a petroleum-based lubricant for a greener alternative, perhaps made from a biofuel. Life cycle analysis is primarily a tool and will reflect whatever the underlying objective is, such as cost-savings or improving efficiency. Therefore, the risk management process must clearly emphasize that **environmental sustainability** be one of the goals for any life cycle comparative exercise.

Sustainable risk management practices must recognize the finite ability of resources on the planet to sustain the population, protect these resources from degradation related to human activities, and ensure that equitable and ethical access to these life-sustaining resources exist now and in the future. Going forward, environmental risk management approaches must evolve to address more global-scale environmental hazards, encompass cooperative agreements between nations, and be adaptable to work in a variety of settings.

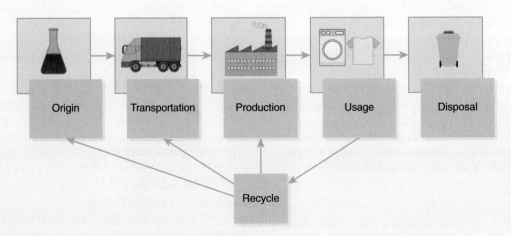

Figure 3.7 Cradle to grave or Cradle once more.

Study Questions

1. Identify characteristics that influence perceptions of the acceptability of an environmental health risk.
2. Provide examples of environmental laws or approaches that demonstrate the risk protection principles of environmental justice, precautionary principle, polluter pays, and sustainability.

References

1. Office of Water. *Drinking water standards and health advisories tables*. United States Environmental Protection Agency. EPA 822-F-18-001. 2018.
2. American Cancer Society. *Lifetime risk of developing or dying from cancer.* Retrieved June 20, 2020 from https://www.cancer.org/cancer/cancer-basics/lifetime-probability-of-developing-or-dying-from-cancer.html. 2020.
3. Sandman, PM. Risk communication: facing public outrage. *EPA J.* 1987;21-22.
4. Starr C. Social benefit versus technological risk: what is our society willing to pay for safety? *Science,* 1969;165:1232-1238.
5. Lowrance W. *Of acceptable risk: science and the determination of safety.* William Kaufman, Inc. 1976.
6. Rowe WD. *An anatomy of risk.* John Wiley & Sons. 1977.
7. Slovic P, Fischhoff B, Lichtenstein S. Rating the risks. *Environment.* 1979;21:14-39.
8. Slovic P. Perception of risk. *Science.* 1987;236(4799): 280-285.
9. Fitchen JM. When toxic chemicals pollute residential environments: the cultural meanings of home and home ownership. *Human Organization,* 1989;48.
10. Covello V. Risk communication. In: H. Frumkin (Ed.). *Environmental Health: From Global to Local,* 2005; 988-1009;34. Jossey-Bass.
11. Denchak, M. (2018). *Flint water crisis: everything you need to know."* Natural Resources Defense Council. Retrieved June 20, 2020 from https://www.nrdc.org/stories/flint-water-crisis-everything-you-need-know
12. U.S. Environmental Protection Agency. (n.d). Plan EJ 2014. 2011. Retrieved June 20, 2012 from https://www.epa.gov/environmentaljustice/plan-ej-2014
13. U.S. Environmental Protection Agency. (n.d.) The U.S. EPA's environmental justice strategic plan for 2016-2020. Retrieved March 12, 2012 from: https://www.epa.gov/sites/production/files/2016-05/documents/052216_ej_2020_strategic_plan_final_0.pdf
14. Hsu T, Rabin RC. Johnson & Johnson to end talc-based baby powder sales in North America. *The New York Times.* https://www.nytimes.com/2020/05/19/business/johnson-baby-powder-sales-stopped.html. 2020.
15. Kriebel D, Tickner J, Epstein P. The precautionary principle in environmental science. *Environ Health Persp.* 2001;109:871-876.
16. Kriebel D, Tickner J. Reenergizing public health through precaution. *Am J Pub Health.* 2001;91(9):1351-1355.
17. Maynard RL. *Late lessons from early warnings: the precautionary principle 1896–2000.* Luxembourg: Office for Official Publications of the European Communities. 2001.
18. European Commission. (n.d.). *REACH.* Retrieved September 2, 2012 from: http://ec.europa.eu/environment/chemicals/reach/reach_intro.htm
19. U.S. Environmental Protection Agency. *History of the resource Conservation and Recovery Act.* Retrieved June 15, 2020 from https://www.epa.gov/rcra/history-resource-conservation-and-recovery-act-rcra
20. United States Environmental Protection Agency. (n.d.). *Superfund: CERCLA Overview.* Retrieved June 15, 2020 from: https://www.epa.gov/superfund/superfund-cercla-overview
21. U.S. Environmental Protection Agency. (n.d.). *Regulatory information by topic: water.* Retrieved November 11, 2012 from https://www.epa.gov/regulatory-information-topic/regulatory-information-topic-water
22. Office of Water, U.S. Environmental Protection Agency. *Consumer confidence report rule: a quick reference guide.* Retrieved June 21, 2020 from: https://nepis.epa.gov/Exe/tiff2png.cgi/P100529A.PNG?-r+75+-g+7+D%3A%5CZYFILES%5CINDEX%20DATA%5C06THRU10%5CTIFF%5C00000518%5CP100529A.TIF. 2009.
23. Yandle B. *Thoughts on the relative merits of cap-and-trade versus emission taxes for controlling carbon emissions.* Property and Environmental Research Center. Retrieved June 20, 2020 from https://www.perc.org/2009/05/27/thoughts-on-the-relative-merits-of-cap-and-trade-versus-emission-taxes-for-controlling-carbon-emissions/ 2009
24. Carson River Subconservancy District. (n.d.). *Carson River Coalition.* Information available at http://www.cwsd.org/carson-river-coalition/

25. Stavins R, Chan G, Stowe R, Sweeney R. *The US sulfur dioxide cap and trade programme and lessons for climate policy.* Retrieved June 21, 2020 from the VOX CEPR Policy Portal https://voxeu.org/article/lessons-climate-policy-us-sulphur-dioxide-cap-and-trade-programme. 2012.

26. Evans M. What is environmental sustainability? *Sustainable Business.* Retrieved June 19, 2020 from https://www.thebalancesmb.com/what-is-sustainability-3157876. 2019.

27. Braungart M, McDonough W. *Cradle to cradle: remaking the way we make things.* Farrar, Straus & Giroux. 2002.

Websites Used as Sources for Table 3.1

U.S. Department of Agriculture

U.S. Department of Agriculture. About FSIS. Available at: www.fsis.usda.gov/About_FSIS/index.asp. Accessed July 23, 2012.

U.S. Department of Agriculture. Agencies and Offices: National Agricultural Statistics Service (NASS) Overview. Available at: www.usda.gov/wps/portal/!ut/p/_s.7_0_A/7_0_1OB?contentidonly=true&contentid=NASS_Agency_Splash.xml&x=7&y=11. Accessed July 23, 2012.

U.S. Department of Agriculture. Agricultural Marketing Service (AMS) Overview. Available at: www.usda.gov/wps/portal/!ut/p/_s.7_0_A/7_0_1OB?contentidonly=true&contentid=AMS_Agency_Splash.xml&x=14&y=10. Accessed July 23, 2012.

U.S. Department of Agriculture. Animal and Plant Health Inspection Service (APHIS) Overview. Available at: www.usda.gov/wps/portal/!ut/p/_s.7_0_A/7_0_1OB?contentidonly=true&contentid=APHIS_Agency_Splash.xml&x=10&y=6. Accessed July 23, 2012.

U.S. Department of Agriculture. Economic Research Service (ERS) Overview. Available at www.usda.gov/wps/portal/usda/usdahome?contentid=ERS_Agency_Splash.xml&contentidonly=true. Accessed July 23, 2012.

U.S. Department of Energy

Energy Information Administration. About EIA. Available at: www.eia.gov/about/. Accessed July 23, 2012.

Office of Civilian Radioactive Waste Management. Available at: http://energy.gov/downloads/office-civilian-radioactive-waste-management. Accessed July 24, 2012.

U.S. Department of Health and Human Services

Agency for Toxic Substances & Disease Registry. ATSDR Background and Congressional Mandates. Available at: www.atsdr.cdc.gov/about/congress.html. Accessed July 23, 2012.

Centers for Disease Control and Prevention. Organizational Chart. Available at: www.cdc.gov/about/organization/pdf/CDC-Photo-Org-Chart.pdf. Accessed July 23, 2012.

Centers for Disease Control and Prevention. Vision, Mission, Core Values, and Pledge. Available at: www.cdc.gov/about/organization/mission.htm. Accessed July 23, 2012.

Food and Drug Administration. FDA Fundamentals. Available at: www.fda.gov/AboutFDA/Transparency/Basics/ucm192695.htm. Accessed July 24, 2012.

National Cancer Institute. NCI Mission Statement. Available at: www.cancer.gov/aboutnci/overview/mission. Accessed July 23, 2012.

National Institute of Environmental Health Sciences. Your Environment, Your Health. Available at: www.niehs.nih.gov/. Accessed July 23, 2012.

National Institutes of Health. Institutes, Centers & Offices. Available at: www.nih.gov/icd/. Accessed July 23, 2012.

National Institutes of Health. Mission. Available at: www.nih.gov/about/mission.htm. Accessed July 23, 2012.

National Institute for Occupational Safety and Health. About NIOSH. Available at: www.cdc.gov/niosh/about.html. Accessed July 23, 2012.

National Toxicology Program. About the NTP. Available at: http://ntp.niehs.nih.gov/index.cfm?objectid=7201637B-BDB7-CEBA-F57E39896A08F1BB. Accessed July 23, 2012.

U.S. Department of Health and Human Services. HHS: What We Do. Available at: www.hhs.gov/about/whatwedo.html/. Accessed July 23, 2012.

U.S. Department of Labor

Mine Safety and Health Administration. MSHA's Statutory Functions. Available at: www.msha.gov/MSHAINFO/MSHAINF1.HTM. Accessed July 24, 2012.

Occupational Safety & Health Administration. About OSHA. Available at: www.osha.gov/about.html. Accessed July 23, 2012.

Independent Executive Agencies

U.S. Consumer Product Safety Commission. About CPSC. Available at: www.cpsc.gov/about/about.html. Accessed July 23, 2012.

U.S. Environmental Protection Agency. About EPA/Our Mission and What We Do. Available at: www.epa.gov/aboutepa/whatwedo.html. Accessed July 23, 2012.

U.S. NRC. About NRC. Available at: http://www.nrc.gov/about-nrc.html. Accessed July 23, 2012.

Private Nonprofit Institutions

Institute of Medicine. About the IOM. Available at: www.iom.edu/About-IOM.aspx. Accessed October 16, 2012.

The National Academies. About Us. Available at: www.nationalacademies.org/about/index.html/. Accessed July 23, 2012.

National Academy of Sciences. Mission. Available at: www.nasonline.org/about-nas/mission/. Accessed July 23, 2012.

National Research Council. Welcome to the National Research Council. Available at: www.nationalacademies.org/nrc/index.html. Accessed July 23, 2012.

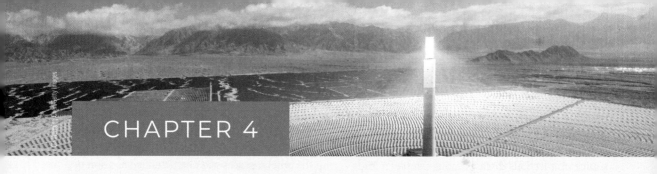

CHAPTER 4

Living with Nature

LEARNING OBJECTIVES

After studying this chapter, the reader will be able to:

- Define or explain the key terms introduced throughout the chapter
- Distinguish among the major types of pathogenic infectious agents
- Explain the distinct and varied ways in which infectious disease can be transmitted
- Describe key strategies for reducing the transmission of infectious diseases
- Describe the health risks associated with natural poisons
- Describe the electromagnetic spectrum and relate it to the distinction between ionizing and nonionizing radiation
- Describe radioactive decay, distinguishing between alpha, beta, and gamma radiation
- Explain how exposure to ionizing radiation is measured
- Describe the key natural sources of exposure to radiation
- Summarize the human health risks of radiation
- Outline the broad range of public health impacts that natural disasters may bring

Increasingly, the natural world is obscured by human modifications to it and elements of *nature* may feel remote from daily life. Nonetheless, humans are not the only species trying to survive on the planet and, in many instances, we are in direct competition with these other planetary passengers for the same resources. At other times we serve *as the food and shelter* for these other species. Prior to continuing this textbook's presentation about how our anthropogenic activities interact with the environment and the resulting impact on our health, this chapter focuses on the natural world and the hazards humans face simply by virtue of living on planet Earth.

- Section 4.1 describes the pathogenic agents responsible for infectious disease and aspects of their transmission. This section also highlights the impact of these infectious agents in terms of human morbidity and mortality and discusses how humans have tried to prevent the large toll that infectious diseases take on our well-being.

- Although brief, Section 4.2 presents information about naturally occurring poisons, including descriptions of some of the venomous creatures that are a reason many people try to avoid nature.

- The electromagnetic radiation spectrum is presented in Section 4.3 with emphasis on the health risks associated with naturally occurring radiation exposure.

- The last section of the chapter, Section 4.4, addresses the public health impact of natural disasters.

4.1 Infectious Disease

Humans exist within ecosystems, which encompass other animals, plants, and microscopic organisms in a complex web of relationships. This close coexistence, which offers many benefits, is also the source of infectious disease among people, a leading cause of global mortality and morbidity.

All animals are habitats for other organisms—the result of millions of years of coevolution. The human body is *host* to many small organisms because it offers sheltered conditions and nutrients that enhance the organisms' reproduction. Many of these organisms are harmless, and some are even helpful. For example, large populations of bacteria in the gut and on the skin ordinarily prevent disease-causing bacteria from establishing colonies. Thus, some relationships between microorganisms and their animal hosts are mutually beneficial; the associations we call **infectious diseases** are those that are troublesome to the animal host.

The term **pathogen** identifies an infectious agent that, when it becomes established in a host organism (i.e., when it infects the host), causes a specific infectious disease in the host. Pathogenic bacteria, for example, cause a large number of distinct diseases in people and other animals. Other factors, such as genetic traits or environmental conditions, may contribute to the risk of illness, but the pathogen is the factor that must be present for a specific infectious disease to occur.

The great variety of symptoms in infectious diseases results from the wide range of processes that can be triggered as a pathogen makes its home in the human body. To give just two examples: The diarrhea caused by some pathogenic *Escherichia coli* bacteria occurs because the bacteria secrete a toxin that stimulates the production of an enzyme, which changes the fluid balance in the intestine[1]; and the chills and fever that characterize malaria occur when, at one point in a complex life cycle, large numbers of parasites are released into the bloodstream by bursting red blood cells.[2]

Death and disability from infectious disease have figured prominently in human experience, and so these diseases have been closely observed for many centuries. Early scientists distinguished among diseases with different symptoms and appreciated that different diseases might have distinct causes. It was well understood by the 16th century, for example, that close contact with a sick person increased the risk of some diseases, including smallpox, leprosy, and syphilis, but not others. For many years, the elusive causal factor for the other diseases was characterized as a sort of atmospheric emanation known as a **miasma**, rising from the Earth (in the 17th-century belief) or from rotting organic matter (in the 19th-century version).[3] For example, miasmas were thought to cause malaria (the name of the disease is derived from the Italian for "bad air").

From the early 19th century, scientists who believed that diseases could be caused by germs were still in the minority. Although microbes were first observed under the microscope in the 17th century, evidence that they caused disease only accumulated slowly. But in 1876, everything changed: Scientist Robert Koch isolated the anthrax bacterium and demonstrated that it produced the disease in cattle. By the end of the 19th century, scientists had documented the infectious agents of typhoid fever, leprosy, malaria, tuberculosis, cholera, diphtheria, tetanus, plague, and other illnesses.[3]

Present scientific understanding of infectious disease is extensive and sophisticated, yet much is still unknown about the complex and ever-evolving relationships among human beings, pathogens, and the environment. Although humans have developed systems to manage infectious disease, we are unlikely to ever control it.

Types of Pathogenic Agents

Several types of infective agents act as human pathogens. **Worms** are multicellular organisms that can be as small as 1 mm in diameter* but can range to more than 1 m in length (see **Figure 4.1**). Worms are not microorganisms; even the smallest are visible to the naked eye. Parasitic worms are also known as helminths.

---

*1 millimeter (mm) = 0.001 meter (m); 1 micron = 0.001 millimeter; 1 nanometer = 0.001 micron.

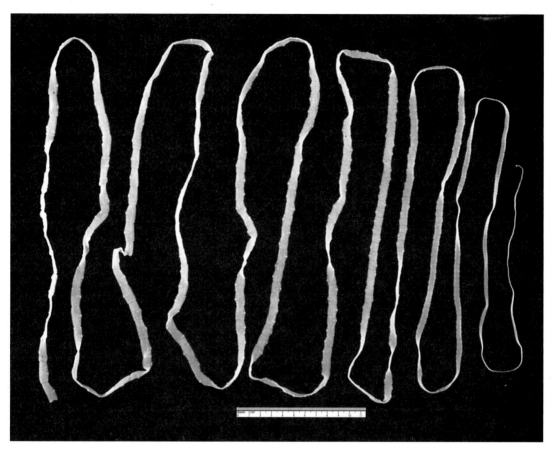

Figure 4.1 Usually ingested in an immature form in undercooked meat, the *Taenia saginata* tapeworm frequently reaches 15 feet in length and can live for years in the small intestine.

Courtesy of CDC Public Health Image Library. ID# 5260. Content provider CDC. Available at: http://phil.cdc.gov/phil/home.asp. Accessed October 3, 2012.

Protozoa are single-celled organisms. These microorganisms are approximately 10 microns in diameter—1/100th the diameter of a small worm—and were some of the first organisms seen under a microscope. A protozoan cell has a true nucleus that contains DNA, and most protozoa can move actively about in the environment. Among the illnesses caused by protozoan parasites are malaria and cryptosporidiosis, a disease that affected more than 400,000 people in a 1993 waterborne disease outbreak in Milwaukee. Pathogenic worms and protozoa are **parasites**: They must spend at least a small part of their life cycle inside an animal host, on which they depend for certain benefits but to which they give no benefit.

Like protozoa, **bacteria** are single-celled organisms. With a typical diameter of about 1 micron, bacteria are smaller than protozoan parasites (see **Figure 4.2**). They lack a true nucleus with a membrane, instead simply containing a mass or ring of DNA. And, unlike parasites, most bacteria can live their full life cycle outside of the body of a host organism, living in water or soil, for example. Tuberculosis, cholera, tetanus, and Lyme disease are examples of diseases caused by bacteria, as is infection by pathogenic *E. coli*. Some bacteria are aerobic, requiring free oxygen to survive; other species can survive only in an anaerobic environment (an environment lacking free oxygen); and still others can tolerate either condition.

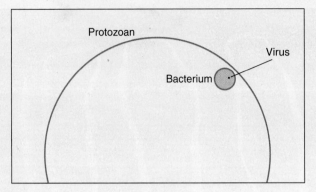

Figure 4.2 Approximate relative size of protozoan, bacterium, and virus.

Some species of bacteria can take on a hardy form, becoming dormant cells with a hard coating; such **bacterial spores** can survive inhospitable conditions such as a dry environment, returning to their active, or vegetative, form when they find themselves in better conditions (e.g., in the human body).

Some bacteria cause injury to cells by invading body tissues and multiplying (infection); others cause injury by secreting a toxin (intoxication). Much of the terminology used to describe bacteria reflects their traditional classification by shape—round (*cocci*), spiral (*spirilli*), or rod-shaped (*bacilli*), like the tuberculosis bacteria in **Figure 4.3**—and their response to laboratory staining techniques.

Certain molds and yeasts, which are single-celled **fungi** slightly larger than bacteria, can also cause human disease. Many fungal infections occur in medical settings or in individuals with weakened immune systems (e.g., from AIDS), but fungi are widespread in the natural environment. The most common fungal diseases worldwide include cryptococcal meningitis, pneumocystis pneumonia, allergic fungal diseases, pulmonary aspergillosis, coccidioidomycosis, histoplasmosis, and fungal eye and skin infections.[4]

Unlike the unicellular pathogens, a **virus**, at about 50 nanometers, is simply a strand of genetic material with a coat of protein. Lacking a cell wall, most viruses do not survive long outside a host organism. A virus cannot reproduce outside the host, but rather uses the host cell's biochemical machinery to make copies of its own genetic material and assemble new viruses. Functionally,

viruses are parasites—they cannot reproduce without the host organism—but the term parasite dates back to an era when viruses were unknown and is more often used to refer to worms and protozoa. Viral pathogens cause influenza, measles, polio, Ebola hemorrhagic fever, dengue fever, and hantavirus pulmonary syndrome, among other illnesses.

Finally, **prions** are simply proteins found on the surface of normal nerve cells of some mammalian species, including humans. These prion proteins exist in normal and abnormal forms, which have the same chemical makeup but different shapes. As is true of all proteins, a prion's shape is a critical part of its identity and affects its function. The shape of the normal prion gives it a weak and flexible structure; the shape of the abnormal prion makes it rigid and nearly indestructible. The abnormal prion also has the special property of inducing nearby normal prions to convert to the abnormal shape, through a mechanism that is not fully understood. When established in the brain, the abnormal prions produce a set of degenerative brain illnesses (encephalopathies). Because abnormal prions form plaques that create holes in the brain, producing a sponge-like appearance at autopsy, these diseases are called transmissible spongiform encephalopathies (TSes). As detailed later in the context of the food supply, prion diseases emerged from relative obscurity in the 1990s when it became clear that abnormal prions could be transmitted to people who ate beef from cattle suffering from "mad cow disease."

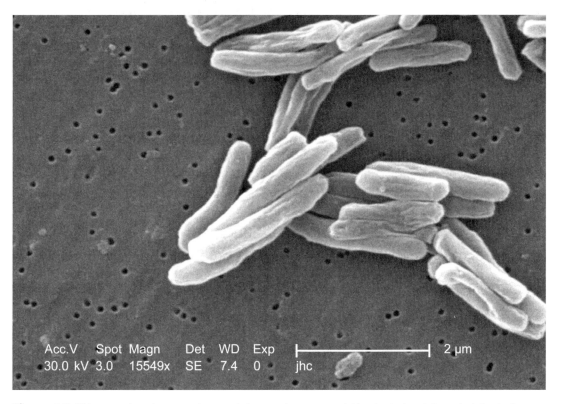

Acc.V Spot Magn   Det WD Exp   2 µm
30.0 kV 3.0 15549x   SE   7.4   0   jhc

Figure 4.3 This scanning electron micrograph image shows several *Mycobacterium tuberculosis* bacteria; as the name suggests, this organism causes tuberculosis.

Courtesy of CDC Public Health Image Library. ID# 8438. Content providers CDC/Dr. Ray Butler; Janice Carr. Available at: http://phil.cdc.gov/phil/home.asp. Accessed October 4, 2012

The Transmission of Infectious Disease

The source of an infectious agent is called the **reservoir**, and is typically thought of as some type of contaminated environmental media, such as bacterial contamination in drinking water. However, the reservoir is often other humans or animal species. An infectious disease that can be transmitted to humans from nonhuman animals, either domestic or wild, is called a **zoonosis**, or a zoonotic disease. Influenza, rabies, and anthrax are all zoonoses. Pathogens are flexible and opportunistic travelers, and so infectious disease is transmitted in many different ways from the source to a susceptible host. Direct transmission occurs mainly by closeness or direct contact, whereas indirect transmission may occur via the fecal–oral pathway; by some environmental medium (including food); or by vector. In the context of infectious disease, the term **vector** (from the Latin verb "to carry") refers to a living transmitter of pathogens.

Transmission Through Closeness or Contact

Microbes can pass from person to person simply through proximity, most often by the sharing of bodily fluids.* For example, coughing and sneezing spray droplets into the air. Droplets from a

---

*Strictly speaking, the term *contagious disease* refers to infectious disease transmitted from person to person through closeness or contact, although in casual usage, it sometimes appears synonymous with *infectious disease*. The term *communicable disease* is used with varied meanings. The terms *contagious disease* and *communicable disease* are not used in this text.

person with an infectious respiratory disease contain pathogens, which can be passed to a nearby person who inhales the suspended droplets during the brief period before they settle out of the air. The global pandemic associated with the COVID-19 coronavirus has made us all acutely aware of this kind of transmission. Diseases transmitted by droplet include respiratory illnesses caused by bacteria (e.g., diphtheria, tuberculosis, and pertussis [commonly known as whooping cough]) or viruses (e.g., influenza, measles, mumps, and rubella [commonly called German measles]). Other pathogens, including streptococcal bacteria, the herpes simplex-1 virus (HSV-1), and the infectious mononucleosis virus, are mainly transmitted by direct oral contact.

Respiratory secretions or saliva can also be passed from person to person via an object in the environment, such as a shared handkerchief, utensil, or computer keyboard. An object that passively transmits pathogens in this way is called a **fomite**. For example, toddlers in daycare transmit disease via fomites by mouthing and sharing toys. Pathogens vary in their capacity to survive such a passage through the environment.

Infectious diseases can also be transmitted via sexual contact. Major sexually transmitted diseases (also called venereal diseases) include the bacterial illnesses syphilis and gonorrhea, as well as the herpes simplex-2 virus (HSV-2, also known as genital herpes) and the human papillomavirus (HPV). Some pathogens that are sexually transmitted, such as the hepatitis B and hepatitis C viruses and the human immunodeficiency virus (HIV) that causes acquired immune deficiency syndrome (AIDS), can also be transmitted via blood. This can occur through medical procedures such as blood transfusions or via syringes acting as a type of **mechanical vector**: Drug users might share syringes, for example, and shortages of new syringes can lead to the reuse of syringes in resource-poor medical settings.

Transmission of diseases through closeness or contact can be reduced mainly through personal behaviors (e.g., covering the nose when sneezing, not sharing utensils, preventing sexual transmission) or by remediating overcrowded conditions. Most of the diseases that can now be prevented by vaccination are diseases transmitted through closeness or contact.

Airborne Transmission of Pathogens

As already noted, pathogens can be transmitted via coughing and sneezing. When this occurs, relatively large droplets are inhaled by a nearby person during the very brief period before the droplets settle out, as is the case for the typical transmission of the flu virus. In contrast, the term **airborne transmission** is reserved for a different phenomenon that does not require close proximity: Some pathogens can be transmitted in **aerosols**, which are very fine liquid droplets or solid particles that stay suspended in air for some time, can be carried for considerable distances on air currents, and when inhaled, can penetrate deep into the respiratory tract.

Airborne transmission is difficult to demonstrate and has been clearly documented for only a few diseases, including tuberculosis and measles.[5] The elusive airborne transmission mechanism was first documented in the 1950s, through an experiment in which guinea pigs were housed in a laboratory above a hospital's tuberculosis ward, and air from the ward was circulated through the guinea pigs' cages.[6] Aerosols can also be created in the cooling towers of large air-conditioning systems (where air is blown through water to cool the water by evaporation) and then carried via ambient air or through air-conditioning ducts.[7] Air-conditioning ducts were the source of the first identified outbreak of the pneumonia-like *Legionella* illness (Legionnaires' disease) at an American Legion convention in 1976. Hantavirus, which causes severe respiratory illness, can be transmitted to people via aerosolized rodent urine or feces.[8]

Fecal–Oral Transmission of Diarrheal Disease

Many diseases transmitted via environmental media are fecal in origin. However, fecal–oral transmission of disease plays out very differently in the more developed and less developed countries. When a person has an infectious diarrheal disease, his or her feces contain pathogens. If another person somehow ingests even a small amount of this fecal matter, he or she is exposed to the pathogens via the **fecal–oral pathway**. In this way, one person's **infectious diarrheal disease** becomes the next person's **disease of fecal origin**; these two terms refer to the same set of diseases. The list of diseases of fecal origin includes cholera and typhoid fever (both bacterial), dysentery (which can be caused either by a bacterium or by a protozoan parasite), the protozoan illnesses giardiasis and cryptosporidiosis, and the viral diseases hepatitis A, norovirus infection, and polio. Both giardiasis and cryptosporidiosis are zoonotic illnesses that affect wild animals and farm animals as well as people.

How does one come to inadvertently ingest fecal pathogens? Much as a fomite can transmit diseases from person to person, usually over short distances, water can act as a passive transmitter of infectious disease organisms through the natural environment, sometimes over very long distances (**waterborne transmission**; see (*a*) and (*b*) in **Figure 4.4**). For example, a community might release untreated sewage into a river from which a downstream community draws its drinking water. This practice remains widespread in less-developed countries and was common in the more developed countries through the early 20th century. For example, for decades, the cities of Detroit, Toledo, Cleveland, and Akron dumped raw sewage into Lake Erie or rivers that flowed into it; and Buffalo dumped its sewage into the river flowing out of the lake.[9] Like lakes and rivers, groundwater is at risk of fecal contamination, and so a drinking water well located downgradient of a privy or a septic system can supply water tainted

by fecal waste. Finally, water at beaches and in swimming pools can be contaminated, with the result that swimmers are exposed via incidental ingestion of the water. (The fecal–oral pathway also runs through food, as described later.)

In the more developed countries, such **waterborne illness** is largely, though not completely, controlled through treatment of both sewage and drinking water (as detailed later in the context of community-level infrastructure). In many less developed countries, however, waterborne illness caused by large-scale fecal contamination of rivers, lakes, and wells is a central fact of life. Diarrheal disease, transmitted by ingesting contaminated water, is the major health impact of such contamination and a leading cause of mortality and morbidity in less-developed countries. Dermal contact carries a different risk: If a person with a skin wound swims or bathes in water contaminated by sewage, the wound can become infected. Left untreated, a serious wound infection may progress to septicemia (blood poisoning).

Although water is the dominant environmental medium in fecal–oral transmission, as indicated by the heavy lines in Figure 4.4, it is not the only one. Uncontrolled fecal waste can also contaminate soil (*c*), a common problem in regions where the latrine (a simple pit, used as a toilet) is widely used for waste disposal, or where fecal waste is simply deposited on the ground. In the industrialized world, exposure to human fecal waste on the ground is mostly limited to recreational activities, such as camping or playing at playgrounds where diaperless toddlers may be present. People can also be exposed to feces of farm animals or pets. In any setting, young children are particularly likely

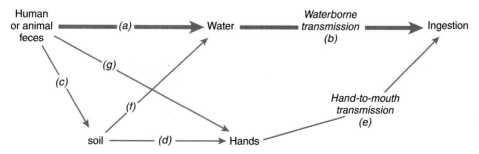

Figure 4.4 Fecal–oral transmission of disease via water, soil, and hands in a setting with no treatment of sewage or drinking water.

to have these exposures because they spend time playing on the ground—getting soil on their hands (*d*) and putting their hands into their mouths, resulting in **hand-to-mouth transmission** of pathogens (*e*). Adults' hands, too, can convey pathogens along the fecal–oral pathway as fingers touch the mouth in eating, smoking, or gesturing. Contaminated soil can also add to the pathogen load of rivers, lakes, or groundwater (*f*).

To prevent direct contamination of the hands with fecal matter (*g*), those who live in more developed countries are routinely taught to wash their hands after using the toilet, changing a baby's diaper, or aiding a sick or disabled person with toileting. The goal of handwashing is not to kill microorganisms but rather to remove them, and this is best accomplished through the use of soap and clean running water, vigorous rubbing for at least 20 seconds, and careful drying of the hands. Despite the growing popularity of hand sanitizers, they do not eliminate all microorganisms, and in fact are ineffective if hands are clearly dirty.[10] In less-developed countries, facilities for effective handwashing may not be readily available.

The Composting Toilet

In some less-developed countries where fecal–oral transmission is a prominent cause of illness, an innovative approach to sanitation is gaining traction. The composting toilet does not require running water, but it is much more than a latrine. It is designed to convert human waste into a stable compost, given adequate time and space in a ventilated composting chamber.

There are two basic variations on the composting toilet: batch systems and continuous systems. A batch (double-vault) composting toilet has two holding tanks side by side. One vault is used until it is full, and then the toilet stool is moved to the second vault. The waste in the first vault slowly dries out so that it can be removed and disposed of or used as fertilizer. A batch composting toilet produces unpleasant odors as fecal waste accumulates because the composting chamber is usually vented passively, typically with a 2-inch pipe. However, the batch composting toilet is less expensive to build than the continuous composting toilet. In a continuous (single-chamber) composting toilet, such as the ReSource Composting Toilet,[1] waste falls into a single tank, and coarse sawdust or wood shavings are periodically added into the composting chamber, adding carbon and helping to maintain the aerobic environment needed for decomposition. The composting chamber is vented, usually with a 4- or 6-inch ventilation stack equipped with a low-voltage electric or solar exhaust fan (see **Figure 4.5**). In the aerobic environment of the tank, bacteria digest the organic wastes, much as in garden compost. The compost is not removed for several years, and over time, pathogens die off, simply losing out in the competition with composting organisms. The tank has an inspection door near the top and another door at the bottom through which finished compost is removed. This compost, which does not carry the chemical burden found in municipal sewage sludge, can be safely used as fertilizer.[2] Urine undergoes nitrification inside the composting tank; within a few days, it becomes an odorless, nitrogen-rich liquid fertilizer that moves through a filter at the bottom of the tank and drains into a separate storage unit below the composting tank. If properly built and vented, a continuous composting toilet is virtually odorless.

In less-developed countries, the centralized sewer model is a particularly poor fit. As detailed later in the context of municipal sanitation, sewage systems are expensive to build and maintain; they create a byproduct known as sludge, which must be disposed of; and they use enormous quantities of water. In less-developed countries, where fecal contamination of drinking water affects a large share of the population and where most of the world's 1.8 million annual deaths from fecal disease occur,[3] the composting toilet offers the potential for dramatic improvements in health and comfort at relatively low cost. Moreover, it is a sustainable approach to sanitation on a global scale, unlike the use of water to carry sewage to municipal treatment facilities.

1. Resource Institute for Low-Entropy Systems. (n.d.). Technology. Retrieved August 29, 2012 from www .riles.org/tech.htm

2. Rockefeller A, Goodland R. What is environmental sustainability in sanitation? In: Goodland R., Orlando L, Anhang J., eds. *Towards Sustainable Sanitation*. The International Association of Impact Assessment. 2001.

3. World Health Organization. Statistical Annex. (2004). World Health Report 2004 – Changing History.

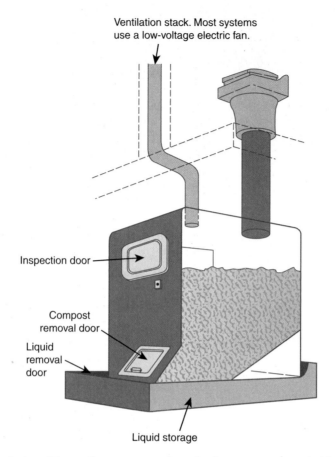

Ventilation stack. Most systems use a low-voltage electric fan.

Inspection door

Compost removal door

Liquid removal door

Liquid storage

Figure 4.5 The design of the continuous composting toilet features a separate holding area for liquid waste, doors to inspect and remove compost and liquid, and a ventilation stack. When properly built and vented, a continuous composting toilet is odorless.

Courtesy of Clivusmultrum Incorporated.

Transmission of Nonfecal Organisms Found in Water or Soil

Although many pathogens found in water or soil are of fecal origin, these media are also natural reservoirs for many nonfecal pathogens. Just two nonfecal pathogens are described here, chosen simply to demonstrate the broad range of ways by which pathogens can be transmitted.

Guinea worm disease (dracunculiasis) is a waterborne parasitic illness. When a person drinks water containing Guinea worm larvae, the parasite matures in the body. Ultimately, a worm

up to three feet long emerges through a skin wound, usually when the skin is immersed in water. The worm immediately spills larvae back into the water, restarting the cycle of disease.[11] Guinea worm disease was once widespread in sub-Saharan Africa but is now uncommon, largely because of the widespread use of simple methods to filter water (see **Figure 4.6**)—a public health success story.

Soil is also a natural reservoir for several pathogens important to human health. Spores of the bacterium *Clostridium tetani*, which causes tetanus (lockjaw), are widespread in soil and

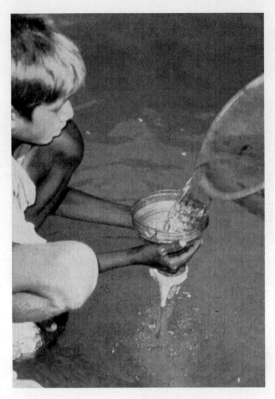

Figure 4.6 Use of a simple strainer like the one being demonstrated here—a metal funnel and a piece of filter cloth—can filter out water fleas that carry the larval Guinea worm parasite.

Courtesy of CDC Public Health Image Library. ID# 8206. Content provider CDC. Available at: http://phil.cdc
.gov/phil/home.asp. Accessed October 4, 2012.

can survive there under dry conditions for many years. People are most commonly exposed to *C tetani* via a skin wound. For example, a deep puncture wound from stepping on a rusty nail can result in a tetanus infection—not from the nail or the rust, but from bacteria in soil that the nail embeds into the wound. In less-developed countries, newborns and their mothers are at risk of tetanus infection because of unhygienic birthing conditions. The bacterium produces a neurotoxin that causes muscle spasms, beginning in the head and neck. Spores of the anthrax bacterium, *Bacillus anthracis*, are also widespread in soil.

Foodborne Transmission

Any infectious illness transmitted in food is a **foodborne illness**. In a setting without sewage treatment or drinking water treatment, several fecal–oral exposure pathways lead through food— see the heavy line labelled (*l*) in **Figure 4.7**; this figure adds **foodborne transmission** of fecal disease (in black) to the pathways depicted in Figure 4.4. As shown in Figure 4.7, water tainted by human sewage may be used in the preparation of food (*h*), or small amounts of contaminated soil may be present on some foods (*i*), such as vegetables. Unwashed hands, or hands washed in unclean water, can also compromise the cleanliness of food preparation (*j*).

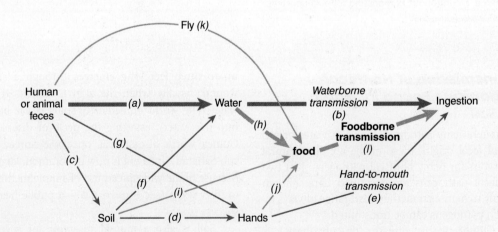

Figure 4.7 Addition of foodborne transmission to basic fecal–oral transmission of disease, in a setting with no treatment of sewage or drinking water.

Finally, the common housefly, by landing first on fecal waste and then on food, can transfer bacteria and protozoan parasites that cling to its feet (*k*). Unlike the inanimate fomite, the housefly is a living transmitter of pathogens—a vector. Still, its function is strictly mechanical—it plays no biological role in the life cycle of the pathogen— and so is also termed a mechanical vector. This type of transmission can be reduced by screening the vents of privies to prevent flies from entering the waste pit, by putting screens in windows and doors, and by covering food.

In a setting without treatment of sewage or drinking water, human fecal contamination so dominates foodborne illness that it is difficult to separate out other sources of food contamination. In contrast, in more developed countries, because fecal wastes are generally controlled and tap water is generally clean, both human fecal contamination and other sources of foodborne illness are often readily identifiable.

Despite the routine treatment of both wastewater and tap water in more developed countries, food is sometimes contaminated by human fecal matter. For example, shellfish can be contaminated by sewage waste before being harvested and might also be eaten raw so that pathogens survive the trip to the table. More often, human fecal contamination of food occurs when someone fails to wash his or her hands thoroughly after using the toilet and before preparing food. Such handwashing is not only important at home but also in food service settings. This is why local health codes require restaurant workers to wash their hands after using the toilet and before returning to work. Noncompliance with these procedures can result in transmission of an illness such as hepatitis A from one worker to a number of customers before the outbreak becomes apparent and is traced to its source.

But most foodborne illness in the more developed countries is not of human fecal origin. Pathogens can be present on food when we bring it home from the store. For example, small quantities of fecal matter from animals eaten as food, such as poultry or cattle, may contaminate the carcass during processing, and this in turn means that animal fecal pathogens can be present on raw meat when it is purchased. Similarly, nonfecal pathogens can be present on food at the time of purchase. Pathogens present on food can contaminate utensils and other kitchen equipment. Careful washing of fruits and vegetables removes soil that might harbor pathogens; this is particularly important if a food is to be eaten raw.

Even human skin is a potential source of pathogens, especially if a person has infected cuts or sores on the hands; thorough handwashing is important even if no infection is present. And control of mechanical vectors, such as houseflies or cockroaches (see **Figure 4.8**), which are attracted to food and can carry pathogens on their feet, is also important.

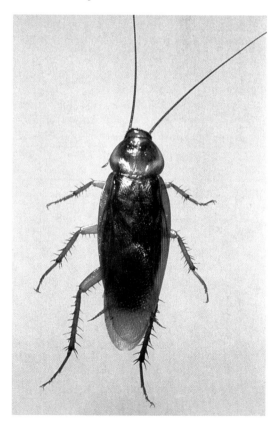

Figure 4.8 Cockroaches, which are widespread household pests, can serve as mechanical vectors in the transmission of foodborne pathogens.

Courtesy of CDC Public Health Image Library. ID# 6319. Content provider: CDC. Available at: http://phil.cdc .gov/phil/home.asp. Accessed October 4, 2012

Some Important Foodborne Pathogens in More Developed Countries. When we think of foodborne illness, we tend to think of vomiting and diarrhea, and indeed these are common symptoms. But in fact, foodborne pathogens cause a range of symptoms and do so by a range of mechanisms. Some foodborne pathogens cause symptoms in the host simply through **infection**—for example, by invading tissues or causing inflammation. Other species produce toxins that cause the symptoms of foodborne illness; this type of illness is called **intoxication**. Usually, intoxication occurs when pathogens produce a toxin in food, which is then eaten, but some pathogens produce toxins in the body after food is eaten. Six important foodborne pathogens in the United States are described briefly here and their key characteristics are summarized in **Table 4.1**.

Table 4.2 presents the overall incidence of, and risk of death from, the first four of these illnesses. *Listeria* is the most fatal of these infections; approximately 13% of cases died.

Nontyphoid **Salmonella** species (i.e., excluding *Salmonella typhii*, which causes typhoid fever) are common in the feces of poultry and, therefore, often contaminate raw poultry during processing. When people become sick from *Salmonella*-contaminated poultry, it is usually for one of two reasons: Either the poultry was not cooked to a high enough temperature to kill organisms; or alternatively, the bird was properly cooked but it was contaminated after cooking by an implement or a surface that had been in contact with the raw bird. This is known as **cross-contamination** of cooked food by raw food. If the recontaminated cooked bird is then allowed to sit for long enough at room temperature, the bacterial population will increase dramatically. Illness from nontyphoid *Salmonella*, which causes vomiting and diarrhea, occurs only after ingesting a very large number of organisms.[12]

Like *Salmonella*, **Campylobacter** species are common contaminants of raw poultry.[12] Analyses of poultry products purchased in stores show that *Campylobacter* and *Salmonella* are widespread in both conventionally and organically grown poultry, but the strains present in the conventionally grown poultry are much more likely to be resistant to common antibiotics.[13,14]

Although nontyphoid *Salmonella* and *Campylobacter* are the two most common foodborne pathogens in the United States, they are not usually

Table 4.1 Key Characteristics of Some Common Foodborne Pathogens

Pathogen	Common Source	Common Food	Aerobic/ Anaerobic	Spore-forming?	Toxin-producing?
Salmonella species	Poultry/fecal	Poultry	Aerobic	No	*
Campylobacter species	Poultry/fecal	Poultry, raw milk	Aerobic	No	No
Listeria monocytogenes	Widespread in environment	Raw milk, soft cheeses	Aerobic	No (but hardy)	No
Escherichia coli O157:H7	Cattle/fecal	Ground beef, leafy greens	Aerobic	No	Yes (produced in the body)
Staphylococcus aureus	Human skin	Ham salad, chicken salad	Aerobic	No	Yes (heat stable)
Clostridium botulinum	Soil	Home-canned food	Anaerobic	Yes	Yes (heat sensitive)

Salmonella has traditionally been thought not to produce a toxin, but recent evidence suggests that it does, although not as the primary mode of infection.

Data from U.S. Food and Drug Administration. *Bad Bug Book: Foodborne Pathogenic Microorganisms and Natural Toxins.* 2nd ed. Available at: www.fda.gov /downloads/Food/FoodSafety/FoodborneIllness/FoodborneIllnessFoodbornePathogensNaturalToxins/BadBugBook/UCM297627.pdf. Accessed November 11, 2012.

Table 4.2 Estimated Overall Incidence and Case-Fatality Ratio* for Four Foodborne Illnesses in the United States in 2015

	Incidence per 100,000 Population	Case-Fatality Rate (%)
Campylobacter	17.12	0.2
Salmonella	16.63	0.4
E. coli O157:H7	3.12	0.6
Listeria	0.23	12.9

*In infectious disease, the term *case-fatality rate* compares the number of deaths among reported cases to the number of reported cases, calculated as: (number of deaths/number of cases) × 100.

Data from Centers for Disease Control and Prevention. Infection with Pathogens Transmitted Commonly Through Food and the Effect of Increasing Use of Culture-Independent Diagnostic Tests on Surveillance — Foodborne Diseases Active Surveillance Network, 10 U.S. Sites, 2012–2015, Available at: https://www.cdc.gov/mmwr/volumes/65/wr/mm6514a2.htm#T1_down Accessed June 25, 2020.

fatal to those who are made ill (see Table 4.2). In contrast, **Listeria monocytogenes** is the least common of the six illnesses described here but by far the most fatal. *Listeria* organisms are widespread in mammals and birds and also in soil. Among non–spore-forming organisms, *Listeria* is unusually resistant to heat, cold (it can multiply in refrigerated foods), and drying.[12] *Listeria* has been documented in many types of foods, but is most associated with raw milk and soft, ripened cheeses. This foodborne pathogen causes serious illness, with symptoms including septicemia (blood poisoning) and meningitis; pregnant women can suffer spontaneous abortion or stillbirth.[12]

One pathogen of particular concern in recent years is a strain of the bacterium *E. coli*. There are hundreds of strains of *E. coli*, many of which are normally present in the human gut. The strain known as **E. coli O157:H7** can be present in the intestines of healthy cattle and can contaminate meat during processing. In people, *E. coli* O157:H7 produces a toxin after colonizing the intestines, and the toxin damages the lining of the intestine, causing bloody diarrhea, sometimes severe. In some people, especially in children under 5 years old and the elderly, the infection also causes destruction of red blood cells and kidney failure; this complication, called hemolytic uremic syndrome, can be fatal.[15] The most common vehicle for illness from *E. coli* O157:H7 is

ground beef. Although adequate cooking does kill this pathogen, the heat must reach the organisms wherever they have been left by processing, and it is harder to heat the interior of a hamburger than the surface of a steak. Moreover, ingesting as few as 10 organisms can cause illness.[12] Among *E. coli* O157:H7 outbreaks from 2003 through 2012 for which it was possible to document the route of transmission (approximately two-thirds of all outbreaks), ground beef was the culprit in 55% and produce in 21%.[16]

Staphylococcus aureus (commonly called *staph*) is a normal inhabitant of human skin but is present in very large numbers in boils and other sores or cuts and is usually passed to food through poor hygiene* practices on the part of someone preparing food. Ham salad and chicken salad are common vehicles for staph illness because contamination occurs after cooking, in handling the meat. If the meat then sits at room temperature (e.g., on a buffet), the organisms multiply and produce a toxin, which causes illness. Because the toxin is heat resistant, reheating food (such as a

---

*In this text, the term *hygiene* is used in the sense of cleanliness, mainly as it relates to infectious disease risks. Historically, this term was used broadly to refer to public health as the science of preventing disease and maintaining health, and this usage survives in the term *industrial hygiene* as a synonym for *occupational health*.

sliced cooked ham) will not prevent illness. Staph causes gastrointestinal illness.

Poisoning by ***Clostridium botulinum*** is commonly known as botulism. *Clostridium* is an anaerobic, spore-forming organism that produces a toxin, which can be denatured by heat. *Clostridium* is widespread in the soil in the environment and may, therefore, be present on vegetables, for example. Historically, the classic vehicle for botulism was home-canned food, which was once more common than it is today. If green beans, for example, are inadequately heated during canning, spores can survive the canning process and germinate in the anaerobic environment of the can, producing a toxin. Although the toxin can be denatured by heat, this requires boiling for some time; if the food is only quickly reheated, the toxin causes illness. Botulinum toxin is a potentially fatal neurotoxin; early symptoms include weakness, vertigo, and difficulty swallowing and breathing.[12] *Clostridium botulinum* spores (sometimes present in honey) do not germinate in the adult gut but can germinate in the gut of infants, and infant botulism can be fatal.[12]

Finally, **scombroid poisoning** (not listed in Table 4.1) is caused by a toxin produced by certain types of bacteria, acting on certain amino acids in foods, when conditions of time and temperature are not adequately controlled. Scombroid poisoning is most associated with the spoilage of fish, especially tuna and related fish (e.g., mahi mahi, bluefish, sardines, mackerel, amberjack, and abalone), but it has also been tied to the production of Swiss cheese.[17] Once the toxin is formed, it is not inactivated by cooking, canning, or freezing; the symptoms, which sometimes require hospitalization, can include a drop in blood pressure, headaches, vomiting, and diarrhea.[17]

Vectorborne Transmission

A host species that transmits an infectious disease to another host species is called a **biological vector** of the disease, and a disease that is transmitted in this way is called a **vectorborne disease**. (Diseases that might be transmitted by a mechanical vector such as a housefly, which is not a host species, are not considered vectorborne diseases.)

Many biological vectors are **arthropods**, a group that comprises insects (e.g., mosquitoes, flies, lice, and fleas) and arachnids (including ticks, mites, and spiders). However, mammalian hosts, such as rodents, can also transmit diseases to people.

Many arthropods transmit disease among larger animals by taking blood meals from them (see **Figure 4.9**). A virus transmitted in this way is called an arthropod-borne virus, or **arbovirus**. For example, the West Nile virus, which can cause encephalitis, infects humans, birds, and certain species of mosquito. When one of these mosquitoes bites an infected bird, it draws blood that contains the virus. In the mosquito, the virus migrates to the saliva glands, and when the mosquito later bites another bird (or a person), the mosquito injects saliva containing viruses into the new host. Thus, a biological vector, such as a mosquito, functions differently from a mechanical vector, such as the housefly, which passively deposits pathogens that are stuck to its feet. Some biological vectors are themselves made ill by the pathogens they transmit, but most are not. Dengue fever (also known as *breakbone* fever for the extreme pain it causes) is another arbovirus disease, carried by mosquitoes between people and monkeys.

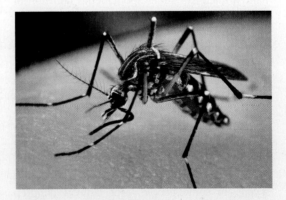

Figure 4.9 An *Aedes aegypti* mosquito, the vector for dengue fever, takes a blood meal from a human host.

Courtesy of CDC Public Health Image Library. ID# 9252. Content providers CDC/Prof. Frank Hadley Collins, Dir., Cntr. for Global Health and Infectious Diseases, Univ. of Notre Dame. Available at: http://phil.cdc.gov /phil/home.asp. Accessed October 4, 2012.

There are many variations on the basic frame-work of vectorborne transmission by arthropods, reflecting the diverse interconnections that are possible among pathogens and their hosts in eco-systems. For example, a pathogen may require more than one host species to complete its life cycle: The protozoan parasites that cause malaria (*Plasmodium* species) pass through some devel-opmental life stages in humans and others in the mosquito vector (*Anopheles* species). Although the life cycle for Malarial transmission is complex, half a million people still died from this proto-zoan vectorborne disease in 2017, a decline from the almost one million it killed annually a decade before.[18] Alternatively, the vector may require multiple hosts to complete its life cycle, with the pathogen merely along for the ride. For example, Lyme disease is caused by a bacterium (*Borrelia burgdorferi*) that is found in the blood of the tick vector (see **Figure 4.10** and **Figure 4.11**). A tick larvum, after taking a blood meal (usually from a bird), molts into a nymph; which, after taking a blood meal (usually from a mouse or a person), molts into an adult tick; which, after taking a blood meal (usually from a deer or a person), pro-duces eggs that hatch into larvae. At any stage of the tick's life, the bacterial pathogen can be passed to a new host when the tick takes a blood meal.

In contrast, the insect vector for typhus (the body louse) simply moves from person to person through close proximity (explaining why this disease, which was once common, most often afflicted armies, prisoners, and others living in crowded conditions). The bacterial pathogen *Rickettsia prowazekii* is not passed via the bite of the louse, but rather is present in the louse's feces. The louse leaves bites and feces on the skin of its human victim. The bites are itchy, and by scratch-ing, the victim rubs the louse feces into the bites. The rickettsial infection is fatal to the louse.

Arthropod vectors transmit many other illnesses, including two that have historically appeared as large-scale epidemics: plague (a bac-terial illness transmitted by rat fleas) and yellow fever (a viral illness transmitted by mosquito). Two parasitic vectorborne diseases that, like

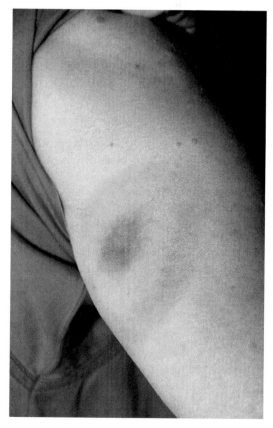

Figure 4.11 The "bulls-eye" rash around a tick bite on this woman's arm is characteristic of the infection known as Lyme disease.

Courtesy of CDC Public Health Image Library. ID# 9873. Content providers CDC/James Gathany. Available at: http://phil.cdc.gov/phil/home.asp. Accessed October 4, 2012.

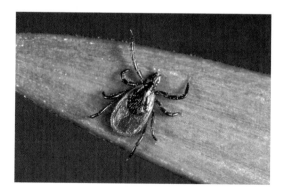

Figure 4.10 The black-legged tick (*Ixodes scapularis*), shown here on a blade of grass, transmits Lyme disease among a number of mammalian hosts, including humans.

Courtesy of CDC Public Health Image Library. ID# 1669. Content providers CDC/Michael L. Levin, PhD. Available at: http://phil.cdc.gov/phil/home.asp. Accessed October 4, 2012 malaria, cause much morbidity in warm climates are onchocerciasis (river blindness), caused by a parasitic worm and transmitted by black flies, and African sleeping sickness, caused by a protozoan parasite and transmitted by tsetse flies.

Bedbugs, known for the itchy bites they leave behind, were a familiar nuisance worldwide before the era of synthetic organic pesticides. But in the more developed nations, three generations have known of bedbugs only through a bedtime nursery rhyme. That's changing, as bedbugs make a comeback. Although the presence of more than 40 pathogens has been documented in bedbugs, and it is plausible to think that they may transmit disease, it has not been documented that these bugs act as disease vectors.[19] The reasons for bedbugs' resurgence are also not completely clear but seem likely to include global travel, the bugs' resistance to some pesticides, and the use of pesticide baits (which do not attract blood-sucking insects) in lieu of sprays. A 2005 survey of 34 pest control operators in Toronto found that the great majority of the infestations treated were in single-family homes (70%) and apartments (18%); infestations were also reported at about one-third of the shelters in the city.[20] More recently, infestations at hotels, including some luxury hotels, have made headlines.

Although most vectorborne transmission is by arthropod vectors, nonarthropod vectors can also transmit disease via bite. For example, a raccoon or squirrel infected with rabies carries the virus in its saliva and can transmit it to a person by biting. Rats transmit a number of diseases to humans, including hantavirus pulmonary syndrome and plague, leptospirosis, rat-bite fever, Salmonellosis, and tularemia.[21]

Vectorborne transmission is commonly managed using two basic approaches. One is to prevent contact between vectors and people; for example, people can choose clothing that minimizes the risk of contact with ticks, use screens or nets to prevent contact with mosquitoes, or use insect repellents to drive pests away. The other approach is to reduce the vector population. This is usually accomplished either through the use of pesticides or by modifying the environment—for example, draining a swamp to reduce mosquito populations or managing rubbish to reduce rodent populations. A more technically sophisticated approach, known as the sterile insect technique, is to create sterile male insects in the laboratory, usually by irradiation, and then release them into the environment. Because no offspring result when these sterile males mate with females, the insect population is reduced. However, if this technique is to work, the sterilization method must not affect the males' ability to mate, and this has been a key technical challenge of using irradiation for this purpose. To address this problem, newer methods are being developed for creating genetically engineered male mosquitoes that are sterile but whose capacity to mate is unimpaired.[22] This approach requires the release of large numbers of genetically modified insects into the environment, with largely unknown consequences.

Pest control is also important in agriculture, not only because insects and rodents eat crops, but also because plant pests (commonly known as weeds) can take nutrients and sunlight away from crops. Given that many of the same approaches are used to manage both disease vectors and agricultural pests, the discussion of pests and pest control is deferred to the next chapter to provide a unified treatment in the agricultural context.

A Complex Web of Transmission

For the purpose of introducing basic concepts of infectious disease, this chapter has described transmission by closeness or contact, by currents of air, by polluted water or soil, by food, and by mechanical or biological vector, as if these were all quite distinct. Yet, in functional terms, it is clear that a sneeze, a handshake, a child's toy, a sexual encounter, aerosolized fecal matter, a polluted river, a housefly, a raw oyster, undercooked poultry, a tick, and a rabid squirrel all play fundamentally similar roles in transmitting disease. In natural settings, infectious agents are transmitted by varied and flexible means, blurring any neat distinctions that might be drawn. Further, there is increasing concern that pathogens might be deliberately transmitted—that is, used as weapons, called **bioweapons**—on a larger scale than has been seen in the past.

The transmission of anthrax illustrates the complexities of disease transmission. This zoonotic disease occurs mostly in large herbivores including cattle, sheep, and goats. Infected animals shed spores in urine and feces, and other animals become infected by ingesting spores in soil while grazing. Anthrax spores can persist in soil for decades and are dispersed in the environment by wind. Spores are also thought to be effectively dispersed on the feathers of vultures and other scavenging birds that have fed on infected carcasses.[23] Most human exposure to anthrax spores occurs through close contact with an animal or its hide or wool. Most often, the spores enter via a skin wound; less frequently, but more fatally, spores are inhaled. People can also become ill by eating the meat of an infected animal. Last but not least, if anthrax spores can be effectively aerosolized for greater airborne dispersion, they can be used by terrorists as a weapon—an act of **bioterrorism**. This complex picture of anthrax transmission combines elements of transmission by biological vector (cow or sheep); by closeness or contact (with the animal's hide or wool);

by mechanical vector (vulture); by soil, feces, or food; and perhaps even by intent.

The web of infectious disease transmission is not only complex but also ever-changing. Scientists now recognize a set of **emerging (or reemerging) infectious diseases**—illnesses that have only recently been identified or are making an unexpected comeback. HIV/AIDS, the H5N1 avian influenza, Ebola hemorrhagic fever, severe acute respiratory syndrome (SARS), bovine spongiform encephalopathy and the associated illness in humans, dengue fever, hantavirus, *E. coli* O157:H7, and drug-resistant malaria are all in this group. Within a few decades, AIDS emerged from obscurity to become a global health threat of enormous proportions. At any time, the constant shuffling of the genome for a virus can produce a variant that is readily transmissible among humans, and when this happens, infected travelers are likely to spread it around the world before they know they are sick. These emerging diseases serve as a reminder that pathogens and vectors are resilient and flexible and that the effects of human activities can ripple through a global ecosystem.

COVID-19

At the end of 2019, residents in Wuhan, China, experienced an outbreak of a respiratory disease of unknown etiology that killed more than 1,800 and infected over 70,000 within the first 50 days.[1] As of late December 2020, almost 67.7 million cases and 1.5 million deaths globally have been identified.[2] The similarity between the symptoms experienced by the extremely ill cases now to the Severe Acute Respiratory Syndrome (SARS) outbreak in 2003 led researchers to confirm that this new disease was also caused by a type of coronavirus now called SARS-CoV-2. The name *corona* refers to the crown-like spikes on the outer surface of the virus that help it attach to a host's cell membrane receptors, thus hijacking the cell to reproduce more virus. Compared with the previous SARS outbreak that infected 8,000 people across 26 countries with a case-fatality rate of 9%, this new disease, named COVID-19, has spread across more than 109 countries with a mortality rate of about 3%.[1] The less deadly a disease, especially if there are many asymptomatic infected individuals, the more the disease may be successfully transmitted.

The outbreak in Wuhan appeared to emerge from a large market where live animals were sold, including bats, a recognized reservoir for the previous SARS coronavirus as well as the Middle East Respiratory Syndrome Coronavirus (MERS-CoV)[1]. Initially, researchers focused on those who had either eaten bats sold from this market or ate snakes that fed on bats. However, subsequent research suggests that the transmission within the marker was already human-to-human, perhaps from someone exposed previously to the bat viral reservoir. Although all evidence strongly suggests that bats were the primary zoonotic host, more work needs to be completed to confirm if an intermediate zoonotic source was involved.[1] As of the time of this writing, the World Health Organization (WHO) has not found any evidence to support the suggestion that the virus was introduced to others shopping at the market from an infected

(continues)

researcher at a nearby lab that studies these bat viruses—evidently, the virus detected in cases does not contain the type of genomic sequences that are typically embedded in viruses created in the lab.[3]

Regardless of its origin, the rapid spread of this novel coronavirus into a global pandemic has brought human activities around the planet to almost a standstill. Because the primary route of transmission is airborne via aerosols when someone infected speaks, coughs, sneezes, shouts or even *sings*, countries have enacted policies to socially distance their citizens as much as possible. Schools and businesses have been closed, forcing families to learn to work remotely from the shelter of their homes. Shops and restaurants have been ordered closed, resulting in the greatest loss of jobs seen since the depression era of the 1930s. Around the world, nonessential air travel ceased almost entirely for two months.

In settings where staying more than 6 feet apart is not feasible, the wearing of face masks is strongly recommended, although apparently a controversial issue to many Americans. The reason for the outrage over masks may reflect the fact that masks were initially reserved for medical workers overwhelmed with patients and very limited supplies. Also, the majority of people fed up with being homebound and feeling economically vulnerable will probably never know they are infected unless they are tested, meaning that wearing face masks is strictly to prevent the spread to someone vulnerable to experiencing a more serious outcome from infection.

The fact that this coronavirus may be transmitted so easily means that any reports regarding the number of positive cases most likely underestimates its true prevalence. Unless someone feels poorly enough to go get a test or has been told to test because of recent contact with someone with a positive test, the actual rates of active cases may be 20 times higher than the data show. Furthermore, as antibody testing increases, which can indicate whether someone ever had an infection of the disease, the prevalence rates may increase tenfold.[4]

As the origin and true extent of the COVID-19 pandemic remains unclear, there is reason for some optimism about a preventive vaccine within another year that would relegate this virus onto the list of manageable environmental health concerns. However, the overwhelming impact that this little microorganism has had should warn us not to ever grow complacent about hazards associated with infectious disease.

1. Shereen, M.A., Khan, S., Kazmi, A., Bashir, N., & Siddique, R. (2020). COVID-19 infection: Origin, transmission and characteristics of human coronaviruses. *Journal of Advanced Research*, 24:91-98. https://doi.org/10.1016/j.jare.2020.03.550
2. New York Times. (n.d.) *Coronavirus World Map: Tracking the Global Outbreak*. Retrieved December 8, 2020 from: https://www.nytimes.com/interactive/2020/world/coronavirus-maps.html
3. World Health Organization. (2020). *Coronavirus disease 2019 (COVID-19) Situation Report – 94*. Retrieved June 26, 2020 from https://www.who.int/docs/default-source/coronaviruse/situation-reports/20200423-sitrep-94-covid-19.pdf?sfvrsn=b8304bf0_4
4. Park, A. (2020). CDC Head Estimates U.S. Coronavirus Cases Might be 10 Times Higher Than Data Show. *Time*. Retrieved June 26, 2020 from: https://time.com/5859790/cdc-coronavirus-estimates/

The Body's Defense Against Pathogens

The body's immune system distinguishes substances that are "self" from those that are foreign, such as bacteria and viruses. The first time the body is exposed to such a foreign substance (called an antigen), the immune system responds by mounting a counterattack. This immune response includes the production of special proteins (antibodies) and cells to eliminate the antigen. The person experiences the disease, but if he survives, he is protected against the same disease in the future because his immune system is now prepared to respond effectively. Such immunity, produced by one's own immune system, is called active immunity, and it is usually permanent.

A vaccine is an antigen preparation that is administered to a person—by injection, by mouth, or by nasal spray—to produce an immune response while bypassing illness. The antigen in a vaccine has been modified so that it does not cause illness (e.g., bacterial cells in the vaccine may be dead or weakened), although it still evokes the immune response. An individual who has been vaccinated is protected against the disease in the future, without ever having actually been ill. This,

Immune Malfunction

Sometimes the body's immune system fails and mounts an unnecessary response to a substance that is foreign but not harmful; such a substance is called an **allergen**, and the abnormal response is **allergy**, a type of immune disease. Many common substances can act as allergens, including pollens, molds and mold spores, animal dander, dust mites, and cockroach droppings.

On first exposure to a specific allergen, a person who is genetically predisposed to allergy produces allergen-specific antibodies that become concentrated in the respiratory tract. This series of events is called **sensitization**: From this point forward, whenever the body is presented with this allergen, the antibodies will cause the release of chemical mediators (e.g., histamine), which in turn produce the symptoms of an allergic reaction. Depending on the mediators and where they act, the reaction can be in either the upper airway (nose and throat) or the lower airway.

In the upper airway, exposure to a specific allergen—in a person who has previously been sensitized to the allergen—triggers an attack of **allergic rhinitis** ("hay fever"), with symptoms of sneezing, runny nose, and watery eyes. These symptoms can persist for some time—for example, during the season when certain pollens or molds are widespread. Events in the lower airways are more complicated. Here, exposure to a specific allergen—in a person who has previously been sensitized to the allergen and who has asthma as a chronic underlying condition—triggers an asthma attack. **Asthma** is an immune illness in which the bronchi (the two major airways that serve the two lungs) are chronically inflamed and also hyperreactive. That is, they are prone to sudden muscle constriction that reduces the diameter of the bronchi (an effect known as **bronchoconstriction**), which in turn reduces the flow of air to and from the lungs. An **asthma attack** is an acute flare-up of the chronic condition, with increased inflammation and bronchoconstriction as well as an overproduction of thick mucus. Together, these changes produce symptoms of coughing, wheezing, and shortness of breath. An asthma attack can be extremely debilitating or even fatal. In a person with chronic asthma, acute attacks can be triggered not only by exposure to an allergen but also by exposure to a simple respiratory irritant such as cigarette smoke, chemical fumes, fragrances, irritating air pollutants, or even cold air. Allergy and asthma, although often expressed in the respiratory system, are fundamentally immune conditions, and noninhalation exposures can be important, as can nonrespiratory reactions. For example, an allergic reaction to eating peanuts (an ingestion exposure) can include asthma symptoms. Much more is known about allergic sensitization and asthma triggers than is known about the root causes of chronic asthma.

Sometimes, the body's immune system fails even more dramatically and no longer recognizes itself, initiating a maladaptive attack on its own cells resulting in an **autoimmune disease**. In the case of Type 1 Diabetes (T1D), the immune system destroys the cells in the pancreas that create insulin. Although the underlying cause for most autoimmune diseases is thought to be primarily genetic, recent epigenetic research suggests that environmental exposures also play a role in triggering the onset of these diseases. For example, mild childhood viral infections have been identified as such a trigger associated with T1D.[1] During the past two decades, cases of Celiac disease have surged, a condition where the body attacks the intestinal lining when gluten-rich food is ingested, and modern food production has seen a large increase in the use of gluten as a bulking agent and preservative.[2]

The "hygiene hypothesis" has emerged as a possible explanation of the causes and rising prevalence of these maladaptive immune conditions.[3] This hypothesis suggested that today's children are on the whole less exposed to bacteria and viruses than children were in the past, because they live in cleaner houses, have fewer siblings, have less contact with animals, and receive vaccines. The idea is that the cells in the immune system do not develop and learn to differentiate self from truly foreign pathogenic agents without these "dirtier" environmental exposures. Much of the human immune system does develop after birth. Therefore, the thinking goes, when a hygienic environment reduces the immune system's exposure to pathogens, a paradoxical effect is an increase in autoimmune and allergic diseases.

1. Jerram ST, Dang MN, Leslie RD. The role of epigenetics in type 1 diabetes. *Curr Diab Rep*. 2017;17:89.

2. Offord C. The celiac surge. *The Scientist*. 2017. Retrieved June 27, 2020 from https://www.the-scientist.com/features/the-celiac-surge-31438

3. Okada H, Kuhn C, Feillet H, Bach JF. The 'hygiene hypothesis' for autoimmune and allergic diseases: an update. *Clin Exp Immunol*. 2010;160:1–9.

too, is active immunity, produced by one's own immune system.

Alternatively, a person may acquire passive immunity from a vaccine that contains antibodies—ready-made protection against attack—rather than antigens. From a public health perspective, the larger goal in vaccinating an individual is not only to keep that person from getting sick but also to keep him or her from spreading disease to others. Herd immunity refers to the practical protection experienced by a community when enough of its members have immunity against a disease so that it becomes difficult to maintain a chain of infection. Put simply, the higher the proportion of those in the group who are immune, the less likely that a sick person will transmit the disease to someone who is vulnerable. The proportion of the group that must be immune to achieve herd immunity depends upon how readily the disease is passed from one person to another, as well as upon environmental factors such as crowding. By coupling the effects of aggressive vaccination and herd immunity, a disease can actually be eradicated—a goal that has been achieved for smallpox and is now being eyed for Guinea worm disease and polio.[24,25]

The term vaccine-preventable diseases refers to the set of diseases for which a vaccine is presently available. The U.S. Centers for Disease Control and Prevention (CDC) lists the following vaccine-preventable diseases as illnesses that once killed or disabled many U.S. children and adolescents in the United States[26]:

- Diphtheria
- Haemophilus influenzae type B
- Hepatitis A
- Hepatitis B
- Influenza
- Measles
- Meningococcal disease
- Mumps
- Pertussis (whooping cough)
- Pneumococcal disease
- Polio
- Rotavirus
- Rubella (German measles)
- Tetanus (lockjaw)
- Varicella (chickenpox)

Vaccines have also been developed for Lyme disease, rabies, typhoid fever, anthrax, and other diseases. Developing effective vaccines for some other diseases has proven to be quite challenging, such as is the case for Dengue and Malaria.

Over the centuries, people have worked hard to prevent transmission of disease, often without understanding these basic processes of transmission. For example, before the microbial causation of disease was widely understood, two main strategies were used to control or prevent infectious disease.[3] One was quarantine—the practice of isolating sick or potentially sick persons so that they could not infect others. Quarantine addressed the fear of person-to-person transmission. The word itself derives from the 14th-century Venetian practice of requiring ships to wait at anchor in port for 40 days before anyone was allowed to disembark. Modern terminology distinguishes between **isolation** (the separation of persons who have an infectious illness) and **quarantine** (the separation of persons who have been exposed to an infectious agent and may become ill).[27] Isolation and quarantine are useful mainly in preventing transmission of disease through closeness or contact.

The second main strategy, beginning in the early 19th century, was **sanitation**—specifically, the removal of decaying organic matter, sometimes even extending to the draining of swamps—to prevent miasmas from rising out of this matter. In the name of sanitary reform, public sewer systems were built and procedures were set up to remove garbage from cities. This sanitary reform movement laid the foundation for the field of environmental health. Although they rested on a misunderstanding of disease causation, sanitary reform measures provided a substantial benefit to public health by reducing sources of exposure to fecal matter and to insect and rodent vectors of disease.[3]

In the 20th and 21st centuries, isolation/quarantine and environmental interventions including sanitation have been supplemented by modern tools for infectious disease control, which attack pathogens directly. Vaccination and the use of **antibiotics** (pharmaceuticals that kill or inhibit bacteria) and antifungal medications have become central to the battle to control infectious disease.

Surprisingly, although vaccination against smallpox was adopted rapidly after it was introduced in 1796, almost 100 years passed before vaccines for any other diseases were developed. Today, vaccines for more than 20 diseases are in use.

Although antibiotics remain an important weapon in the battle against infectious disease, bacterial resistance to antibiotics is a growing problem. Over time, a population of bacteria can become largely resistant to a specific antibiotic if, at the outset, some of the bacteria have a genetic makeup that confers resistance. This is the familiar phenomenon of "survival of the fittest," as occurs in natural selection, except that in this case, the selection factor is a man-made antibiotic. With the widespread use of antibiotics in both humans and animals, such **antibiotic resistance** has become a major public health concern. For example, such drug resistance has created challenges in the treatment of tuberculosis, HIV/AIDS, and malaria. Of particular concern at present is a virulent antibiotic-resistant strain of *Staphylococcus aureus*. Known as **methicillin-resistant *Staphylococcus aureus* (MRSA)**, the strain is also resistant to related antibiotics, including penicillin and amoxicillin. MRSA is widespread in hospitals and commonly found on the hands of healthcare workers, and most cases of MRSA are associated with invasive procedures in a healthcare setting, leading to infections of surgical wounds or of the bloodstream, for example.[28]

Population-Level Impacts of Infectious Disease

For human beings, infectious disease is an integral part of life and a common cause of death. Infectious diseases cause death directly and also indirectly by increasing the risk of certain cancers.

Global Patterns of Infectious Disease Mortality

Although there are a great number of human pathogens, a relatively well-defined set of illnesses account for most deaths from infectious disease worldwide—a total of approximately 7 million deaths in 2016.[29] The burden of death from respiratory infections (40% of infectious disease deaths), diarrheal disease (20%), HIV/AIDS (14%), tuberculosis (18%), and malaria (7%) is particularly heavy. Among deaths from childhood diseases (which account for 4% of all infectious disease deaths), pertussis (whooping cough) and measles together account for more than 80% of deaths, and most others are from tetanus. Malnutrition contributes heavily to infectious disease mortality: WHO estimates that malnutrition is a factor in more than one-third of childhood deaths worldwide.[30]

By the 1960s and 1970s, experts in the United States and other more developed countries were riding a wave of optimism, believing that infectious disease was no match for modern medicine. But by the end of the century, that optimism had been deflated by the emergence of new diseases, the reemergence of old ones, and the stubborn hold of infectious disease as a major cause of mortality and morbidity in much of the world.

Simple mortality statistics, of course, cannot capture the full impact of infectious disease in morbidity and in economic and social costs. Even so, mortality patterns reveal much about the burden of ill health and about disparities in that burden. Worldwide, 20% of all deaths were from infectious disease in 2016, the most recent year for which detailed infectious disease mortality statistics are available. In most regions of the world, chronic diseases cause the majority of deaths. However, in Africa, more than half of all deaths are caused by infectious diseases, and almost one-third of deaths in Southeast Asia and the Eastern Mediterranean are still attributed to infections.[29]

Infectious Disease as a Cause of Cancer

The International Agency for Research on Cancer (IARC), which not only evaluates the carcinogenicity of chemical and physical hazards but also of infectious agents, has designated several pathogens as known, or probable, human carcinogens. An infection can increase cancer risk through various mechanisms—for example, through chronic irritation, resulting in cell proliferation and increased opportunity for mutation.

Known infectious causes of cancer were estimated to account for about 15% of cancers worldwide in 2018.[31] Taken as a group, the less developed countries had a higher incidence of infectious disease than the more developed countries, and fully 30% of cancers in the lower-income nations, but only 5% of cancers in the more developed countries in the same year, were estimated to be attributable to infectious causes.[31] The *Helicobacter pylori* bacteria is thought to be responsible for 90% of all global stomach cancer cases, half of which occur in China. In addition to this bacteria, hepatis B virus, hepatitis C virus, and human papillomavirus are thought to be responsible for every 9 of 10 cancers caused by an infectious agent.[31]

U.S. Regulatory Framework for Managing Infectious Disease Risk

In the United States today, the U.S. Food and Drug Administration is responsible for ensuring the safety and effectiveness of vaccines. The CDC develops disease-specific guidelines for the vaccination of children and adults and provides these recommendations to the states. The individual states can then adopt the recommendations requiring children to have immunizations before entering school in the state. States also set rules for exemptions from the vaccination requirements—for example, for medical or religious reasons. Similarly, each state is responsible for isolation and quarantine within its own borders.

At the national level, the CDC has the authority under the U.S. Public Health Service Act to use isolation or quarantine to prevent infectious diseases from being brought into the country. There are limitations on this power; however, and it has rarely been invoked. In addition to its FoodNet program, the CDC also conducts infectious disease surveillance for a list of nationally notifiable diseases, using data collected voluntarily by the states. Finally, the CDC investigates epidemics and foodborne disease outbreaks and does research and public education on infectious disease.

At the international level, the WHO conducts infectious disease surveillance and prevention programs and responds to outbreaks.

4.2 Poisons in Nature

Several types of poisons, produced by animals, plants, algae, or fungi, can cause illness in people. For example, nature arms some animals with poisons, which they use mainly to defend against predators or to subdue their own prey, usually by biting or stinging.[32] Some of the best known among the many species of venomous snakes worldwide are the cobra, viper, copperhead, diamondback rattlesnake, and coral snake. Some scorpions and spiders (e.g., the black widow and brown recluse; see **Figure 4.12**) are also venomous, as are some marine creatures, including stingrays and scorpionfishes.

Both the medicinal and poisonous properties of plants have long been recognized. Many plants cause gastrointestinal upset or minor skin irritation (e.g., poison ivy), and some have more serious health effects. Because of exposures through foraging, livestock often suffer the effects of plant toxins. Of particular note for human risk is the castor bean plant, whose seeds contain **ricin**, a toxin so potent that eating a mere five or six seeds can be fatal to a child.[33]

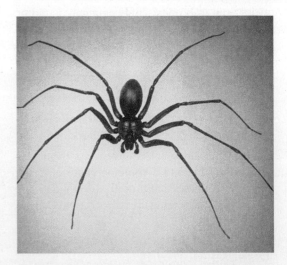

Figure 4.12 The venomous brown recluse spider—including legs, about the size of a U.S. quarter—is found in several south-central states in the United States.

Courtesy of CDC Public Health Image Library. ID# 6268. Content providers: CDC/Andrew J. Brooks. Available at: http://phil.cdc.gov/phil/home.asp. Accessed October 4, 2012

Some organs of the **pufferfish** (also called fugu, blowfish, and several other names) contain potent neurotoxins—tetrodotoxin, saxitoxin, or both—that may cause death from progressive paralysis that impairs respiration.[34,35] In Japan, where this fish is considered a delicacy, some fish cutters are specially trained to remove the organs that contain the toxins, without contaminating the rest of the fish. However, depending on the location where pufferfish are caught off the U.S. Atlantic coast, the entire fish (rather than only certain organs) can be toxic, and the U.S. Food and Drug Administration advises consumers to eat pufferfish only from sources known to be safe.[35]

When eaten as food, both animals and plants can serve as the vehicles for toxins produced by smaller organisms such as algae or fungi. For example, the tiny marine algae known as dinoflagellates, which are near the base of the oceanic food chain, produce toxins. These toxins accumulate up the levels of the food chain, ultimately reaching concentrations in shellfish or finfish tissues that can poison people who eat them.[32] **Paralytic shellfish poisoning** (also called saxitoxin poisoning), which has symptoms ranging from tingling and numbness to respiratory paralysis,[36] occurs most often in people who have eaten mollusks. **Ciguatera poisoning**, marked by gastrointestinal, neurological, and cardiovascular symptoms,[37] is typically caused by eating warm-water reef fish, such as barracuda, grouper, or snapper. During warm weather, dinoflagellate populations in coastal waters can multiply rapidly, giving the water a reddish color, a phenomenon known as "red tide."

Plants, especially grain plants used as food, can serve as the vehicle by which people are exposed to toxins produced by molds or other fungi (**mycotoxins**). For example, the mold *Claviceps purpurea*, commonly known as ergot, is a parasite that affects grains of rye and other cereals in the field. Ergot produces a mycotoxin; the symptoms of ergot poisoning (**ergotism**) include vasoconstriction, especially in the extremities, leading to gangrene. Historically, ergotism was a common and much-dreaded condition, known in the Middle Ages as St. Anthony's Fire because of the characteristic blackened gangrenous limbs.[33]

Unlike ergot, the mold *Aspergillus flavus* grows mainly on crops in storage,[38] affecting especially peanuts and corn. Under favorable conditions, this mold produces **aflatoxins**, which might then be present in food products, including peanut butter. On the whole, storage conditions are much better controlled and less conducive to the growth of mold in more developed countries. In these countries, foods are rarely contaminated with aflatoxins at concentrations high enough to cause acute toxicity, although such outbreaks occur occasionally in less developed countries. More importantly, aflatoxin exposure is associated with increased risk of hepatocellular carcinoma, a common form of primary liver cancer. As mentioned previously, the hepatitis B virus is also a risk factor for hepatocellular carcinoma, and the risk from combined exposure to hepatitis B and aflatoxin is about 60 times greater than the sum of their separate risks.[39,40]

Finally, some mushrooms (which, like molds, are a type of fungus) are poisonous to humans. Many species of mushrooms grow wild, and there is no simple way to distinguish harmless species from poisonous ones. Poisonous mushrooms cause a wide range of symptoms including gastrointestinal and neurological effects, and occasionally death.[41] Worldwide, most deaths from mushroom poisoning are caused by eating *Amanita phalloides*, also called the "death cap."[41]

4.3 Naturally Occurring Radiation

Radiation is a physical hazard—a form of energy that can cause harm to living things. It originates from both natural sources, described here, and from certain human activities, described later. Before describing the major natural sources of exposure to radiation and the associated health risks, it is useful to consider the basics of radiation itself, including the electromagnetic spectrum, radioactive decay, the distinction between ionizing and nonionizing radiation, and the specialized

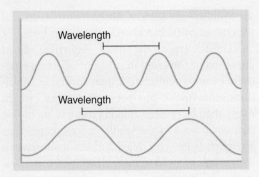

Figure 4.13 Electromagnetic radiation of shorter and longer wavelengths.

period of time (that is, they arrive with greater frequency). For example, gamma radiation is a short-wavelength, high-energy form of electromagnetic radiation (see the following sidebar titled "About the Electromagnetic Spectrum").

Radiation Basics

One source of radiation is the **radioactive decay** of atoms of certain chemical elements, such as uranium.

Radioactive Decay

Chemical elements exist as different **isotopes** (see the following sidebar titled "About Atomic Structure, Chemical Isotopes, and Uranium"). Certain isotopes of some chemical elements, including uranium, are unstable, or **radioactive**. To achieve a more stable configuration, an atom of a radioactive isotope ejects a part of its nucleus; this process is termed radioactive decay. A sample of uranium, in which many atoms are undergoing radioactive decay, emits a steady stream of such particles—that is, radiation.

units for quantifying exposure to ionizing radiation and its biological effects.

In simple terms, **radiation** is energy in transit, in packets, traveling at the speed of light. Electromagnetic radiation varies in wavelength, the distance from one peak to the next (see **Figure 4.13**). The **electromagnetic spectrum** is the full set of distinct types of electromagnetic radiation, arranged in order of wavelength.

Because all electromagnetic radiation moves at the same speed, shorter-wavelength radiation has higher energy: More packets arrive in a given

The particle ejected from the nucleus of an atom during radioactive decay can be either

About the Electromagnetic Spectrum

Electromagnetic radiation emitted from different sources has characteristic wavelengths. Taken together, these types of radiation make up the *electromagnetic spectrum*, which ranges from the very-long-wavelength radiation of power lines (thousands of meters) to the very-short-wavelength cosmic radiation that originates in outer space (less than one-trillionth of a meter).

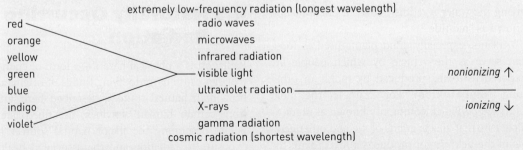

In the middle of the electromagnetic spectrum, infrared and ultraviolet radiation bracket the familiar spectrum of visible light. Sunlight is made up of infrared radiation, visible light, and ultraviolet radiation. Infrared radiation is simply heat; any object that is warmer than its surroundings gives off infrared radiation.

About Atomic Structure, Chemical Isotopes, and Uranium

At their most basic, atoms are made up of three types of particles. In the nucleus are two types of particles that on the atomic scale are relatively massive: protons, which are positively charged; and neutrons, which have no charge. Orbiting around the nucleus are the much smaller electrons, which are negatively charged.

A chemical element is defined by the number of protons in its nucleus; for example, if an atom has 92 protons, it is a uranium atom. But atoms of the same element can have *different* numbers of neutrons in the nucleus; these are different *isotopes* of the element.

As it exists in nature, uranium consists almost entirely of two isotopes. Most uranium is an isotope with 92 protons and 146 neutrons, denoted as uranium-238 (the mass number, 238, is the number of protons and neutrons in the nucleus); most of the remainder, less than 1% of naturally occurring uranium, is uranium-235, which has 92 protons and 143 neutrons.

an alpha particle or a beta particle. An **alpha particle** consists of two protons plus two neutrons. A **beta particle** is an electron, and with the ejection of this negative particle from the nucleus, a neutron is converted to a proton.

Thus, the ejection of either an alpha or a beta particle changes the number of protons in the nucleus, and this in turn changes the chemical element. For example, when an atom of uranium ejects an alpha particle, what is left is an atom with 90 protons. This element is thorium, and we say that uranium "decays into" thorium. Alpha decay, but not beta decay, also changes the mass number (see **Table 4.3**).

Such decays occur in chains, creating new elements in characteristic series. Table 4.3 shows the decay chain for uranium-238. The ejection of an alpha particle (two protons plus two neutrons) is reflected in the mass number, which is reduced by four; the ejection of a beta particle, in contrast, does not affect the mass number.

The rate at which atoms undergo radioactive decay varies widely. As shown in Table 4.3, each radioactive isotope, or **radionuclide**, has a characteristic **half-life**, the time it takes for half of the atoms in a sample of the element to undergo radioactive decay. Half-lives range from microseconds to billions of years. From a public health point of view, the most important radioactive elements in the uranium-238 decay chain are those with short half-lives. Atom for atom, these elements emit the most radiation in a given period of time.

Of particular concern is the decay of **radon** (it indicates that Radon-222 is highlighted in Table 4.3). Because radon is a gas, it is highly mobile in the environment and is readily inhaled. Moreover, radon has a relatively short half-life of about 4 days, and the decay of radon kicks off a series of very rapid breakdowns. In fact, the four isotopes that follow radon in the decay chain are commonly referred to as radon progeny (or, in earlier literature, radon daughters).

The release of an alpha or beta particle is often accompanied by a burst of energy. This energy is **gamma radiation** and travels through space in the form of waves rather than subatomic particles.

Ionizing and Nonionizing Radiation

In public health, it is important to distinguish between ionizing and nonionizing radiation, a functional distinction based on radiation's biological effect. **Ionizing radiation** is radiation that, when it strikes matter, has enough energy to knock an electron out of orbit, creating an ion.* Such ionization can lead to damage to the cells of the body, including the death of cells.

All the products of radioactive decay—alpha and beta particles and gamma radiation—are ionizing forms of radiation. **Cosmic radiation** and **X-rays** are also ionizing. In the electromagnetic spectrum, the dividing line between ionizing and

---

*An ion is an atom that is either missing electrons or has extra electrons and, therefore, has a positive or negative charge.

Table 4.3 The Decay Chain of Uranium-238

| Particle Ejected | | Radioactive Isotope | Half-life | | | |
Alpha	Beta		Seconds	Minutes	Days	Years
X		Uranium-238				4.47 billion
	X	Thorium-234			24.10	
	X	Protactinium-234		1.17		
X		Uranium-234				245,500
X		Thorium-230				75,400
X		Radium-226				1,599
X		Radon-222			3.823	
X		Polonium-218		3.04		
	X	Lead-214		26.9		
	X	Bismuth-214		19.7		
X		Polonium-214	0.000164			
	X	Lead-210				22.6
	X	Bismuth-210			5.01	
X		Polonium-210			138.4	
		Lead-206 (stable)				

Reproduced from Holden N. Table of the isotopes. In: Lide D, ed. *CRC Handbook of Chemistry and Physics.* 84th (2003–2004) ed. Boca Raton, Fla: CRC Press; 2003: 11-50–11-197.

nonionizing radiation falls within the ultraviolet range (see the preceding sidebar titled "About the Electromagnetic Spectrum"). The shortest-wavelength **ultraviolet radiation** (known as UV-C) is ionizing; other ultraviolet radiation (the longer wavelengths, UV-A and UV-B) are not. **Nonionizing radiation**, although it does not have enough energy to knock an electron out of orbit, can cause biological damage; both UV-B and UV-A radiation in sunlight are now recognized as risk factors for skin cancer.

Measuring Exposure to Ionizing Radiation

Two sets of internationally agreed-upon units are used to quantify exposure to ionizing radiation. The first set of units (**Grays**, abbreviated Gy) measures the intensity of a radiologic exposure: the amount of energy delivered per gram of tissue. The second set of units (**Sieverts**, abbreviated Sv) incorporates the **relative biological effectiveness (RBE)** of a radiologic exposure. That is, expressing exposure in Sieverts takes account of the fact that some types of radiation do more damage than others per unit of energy delivered to tissue.[*]

---

[*] Grays and Sieverts correspond to the **rads** and **rems** of older terminology, which is still widely used; 1 Gray = 100 rads; 1 Sievert = 100 rems. One milli-Sievert (1/1000 Sievert) is abbreviated mSv; 1 micro-Sievert (one-millionth Sievert) is abbreviated μSv. Another unit, the **Becquerel (Bq)**, is not a measure of dose but simply of radioactivity: one Becquerel = 1 disintegration per second. (An older unit of radioactivity is the **Curie**.)

Table 4.4 An Example Showing the Relationship Between Dose in Grays and Dose in Sieverts for Alpha, Beta, and Gamma Radiation

Type of Radiation	Description	Dose in Grays	Relative Biological Effectiveness (RBE)	Equivalent Dose in Sieverts
Alpha	2 protons + 2 neutrons	2	10	20
Beta	1 electron	2	5	10
Gamma	High-energy electromagnetic radiation	2	1	2

Relative biological effectiveness is determined largely by the density of ionization along the path taken through tissue by a particle. Because it is relatively massive, an alpha particle (two protons plus two neutrons) causes a dense track of ionizations along its path. A beta particle (an electron), which is much smaller, causes less frequent ionizations along its track. And gamma rays (mere waves of energy) pass through the body, only occasionally dislodging an electron by a direct hit.

Because of their differing RBE, the same dose (expressed in Grays) of alpha, beta, or gamma radiation translates into different doses expressed in Sieverts:

$$\text{dose (Gy)} \times \text{RBE} = \text{dose (Sv)}$$

As a rule of thumb (see **Table 4.4**), the RBE of alpha radiation is about 10 times that of gamma radiation, and the RBE of beta radiation is about five times that of gamma radiation. However,

relative biological effectiveness can be affected by the type of cell or tissue and other factors.

The impact of radiation exposure also depends upon whether the radiation is delivered to the interior of the body by ingestion or inhalation, or to the exterior of the body (i.e., to the skin). Alpha, beta, and gamma radiation are all internal hazards—that is, they cause ionizations if they are delivered directly to vulnerable internal cells (see **Table 4.5**). As an internal exposure, alpha radiation causes the most damage because its track of ionizations is so dense, and gamma radiation causes the least damage.

If radiation exposure comes from outside the body, it is a different story. An alpha particle, with its dense track of ionizations, gives up its energy over such a short distance that it does not even penetrate through the layer of dead cells on the surface of the skin. As a result, alpha radiation is not hazardous as an external exposure. A sheet of

Table 4.5 Key Characteristics of Alpha, Beta, and Gamma Radiation

Type of Radiation	Description	Internal Hazard?	External Hazard?	Effective Shielding	Examples of Emitters
Alpha	2 protons+ 2 neutrons	Yes	No	Dead skin cells, paper	Uranium-238, radon and progeny
Beta	1 electron	Yes	Yes	Aluminum, plastic	Strontium-90, iodine-131
Gamma	High-energy electromagnetic radiation	Yes	Yes	Lead, concrete	(Often accompanies alpha or beta)

paper would also shield against alpha radiation. Beta radiation passes through the skin, but does not penetrate deep into the body; a thin sheet of plastic or aluminum shields against beta radiation. Gamma radiation passes completely through the body, and a dense material like lead or concrete is needed to protect against it.

All the products of radioactive decay—alpha, beta, and gamma radiation—are ionizing radiation. That is, they have the capacity to create biologically active charged ions by knocking electrons out of orbit. Because much of the human body is water, ionizing radiation often strikes water in tissues, creating ions that react with cellular compounds.

Radiation Health Impacts and Exposures

Scientists distinguish between high-level and low-level exposures to ionizing radiation. A high-level exposure is defined as a whole-body dose of one Sv or greater, occurring within minutes or hours. Such exposures occur mainly in industrial accidents, including nuclear power plant accidents, or with exposure to nuclear weapons blasts; since the two instances when nuclear weapons were used near the end of World War II, such high-level exposures have been rare. Exposures that are not considered high-level exposures encompass a considerable range, including both natural (background) exposures and certain anthropogenic exposures. Low-level exposures are defined on the order of mSvs, compared to Svs.

High-level exposure to ionizing radiation causes three well-known syndromes, all caused by the death of cells, which together are known as **radiation sickness**. Cell death in the central nervous system (the brain and spinal cord) leads to stupor and loss of coordination. Cells that are forming and dividing rapidly are particularly susceptible to the effects of ionizing radiation. In the gastrointestinal tract, cells die and are sloughed off, resulting in massive destruction of the gut. The bone marrow stops producing blood cells, leading to hemorrhage, anemia, and decreased resistance to infection. High-level exposure to ionizing radiation is frequently fatal. A whole-body dose of

100 Sv is fatal within 48 hours, and a whole-body dose of 2.5 to 5 Sv may be fatal within weeks.[42] People who survive a high-level exposure to ionizing radiation are subject to increased cancer risk afterward.

Chronic low-level exposure to ionizing radiation, rather than causing cells to die, causes damage to DNA. In adults and children, including unborn children, this damage results in an increased risk of later developing cancer via mechanisms described earlier. The fetus and young child are most susceptible to ionizing radiation because more cell division and tissue differentiation are occurring in their bodies.

Natural Sources of Exposure to Radiation

Simply by living on planet Earth, human beings are exposed to radiation—from the sun, from outer space, and from the Earth itself—and these exposures carry certain health risks.

People are exposed more or less continuously to naturally occurring radiation, both nonionizing and ionizing. Nonionizing UV-A and UV-B radiation are present in sunlight, for example, and this exposure varies with latitude. Cosmic radiation is a form of ionizing radiation that originates in outer space. Most, but not all, incoming cosmic radiation is screened out by the atmosphere, and thus exposure varies with altitude; for example, exposure to cosmic radiation is greater in Denver than in Boston. Ionizing radiation is also emitted by minerals, such as uranium and thorium in rocks and soil.

Internal exposures to naturally occurring ionizing radiation also occur, mostly by inhalation of radon (including exposure to radon progeny), ingestion of water in which radon is present due to local geology, and ingestion of food. Exposures through food occur because plants take up radioactive elements from soil, animals eat plants, and people in turn consume both plants and animals.

On average, inhalation of radon is the greatest single natural source of exposure to ionizing radiation. This is because radon, as a gas, is highly mobile; and also because it begins a series of rapid breakdowns, as described previously. As a global average, radon is estimated to account for about half of exposure to ionizing radiation from natural sources; however, it is not unusual for radon to be the dominant source of exposure to ionizing radiation, driving a higher-than-average total.[43]

The highest exposures to radon, although it is a natural hazard, occur in the context of human modifications to the natural environment—for example, occupational exposures in underground mining. Outside of mining, exposure to radon mainly occurs as a result of its accumulation in indoor settings[43] and depends not only on local geology, but also on building styles—for example, choice of building materials, airtightness of construction, and the presence of basements.

Human Health Impacts of Naturally Occurring Radiation

Exposure to ionizing radiation carries an increased risk of several cancers, and exposure to the nonionizing radiation in sunlight carries some risk of skin cancer as well as damage to the eyes.

Ionizing Radiation. The International Agency for Research on Cancer (IARC) classifies ionizing radiation as a known human carcinogen (Group 1). Like other cancer risks, the risk of cancer from ionizing radiation is understood to have no threshold; that is, any dose greater than zero carries some risk. However, because most exposures to naturally occurring ionizing radiation are very low, their effects in populations are difficult to establish through epidemiologic studies, and for this reason, studies of highly exposed atomic bomb survivors are of special importance. Research on underground uranium miners, discussed elsewhere in the context of the nuclear fuel cycle, provides further insight into the effects of radon exposure.

Intensive study of survivors of the 1945 atomic bomb blasts at Hiroshima and Nagasaki has yielded much of what we know about the specific health risks of exposure to ionizing radiation. This large group (originally about 120,000) included both males and females of all ages, with acute whole-body exposure at various distances from the blasts. Analyses of this group have documented statistically significant associations between exposure to ionizing radiation and risk of leukemia; cancers of the breast, thyroid, ovary, bladder, lung, colon, liver, and stomach; and nonmelanoma skin cancer.[44] Because ionizing radiation's effect has no threshold, lower-level exposures are also known to carry some risk of these cancers.

Low-level exposure to ionizing radiation in utero has effects in addition to the later risk of cancer.[45] Very early in pregnancy, even low exposure may cause a failure of the embryo to implant in the uterine wall, and exposure in weeks 2 through 15 may result in major malformations, growth retardation, or reduction of IQ, potentially severe.[45]

Nonionizing Radiation. A large volume of epidemiologic research shows that three types of skin cancer—basal cell carcinoma, squamous cell carcinoma, and malignant melanoma—are associated with exposure to the sun; specifically, to UV-A and UV-B radiation in sunlight.[46] Both **squamous cell carcinoma** and **basal cell carcinoma** originate in cells of the outer skin layer, the epidermis: Squamous cells are the most superficial cells, and basal cells are deeper in the epidermis. **Malignant melanoma** is a cancer of melanocytes, cells in the skin that produce pigment (melanin).

Squamous and basal cell carcinoma are much more common than malignant melanoma, but malignant melanoma is far more fatal. For example, in 2010 in the United States, there were more than 1 million new cases of nonmelanoma skin cancer, but only 76,250 new cases of malignant melanoma; yet malignant melanoma accounted for more than 9,000 deaths that year, compared with fewer than 1,000 deaths from nonmelanoma skin cancer.[47,48]

Fair skin color is a risk factor for all three types of skin cancer, especially for malignant melanoma.[46] The effect of sun exposure is also reflected in incidence patterns of squamous and basal cell cancer: Incidence is higher at lower (sunnier) latitudes, and these cancers occur more frequently on exposed parts of the body.[46] High exposure to sunlight early in life appears to pave the way for later skin cancer.

Cancer is not the only health effect associated with exposure to ultraviolet radiation. Exposure of the eyes to ultraviolet radiation in sunlight is associated with an increased risk of cataracts.[49] The WHO estimates that up to 20% of cataracts worldwide are attributable to exposure to ultraviolet radiation,[50] a risk that could be substantially reduced with relatively simple preventive measures. Finally, exposure to UV radiation can suppress the functioning of the immune system, making people more susceptible to infectious diseases.[51]

In view of all these hazards of exposure to natural ultraviolet radiation, it is important to remember that UV radiation also triggers the synthesis of vitamin D, an essential nutrient, in the skin. In this way, exposure to sunlight is healthful, and overprotection from the sun, especially in higher-latitude locations, can deprive the body of a natural source of vitamin D.

4.4 Natural Disasters

The most visible natural hazards are physical hazards that strike down large numbers of people in a relatively short time. Hydrometeorological disasters include events such as heat waves, drought, fires, floods, and storms. Storms include dust, snow and ice storms in addition to hurricanes, tornados, and cyclones. Geophysical events, such as earthquakes, landslides, volcanic eruptions, and tsunamis, are another category of natural disasters. Over the last 50 years, the death toll associated with natural disasters has decreased significantly, averaging less than 20,000 per year, compared with one million deaths per year during the early-to-mid 20th Century.[52] Unfortunately, there are still large numbers of fatalities associated with natural disasters in the world's poorest countries that lack a resilient infrastructure to respond to such events.[52] The public health impacts of these emergencies, of course, are also much broader than the fatalities and create a longer-term drain on resources. For example, in the wake of the most recent 50 years' worth of disasters, an estimated 6.6 billion individuals were in need of assistance in the form of food, water, shelter, sanitation, or emergency medical care.[53] The grief and stress that victims of such disasters experience cannot be quantified.

Table 4.6 offers a snapshot of four fairly recent natural disasters. The very high ratio of affected persons to deaths associated with Hurricane Katrina stands out and reflects how the long warning period for hurricanes, in conjunction with the resources of a wealthy country, helped keep the number of deaths low. Yet, because the emergency response was inadequate in an area that included a large city, a much greater number of people were affected.

Table 4.6 A Snapshot of Four Natural Disasters

Type of Disaster, Location	Year	Setting	Number Killed	Number Affected*
Tsunami, Indian Ocean/ Indonesia	2004	Less developed country	226,096	2,321,700
Hurricane (Katrina), United States	2005	More developed country	1,833	500,000
Earthquake, Haiti	2010	Less developed country	222,570	3,700,000
Earthquake and tsunami, Japan	2011	More developed country	20,319	405,719

*In need of assistance in the form of food, water, shelter, sanitation, or emergency medical care.
Data from Centre for Research on the Epidemiology of Disasters. Emergency Events Database (EM-DAT). Available at: www.emdat.be. Accessed March 21, 2012.

About three-quarters of deaths from the 2004 tsunami in the Indian Ocean occurred in the Aceh region at the northern tip of the Indonesian island of Sumatra.[54] Together, Aceh, Sri Lanka, and India accounted for 96% of those killed by the tsunami and similarly, 95% of those needing assistance after the event.[54]

A study of tsunami survivors (internally displaced persons) in Sri Lanka after the tsunami found that mortality was higher among females (17.5%) than among males (8.2%).[54] Furthermore, compared with 20- to 29-year olds (7.4% mortality), children younger than 5 years of age and those 5 to 9 years experienced significantly higher mortality (31.8% and 23.7%, respectively), as did adults older than 50 years (15.3%).[54] In areas of Sumatra that were severely damaged by the tsunami, about two-thirds of the population moved out of the homes they had lived in before the tsunami; most in this group moved beyond the community they had previously lived in, and more than half went to a camp or shelter at least once.[55]

In New Orleans, the environmental impacts of Hurricane Katrina included breached levees and flooding; severe damage to homes and whole neighborhoods; and loss of electricity, with the result that drinking water could not be pumped and sewage treatment plants could not operate. Katrina also brought home the profound impact of social and economic characteristics in a population coping with a natural disaster. Those with fewer financial resources, who had less access to communication devices and whose personal networks tended to be local, were less likely to hear about the impending crisis in sufficient time and less able to leave the city and find a place to stay.[56] These lower-income residents of the city were also more likely to be African American. The elderly and those with chronic health conditions were also more likely to remain in the city.[56] This inability to evacuate led to the disaster-within-a-disaster for those who took shelter in the Superdome sports arena, where they camped, without air conditioning or showers, as garbage rotted and toilets overflowed with waste.

Since Katrina, researchers have documented concentrations of lead in the soil of some New Orleans neighborhoods that are more than one-third higher than concentrations reported in the same census tracts before Hurricane Katrina.[57] Furthermore, soil samples at more than one-quarter of homes with bare soil showed concentrations of lead in soil more than three times the federal standard. Given that no sociodemographic pattern in lead concentration was found, the researchers hypothesize that the widespread contamination may be due to the post-Katrina demolition of old housing across many neighborhoods, rich and poor.[57]

The January 2010 earthquake in Haiti leveled the capital city of Port-au-Prince and severely damaged the country's already-weak infrastructure. About 10 months after the earthquake, the first cholera outbreak in Haiti in more than a century was documented; over the next 11 months, 378,638 cases of cholera were reported, and 5,592 deaths were ultimately attributed to the disease.[53] In addition to rebuilding the infrastructure for sanitation and drinking water treatment to prevent further waterborne disease outbreaks, much of the work in Haiti has focused on removing rubble and providing temporary shelter and schools.[58]

Because the 2011 earthquake and tsunami in Japan severely damaged the Fukushima nuclear power reactor, the full aftermath has yet to be calculated. (Damage to the reactor, and the effects of this damage, will be taken up elsewhere in the context of nuclear power safety.) The tsunami itself killed many thousands and essentially wiped out the built environment of Northern Japan. It left behind enormous quantities of debris—containing an unknown set of chemicals from industrial facilities, including oil refineries—much of which, 1 year later, had been cleared away. More debris was swept into the Pacific Ocean and began to drift slowly eastward. Some of the tsunami debris is expected to join the rotating mass of floating ocean trash known as the North Pacific Gyre, but some has already reached North America, and more is expected over the next year or two. In Northern Japan, electricity remains rationed, limiting the use of air conditioning, lighting, and mass transit.[59]

In the United States, the Federal Emergency Management Agency (FEMA) is responsible for emergency preparedness and response. Hurricanes, which in most years kill more people in the United States than any other natural disaster, are forecast by the National Hurricane Center with the goal of helping communities to minimize their losses by preparing for these storms. On a global scale, the WHO, the health agency of the United Nations, mitigates the environmental health impacts of natural disasters by providing shelter, sanitation and clean water, food, pest control, and health care. In addition, because refugees and internally displaced persons are often especially vulnerable to the effects of natural disasters, the Office of the U.N.'s High Commissioner for Refugees (UNHCR) may play a role in the agency's response to disaster, even though disaster relief is not formally part of its mandate.

Study Questions

1. Describe three distinct ways in which infectious disease is routinely transmitted via the hands, giving an example of a pathogen for each.
2. Identify a factor you could change to reduce your risk, or your family's risk, of infectious disease, explaining why this change would be effective.
3. Describe the health connection between infection and cancers.
4. In the event of a viral outbreak in a U.S. state, under what conditions do you think it would be appropriate for the state government to use quarantine and/or isolation to control the outbreak?
5. Identify factors that influence the emergence or reemergence of an infectious disease.
6. Explain why radon stands out as an important source of exposure to naturally occurring ionizing radiation.

References

1. Black RE. Escherichia coli diarrhea. In: Wallace RB, Doebbeling BN, eds., *Maxcy-Rosenau-Last Public Health & Preventive Medicine,* [14th edition] Appleton & Lange. 1998:243-245.
2. Kachur SP, Bloland PB. Malaria. In: Wallace RB, Doebbeling BN, eds. *Maxcy-Rosenau-Last Public Health & Preventive Medicine,* [14th edition] Appleton & Lange. 1998: 313-326.
3. Rosen G. *A History of Public Health.* Expanded edition. Originally published in 1958. The Johns Hopkins University Press. 1993.
4. The Fungal Research Trust. (2011, June). *How Common Are Fungal Diseases?* Fungal Research Trust 20th Anniversary meeting, London, UK. Retrieved June 20, 2012 from https://www.fungalinfectiontrust.org/How%20 Common%20are%20Fungal%20Diseases5.pdf
5. Roy CJ, Milton DK. Airborne transmission of communicable infection—the elusive pathway. *NEnglJ Med.* 2004;350:1710.
6. Riley RL. Aerial dissemination of pulmonary tuberculosis. *Am RevTuber Pulmon Dis.* 1957;76(6):931-941.
7. Breiman RF, Butler JC. Legionellosis. In Wallace RB, Doebbeling BN, eds. *Maxcy-Rosenau-Last Public Health & Preventive Medicine,* [14th edition] Appleton & Lange. 1998:246-248.
8. U.S. Centers for Disease Control and Prevention. Transmission: how people get hantavirus infection. Retrieved April 30, 2012 from www.cdc.gov/hantavirus /hps/transmission.html
9. Ellms JW. Lake Erie and the Niagara River. *Am J Public Health.* 1927;17:457-459.
10. U.S. Centers for Disease Control and Prevention. When and how to wash your hands. Retrieved September 1, 2020 from www.cdc.gov/Features/HandWashing/
11. Hopkins DR. Dracunculiasis. In Wallace RB, Doebbeling BN, eds. *Maxcy-Rosenau-Last Public Health & Preventive Medicine,* [14th edition] Appleton & Lange. 1998:254-255.
12. U.S. Food and Drug Administration. Foodborne Pathogenic Microorganisms and Natural Toxins Handbook. Retrieved March 3, 2012 from https://www .fda.gov/food/foodborne-pathogens/bad-bug-book -second-edition
13. Cui S, Ge B, Zheng, J, Meng J. Prevalence and antimicrobial resistance of *Campylobacter* spp. and *Salmonella* serovars in organic chickens from Maryland retail stores. *Appl Environ Microbiol.* 2005;71:4108-4111.

14. Luangtongkum T, Morishita T, Ison A, Huang S, McDermott PF, Zhang Q. Effect of conventional and organic production practices on the prevalence and antimicrobial resistance of *Campylobacter* spp. in poultry. *Appl Environ Microbiol.* 2006;72:3600-3607.

15. U.S. Centers for Disease Control and Prevention. *Escherichia coli* O157:H7 infection associated with drinking raw milk—Washington and Oregon, November—December 2005. 2007;56(08):165-167.

16. Heiman KE, Mody RK, Johnson SD, Griffin PM. & Gould LH. *Escherichia Coli* O157:H7 Outbreaks in the United States, 2003–2012. *Emerg Infect Dis.* 2015;21(8): 1293-1301.

17. U.S. Food and Drug Administration. *Bad bug book: handbook of foodborn pathogenic microorganisms and natural toxins.* 2006. Retrieved October 1, 2020 from https://www.fda.gov/files/food/published/Bad-Bug-Book-2nd-Edition-%28PDF%29.pdf

18. World Health Organization, Global Health Observatory (GHO) data. Number of malaria deaths: Estimated deaths, 2010–2017. Retrieved June 27, 2020 from https://www.who.int/gho/malaria/epidemic/deaths/en/

19. Delaunay P, Blanc V, Del Giudice P, et al. Bedbugs and infectious diseases. *Clin Infect Dis.* 2011;52(2):200-210.

20. Hwang SW, Svoboda TJ, De Jong IJ, Kabasele KJ, Gogosis E. Bed bug infestations in an urban environment. *Emerg Infect Dis.* 2005;11(4):533-538.

21. U.S. Centers for Disease Control and Prevention. Diseases directly transmitted by rodents. Retrieved March 12, 2012 from www.cdc.gov/rodents/diseases/direct.html

22. Nolan T, Papathanos P, Windbichler N, et al. Developing transgenic *Anopheles* mosquitoes for the sterile insect technique. *Genetica*, 2011;139:33-39.

23. The Center for Food Security & Public Health; Institute for International Cooperation in Animal Biologics. Anthrax. Retrieved July 18, 2006 from https://www.tchd.org/DocumentCenter/View/1599/AnthraxISU

24. The Carter Center. Guinea worm disease eradication. Retrieved February 3, 2012 from https://www.cartercenter.org/health/guinea_worm/index.html

25. Global Polio Eradication Initiative. Polio now. Retrieved March 15, 2012 from www.polioeradication.org/Dataandmonitoring/Poliothisweek.aspx

26. The Carter Center. Guinea worm eradication program. Retrieved March 15, 2012 from https://www.cartercenter.org/health/guinea_worm/index.html

27. U.S. Centers for Disease Control and Prevention. History of quarantine. Retrieved July 13, 2006 from www.cdc.gov/ncidod/dq/history.htm

28. U.S. Centers for Disease Control and Prevention. Methicillin-resistant *Staphylococcus aureus (MRSA)*. Retrieved March 20, 2008 from https://www.cdc.gov/mrsa/healthcare/index.html

29. World Health Organization. The top 10 causes of death in 2016. 2018. Retrieved June 25, 2020 from https://www.who.int/news-room/fact-sheets/detail/the-top-10-causes-of-death

30. World Health Organization. Children: improving survival and well-being. Retrieved March 19, 2012 from www.who.int/mediacentre/factsheets/fs178/en/index.html

31. American Cancer Society, The Cancer Atlas. Risk Factors: Infections. 2019. Retrieved June 26, 2020 from https://canceratlas.cancer.org/risk-factors/infection/

32. Russell FE. Toxic effects of animal toxins. In: Klaassen CD, ed. *Casarett & Doull's Toxicology: The Basic Science of Poisons*, [5th edition]. McGraw-Hill. 1996:801-839.

33. Norton S. Toxic effects of plants. In: Klaassen CD, ed. *Casarett & Doull's Toxicology: The Basic Science of Poisons*, [5th edition]. McGraw-Hill. 1996:841–853

34. U.S. Food and Drug Administration. Bad bug book: foodborne pathogenic microorganisms and natural toxins handbook. Retrieved March 19, 2012 from https://www.cdc.gov/mrsa/healthcare/index.html

35. U.S. Food and Drug Administration, Center for Food Safety and Applied Nutrition. Advisory on puffer fish. Retrieved October 3, 2012 from https://www.fda.gov/food/alerts-advisories-safety-information/advisory-puffer-fish

36. U.S. Food and Drug Administration. Foodborne pathogenic microorganisms and natural toxins handbook: various shellfish-associated toxins.

37. U.S. Food and Drug Administration. Foodborne Pathogenic Microorganisms and Natural Toxins Handbook: Ciguatera. Retrieved March 9, 2012 from https://pdf.usaid.gov/pdf_docs/pnado152.pdf

38. Kotsonis FN, Burdock GA, Flamm WG. Food toxicology. In: Klaassen CD, ed. *Casarett & Doull's Toxicology: The Basic Science of Poisons*, [5th edition]. McGraw-Hill. 1996: 909-949.

39. Yu MC, Yuan JM. Environmental factors and risk for hepatocellular carcinoma. *Gastroenterology.* 2004;127(5): S72-S78.

40. National Institute of Environmental Health Sciences. Aflatoxin & Liver Cancer. Retrieved April 30, 2012 from www.niehs.nih.gov/health/impacts/aflatoxin/index.cfm

41. U.S. Food and Drug Administration. Foodborne pathogenic microorganisms and natural toxins handbook: mushroom toxins.

42. Advisory Committee on Human Radiation Experiments. ACHRE Report. How does radiation affect humans? Retrieved September 3, 2012 from https://bioethicsarchive.georgetown.edu/achre/final/intro_9_5.html

43. United Nations Scientific Committee on the Effects of Atomic Radiation (UNSCEAR). UNSCEAR Report to the General Assembly, with scientific annexes. United Nations; 2000;I: Sources and effects of ionizing radiation.

44. National Academy of Sciences.. *Biological Effects of Ionizing Radiation (BEIR) VII: Health Risks from Exposure to Low Levels of Ionizing Radiation.* National Academies Press. 2005.

45. U.S. Centers for Disease Control and Prevention. Radiation and Pregnancy: A Fact Sheet for Clinicians. 2011. Retrieved August 29, 2012 from https://www.cdc.gov/nceh/radiation/emergencies/prenatalphysician.htm

46. Armstrong BK, Kricker A. The epidemiology of UV induced skin cancer. *J Photochem Photobiol B: Biol.* 2001;63(1-2):8-18.

47. National Cancer Institute. Skin cancer. Retrieved June 6, 2012 from www.cancer.gov/cancertopics/types/skin

48. National Cancer Institute. (n.d.). Melanoma. Retrieved March 19, 2012 from www.cancer.gov/cancertopics/types/melanoma

49. McCarty C, Taylor HR. A review of the epidemiologic evidence linking ultraviolet radiation and cataracts. *Dev Ophthalmol.* 2002;35:21-31.

50. World Health Organization. The known health effects of UV. Retrieved October 16, 2017 from www.who.int/uv/faq/uvhealtfac/en/index.html

51. Sleijffers A, Garssen J, Van Loveren H. Ultraviolet radiation, resistance to infectious diseases, and vaccination responses. *Methods,* 2002;28(1):111-121.

52. Ritchie H, Roser M. Natural disasters. *Our World in Data.* 2014. Retrieved June 27, 2020 from: https://ourworldindata.org/natural-disasters#number-of-deaths-from-natural-disasters

53. EM-DAT The International Disaster Database. Centre for Research on the Epidemiology of Disasters. Emergency Events Database (EM-DAT) [data]. Retrieved April 30, 2012 from: http://www.emdat.be/

54. Nishikiori N, Abe T, Costa DG, Dharmaratne SD, Kunii O, Moji K. Who died as a result of the tsunami?—Risk factors of mortality among internally displaced persons in Sri Lanka: a retrospective cohort analysis. *BMCPublic Health.* 2006;6:73.

55. Gray CL, Frankenberg E, Thomas D, Sumantri CS. Tsunami-Induced Displacement in Sumatra, Indonesia. 2009. Retrieved October 17, 2012 from http://paa2009.princeton.edu/papers/90062

56. Fussell E. The long-term recovery of New Orleans' population after Hurricane Katrina. *Am Behav Sci.* 2015;59(10):1231-1245.

57. Rabito FA, Iqbal S, Perry S, Arroyave W, Rice JC. Environmental lead after Hurricane Katrina: implications for future populations. *Environ Health Perspect.* 2012;120(2):180-184.

58. United Nations Department of Public Information. Haiti two years after the earthquake [fact sheet]. 2012. Retrieved June 20, 2012 from https://reliefweb.int/report/haiti/haiti-two-years-after-earthquake-united-nations-response

59. Harmon K. Japan's post-Fukushima earthquake health woes go beyond radiation effects. *Scientific American.* 2012;41.

CHAPTER 5

Producing Food

LEARNING OBJECTIVES

After studying this chapter, the reader will be able to:

* Define or explain the key terms introduced throughout the chapter
* Describe the origins and use of chemical pesticides and their impacts on the environment and human health
* Discuss integrated pest management as an alternative to routine pesticide use
* Discuss the benefits and potential health risks of genetically modified crop plants
* Describe typical livestock production practices in the United States and explain how several emerging health concerns are associated with modern livestock practices
* Describe modern fishing practices, risks to workers, and the future of fishing
* Describe the contribution of agriculture to global resource degradation
* Characterize the modern food supply system and contrast it with the movement toward locally grown food and organic farming
* Describe key approaches to managing the public health risks associated with modern methods of food production
* Describe the U.S. regulatory framework for managing food quality and safety

The competition between species on our planet is perhaps most intense when it comes to food. To survive, not only do humans need to fight off bugs and other larger animals interested in the same food resources but also beat back weeds and plants that compete with our crops for the same soil, water, and sunshine to grow. Any of these other species may be termed a **pest** when they interfere with human agricultural efforts, similar to the term *pathogen* in the last chapter to refer to any unhelpful microorganism. Also, many of these insect pests put human lives at risk as *vectors* for serious infectious diseases.

This chapter begins with the origin of modern chemicals used in agriculture to combat pests (Section 5.1) and discusses the human health effects associated with pesticides. The environmental health impacts of modern practices for the production of crops (Section 5.2), livestock rearing (Section 5.3), and modern fishing (Section 5.4.) are described next, including their impacts on global resources (Section 5.5). Some of the complexities of the modern food supply system (Section 5.6) are contrasted with the movement toward locally grown food and organic farming (Section 5.7). The chapter closes with a description of how we regulate food protection practices (Section 5.8).

5.1 Origin of Modern Pesticides

Humans have been trying to eradicate pests ever since our earliest efforts to find shelter—somewhere to stay dry and rest at night without being bitten or stung. The earliest control efforts were physical, such as slapping or crushing these annoying pests, techniques still resorted to today. Sometimes, the infestation was so extreme that shelters had to be burned to kill off pests. Part of the route that indigenous people in southern California established as they moved on from periodically burning their flea-infested villages still exists today as a major road known as *Alameda de las Pulgas*, or "flea road."

Although a few effective pest control measures were documented in Arabia and China that relied on toxic metals or plant extracts, such chemical-based efforts did not truly emerge until the 18th and 19th centuries in Europe.[1] By this time, urban populations had grown tremendously where many lived close together in unsanitary conditions that favored the growth of pest populations. In addition, these cities relied on larger farming efforts for food that often focused on the production of a single crop, a risky situation if a destructive pest favored that food as well. A famous potato blight in 1848 caused by a fungus resulted in widespread famine in Ireland (refer to **Figure 5.1**) and parts of England and Belgium.[1] During this same time period in France, the wine industry faced destruction from both an insect as well as mildew. And in the colonies, coffee supplies were depleted by another fungal agent. Facing not only hunger but also the loss of their economies, efforts got underway to develop more successful pest control tools.

Inorganic compounds containing toxic metals became widely used to control pests, and some of these are still used today. This group includes lead arsenate, in which arsenic

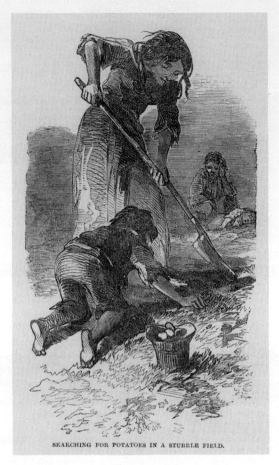

SEARCHING FOR POTATOES IN A STUBBLE FIELD.

Figure 5.1 Hungry children dig for potatoes during the Irish Famine.
© Historia/Shutterstock

is the active ingredient; Bordeaux mixture (copper sulfate and lime), in which copper is the active ingredient; and Paris Green (copper and arsenic), in which both ingredients are toxic. Kerosene and oil were also used as insecticides—when poured into standing water, they form a film on the water's surface that suffocates insect larvae.

Unfortunately, heavy metals are often as toxic to humans as to other species so research into other alternatives intensified. The first generation of organic chemical pesticides were the **organochlorines**, also known as **chlorinated hydrocarbons**. The best-known chemical in this group is dichloro-diphenyltrichloroethane (DDT), whose insect-killing properties were discovered in 1939 by Swiss research chemist Paul Müller; Müller was awarded the Nobel Prize for this discovery in 1948.

Types of Pesticides

A **pesticide** is a chemical used to kill pests. But what is a pest? Essentially, a **pest** is any animal or plant that interferes with human well-being or interests by carrying disease or causing discomfort in people or in the animals we care about; or by competing with people for resources (e.g., locusts that eat crops, or weeds that steal nutrients from them); or by destroying property (e.g., termites or mold); or even simply by being where it is not wanted (e.g., a dandelion in a manicured lawn).

Within the broad category of pesticides, subgroups are defined according to the type of pest they are intended to kill. The major groups of pesticides are **herbicides** (used against plant pests, commonly called **weeds**), **insecticides** (not only used against insects but also arachnids), **fungicides** (used to control fungal growth in the environment, as distinct from fungal infections in people, which are treated with antifungal medications), and **rodenticides** (used to kill rodents). Other types of pesticides, used in smaller quantities, include nematicides (used against nematodes, or roundworms), molluscicides, and poisons used against fish and birds.

More herbicides were sold in 2012 than any other category of pesticide and the agricultural sector accounted for almost 60% of these sales, or over $5 billion in expenditures.[2] Insecticides were the second major type of pesticide sold in 2012, with more sold to the home and garden sector than for commercial agriculture. In fact, 80% of all pesticides purchased by domestic home owners and gardeners were to kill insects. Fungicides expenditures were the third-largest category in 2012, followed by much lower sales of fumigants and other categories, such as nematicides, rodenticides, molluscicides, and poisons used against fish and birds.

Herbicides

Synthetic herbicides have a wide range of chemical structures with considerable overlap in toxic effects, and thus it is simpler to group these chemicals by their effects on different classes of plants. A **selective herbicide** either kills broad-leaved plant species but not plants in the grass family or the reverse. In agriculture, this distinction means that a selective herbicide applied to a field of grain kills weeds but not the crop. Similarly, a selective herbicide applied to a lawn kills only the weeds. Atrazine is the most widely used selective herbicide in U.S. agriculture.[2]

The first synthetic herbicide was 2,4-D, a selective herbicide introduced shortly after World War II and still used in many over-the-counter weed killers. 2,4-D was one of two major ingredients in the defoliant Agent Orange, used by U.S. forces in the Vietnam War. In this context, a selective herbicide was used to kill larger plants—trees and bushes—that provided cover to combatants on the ground, without wiping out all plant life. As described elsewhere in the context of chemical manufacturing, the other key ingredient in Agent Orange, 2,4,5-T, was contaminated with dioxin.

In contrast, a **nonselective herbicide** kills all types of plants. Such an herbicide might be broadly applied, for example, in a railroad yard, to prevent workers from slipping on weeds. Alternatively, a nonselective herbicide can be applied in a targeted fashion to individual weeds—in a lawn, for example. Roundup is a nonselective herbicide used in this way. Before the 1950s, waste oils, salt, and arsenicals were used to kill plants nonselectively.

Some genetically modified crop plants have been designed to be resistant to particular nonselective herbicides, specifically so that these nonselective herbicides can be used in agriculture. For example, the Monsanto Corporation, which produced Roundup, also developed Roundup Ready genetically engineered soybeans, designed to be planted in fields treated with Roundup.

Insecticides

Many insecticides are used against vectors of human or animal disease—most importantly, mosquitoes, but also flies, fleas, ticks, and lice, for example. Insecticides are also widely used in agriculture to keep pests from consuming crops intended as food for people or farm animals. Some insecticides poison a pest when it eats the poison; others poison on contact.

By the mid-1950s, more than 25 organochlorine pesticides were in use in the United States, including chlordane, aldrin, dieldrin, and heptachlor. Worldwide use of DDT from 1950 to 1980 is estimated at more than 40,000 metric tons per year.[3] DDT was used extensively by the U.S. military during World War II to protect troops against disease (see **Figure 5.2**). After the war, DDT, widely viewed as a wonder chemical, was sprayed broadly in communities.

The organochlorine pesticides are nerve toxins: They disrupt the central nervous system, causing convulsions and death. However, their acute toxicity to people is very low, and for this reason it was many years before they were considered a human health problem. These chemicals are very persistent in the environment, are lipophilic, bioconcentrate in fatty tissue, and ultimately biomagnify in the food chain. However, at the time when DDT came into use, these processes were not appreciated, and Müller and others considered DDT's environmental persistence a good thing, since it offered extended protection against insect pests.[4] The organochlorine pesticides' toxicity in wildlife was ultimately brought to light largely through the efforts of Rachel Carson, a naturalist and author of the famous 1962 book, *Silent Spring*. Among other effects, Carson described how DDT softened the shells of bald eagles' eggs, preventing these birds from breeding successfully. The bald eagle is a carnivorous bird at the top of the food chain and also the national symbol of the United States. The effects of DDT on the bald eagle caused a national outcry, and the pesticide was banned in the United States in 1972.

Several other organochlorine pesticides in addition to DDT are now banned in the United States and other more developed countries; the Stockholm Convention on Persistent Organic Pollutants also restricts these chemicals. The Stockholm Convention adopted in 2001 originated as an initiative of the United Nations Environment Programme and is an international agreement on controlling a set of chemicals designated as persistent organic pollutants, commonly referred to as POPs.* The list of chemicals

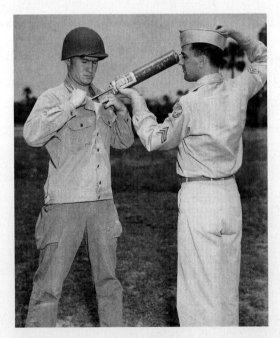

Figure 5.2 A World War II era soldier demonstrates the application of DDT to U.S. army personnel.

---

*The term *persistent organic pollutants* (POPs) originates with the Stockholm Convention (see text). Another term, *persistent, bioaccumulative, and toxic* (PBT) *chemicals*, has been used more recently by the Environmental Protection Agency (EPA) to designate a set of chemicals of regulatory concern. This list has some overlap with the POPs list but includes other organic chemicals as well as the heavy metals lead and mercury. Both terms are often used more loosely as descriptive rather than regulatory names. A more recent coinage, *ubiquitous bioaccumulative toxins*, captures the implications of persistence; however, the term *toxin* typically refers to a substance produced naturally by a plant or animal.

comprises DDT and eight other organochlorine pesticides (aldrin, chlordane, dieldrin, endrin, heptachlor, hexachlorobenzene, mirex, and toxaphene) along with polychlorinated biphenyls (PCBs), dioxins, and furans. By ratifying the agreement, countries commit to eliminate or reduce the release of these chemicals into the environment.

However, DDT usage pits public health practitioners against environmentalists in the context of infectious disease. For about 20 years, DDT was widely used for mosquito control in both more-developed and less-developed regions, until it became clear that bioaccumulation and bioconcentration of DDT threatened the health of both wildlife and humans. DDT and related chemicals are now widely banned as pesticides, but DDT is still used for mosquito control in certain less-developed countries. This practice reflects the very different view of DDT's risks and benefits in countries that are burdened with high rates of malaria and cannot afford newer, more expensive pesticides. In 2006, the World Health Organization approved the use of DDT for targeted indoor spraying of walls and roofs—killing mosquitoes that land there—both in houses and in shelters for domestic animals, and reaffirmed this position in 2009.[5] As of early 2011, about 11 countries, mostly in sub-Saharan Africa, were using DDT in this targeted way.[6]

The second generation of synthetic organic insecticides were the **organophosphates**, originally developed as nerve gases to be used in war. Like the organochlorines, the organophosphates also disrupt the central nervous system by stopping a key enzyme in the nervous system called cholinesterase from working. This category of organic chemicals is often thought preferable to organochlorines because these chemicals do not persist in the environment. However, organophosphates can be very toxic when exposure involves a highly concentrated solution or large amount in the air, causing severe effects, including death. The acute toxicity of organophosphates to people varies widely; for example, parathion is highly toxic to humans, whereas malathion is much less toxic. Other familiar organophosphates

are Diazinon, banned in 2005, and chlorpyrifos which was banned in California for consumer purchase in 2020.

The organophosphates were quickly followed by the **carbamates**, which have a similar chemical action but low short-term toxicity in people. Sevin is an example of a carbamate pesticide widely used for gardens and mosquito control. Although the final carbamate product is not as toxic as organochlorines and organophosphates insecticides, an intermediate product produced during production was responsible for the deadly industrial accident in Bhopal, India, which killed almost 3,000 people immediately (refer to **Figure 5.3**). Its final death toll was debated to be as large as between 15,000 to 20,000.[7] In 1984, a large cloud of toxic methyl isocyanate gas was released from the Union Carbide plant over the surrounding densely populated neighborhoods, causing people to awaken in acute respiratory distress. Subsequent investigations determined that the plant was understaffed and operating with obsolete and substandard safety technology, an unjust situation that has triggered ongoing legal action to this day. As mentioned previously, shock and outrage over Bhopal was also the motivation for the Emergency Planning and Community Right-to-Know Act in the United States.

Natural botanical insecticides have also been used for many years and function primarily

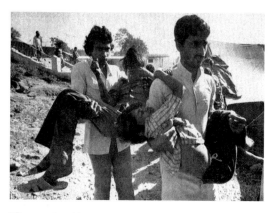

Figure 5.3 Victims of the Bhopal poisonous gas disaster.
© Sondeep Shankar/AP/Shutterstock.

by disrupting the central nervous system. The insecticide **pyrethrum** is extracted from chrysanthemums and most recently, synthetic insecticides called **pyrethroids** (i.e., pyrethrum-like chemicals) have been developed, including permethrin. These pesticides, although based on a natural poison, are extremely potent and consumer products contain only a low dose so that they pose a low acute toxicity to people. Pyrethrum and its synthetic alternatives is often the pesticides of choice in community-level spraying for mosquitoes—for example, to minimize the risk of illness from West Nile Virus. Pyrethroids are also used in agriculture, as mosquito repellents and as head-lice treatments.

Fungicides

Fungicides can be critical in the protection of fruits and also of crops grown in wet conditions. Various inorganic compounds were widely used as fungicides before the era of synthetic organic compounds, and indeed some are still in use. However, today there are many synthetic organic fungicides, of different chemical types, often used in combination. For example, fungicides are commonly used in both cranberry bogs and apple orchards.

Rodenticides

Most rodenticides take the form of baits that attract rodents and kill them when they consume the bait. Many rodenticides, including those that have been on the market the longest, contain an anticoagulant: When a rodent consumes the bait, the chemical causes massive internal bleeding, resulting in death. Some newer products contain poisons that kill in other ways.

Overall, rodenticides are effective in killing rodents; however, they also pose some health risk to both people and wildlife. Most human victims are young children who find a trap and eat the toxic bait. In nature, the unintended victims are animals that eat rodents, including birds of prey, such as hawks and owls, as well as larger mammals, such as foxes and mountain lions. Recent EPA regulations restrict the uses of certain

rodenticides and set requirements for labeling and tamper-resistant packaging.

Limitations of Pesticides

In simple terms, pesticides are effective in killing their targets. However, their broader effectiveness is limited in two key ways, both reflecting the fact that communities of plants and pests are not static but rather dynamic.

First, just as some bacteria are resistant to a specific antibiotic, some pests may have a genetic makeup that confers resistance to a specific pesticide. At the first application of the pesticide, the resistant organisms survive; most susceptible individuals die, although some may somehow escape exposure and survive. As a result of this differential mortality in the two groups, the resistant organisms make up a larger proportion of the population after the pesticide application than they did beforehand. In this way, as the population continues to multiply, its makeup changes: The selection effect is magnified through repeated pesticide applications until most or all of the surviving population carries the genetic trait that confers resistance to the pesticide. Because many pests have lifespans much shorter than our own, the development of such **pesticide resistance** can occur rather quickly in response to this sudden change in the pests' environment—a sped-up version of evolutionary survival of the fittest. Once pests develop resistance to a pesticide, it is no longer useful, and this creates pressure to develop new pesticides. The problem of pesticide resistance is important both in managing infectious disease and in agriculture.

In the agricultural context, a second important limitation on the effectiveness of pesticides is that the crop and the **target pest** (the pest that eats the crop and which the farmer wishes to eliminate using pesticides) do not exist in isolation. Rather, they are part of an ecosystem in which the pest species eats (or is eaten by) other species. These connections cause ripple effects from the use of pesticides. For example, the pesticide may not only kill the target pest but also may kill another species—a bystander in the war between the farmer and the target pest—which happens to serve the beneficial purpose of eating the target pest. If the population of this beneficial species is suddenly reduced, the target pest population can rebound dramatically for a time in the absence of its natural predator, a phenomenon called **target pest resurgence**.[8] Alternatively, the target pest itself may not only eat the crop but also serve the beneficial purpose of eating yet another insect, which is also a pest that eats the crop. In this situation, wiping out the target pest population allows the population of this alternative pest species to explode, and the crop still gets eaten. This phenomenon, in which there is a surge in the population of the secondary pest, is known as a **secondary pest outbreak**.[8]

Human Health Effects of Pesticides

Although many parents worry about the effects of pesticide residue on the food, especially fruit, that their children eat, it is particularly difficult to study the chronic health effects of specific pesticides in people because it is difficult to assess exposure accurately. In addition to the difficulties estimating intake (Americans rarely take in their daily recommended amounts of vegetables and fruit), the relatively small amount of pesticide residue legally allowed to remain on agricultural products tends to dissipate with time and is often removed with simple washing. Many people who work with pesticides, such as farmers or pesticide applicators, are exposed to a changing mix of chemicals, and they may not know what chemicals they are using. There is great variation in pesticide application methods, training, and work practices, including the use of protective gear. Finally, the longer-term effects of a prior acute exposure may be difficult to disentangle from the effects of chronic exposure. In light of these complications, many epidemiologic studies have simply used the farming occupation or agricultural work experience as a surrogate for pesticide exposure. Exposure to pesticides has been linked most clearly to neurologic effects, cancer, and reproductive and developmental outcomes.

The neurologic effects of acute pesticide exposure are well known and include headache, dizziness, nausea and vomiting, muscle weakness, and even convulsions and coma at high exposures.[9,10] The World Health Organization estimates that roughly 30% of suicides globally are by self-poisoning with pesticides.[11] In a number of studies, chronic exposure to pesticides has been associated with deficits in cognitive function (e.g., memory, attention, and visual–spatial processing) and also in psychomotor function (e.g., reaction time).[9,10] There is considerable support in the literature for a link between pesticide exposure and Parkinson's disease, and some evidence of an association with amyotrophic lateral sclerosis (ALS, also known as Lou Gehrig's disease).[9,10]

Among the organochlorine pesticides, DDT, aldrin, dieldrin, chlordane, and others have been shown to cause cancer in animals.[10] Risk of non-Hodgkin's lymphoma is associated with exposure to some herbicides, as well as to organochlorine and organophosphate pesticides,[10] including the insecticide hexachlorocyclohexane, used for sheep dipping.[12] The farming occupation has been linked to increased risk of several cancers, including leukemia, multiple myeloma, soft tissue sarcoma, and cancers of the brain, stomach, and prostate.[10, 13–16] Furthermore, a meta-analysis of mortality data for farmers has documented elevated mortality from multiple myeloma, non-Hodgkin's lymphoma, Hodgkin's disease, and cancers of the brain, stomach, and skin.[17] A review of 28 epidemiologic studies conducted in the same study cohort reported that 19 pesticides were significantly associated with an increased risk of at least one cancer.[18] Emerging epidemiologic evidence suggests that breast cancer risk in older women is linked to prepubertal exposure to DDT.[19]

Reproductive effects have been associated with chronic exposure to some pesticides. In various studies, a woman's history of agricultural work has been linked to increased risk of spontaneous abortion and stillbirth, fetal death, and prematurity.[20] In the 1970s, the now-banned pesticide dibromochloropropane (DBCP), used to kill worms, was found to affect the fertility of male workers in a production plant.[20, 21] A literature review reported evidence suggestive of effects of pesticide exposure on semen quality, as well as DNA or chromosomal damage in sperm.[22] Prenatal pesticide exposure has been linked to some birth defects, including oral clefts.[21] There is some evidence that childhood exposure to pesticides may increase the risk of leukemia and certain brain cancers and may alter thyroid function or have other endocrine-disrupting effects.[23] A review of 21 epidemiologic studies since the late 1990s concluded that there is an association between pesticide exposure and childhood cancer, although a causal link has not been demonstrated[24]; for childhood leukemia, the best-documented link is with mother's occupational exposure to pesticides.[25, 26]

The burden of pesticide exposure weighs more heavily on certain populations, among them pesticide production workers, farmers and their families, and hired farmworkers. In the United States, more than 80% of these farmworkers are men; they are about 50% Hispanic and about 50% foreign-born, and about one-third have less than a ninth-grade education.[27]

Migrant farmworkers are often at special risk from pesticide exposures because they may work with inadequate protection; live in close proximity to agricultural land; lack adequate facilities to wash; be unable to understand hazard warnings in English, whether spoken or printed; and lack health insurance and access to health care. A study of farmworkers in Oregon found that most wore no protective clothing on the job, yet wore their work clothes and boots home, and did not change their clothes within 30 minutes of arriving home,[28] suggesting that they did not appreciate the potential risk to their families. A survey of 300 migrant farmworkers in Eastern North Carolina found that those without a visa for seasonal agricultural work were significantly less likely to be told by their supervisor when pesticides were applied, or when the no-reentry interval had ended, and significantly more likely to have worked in a field adjacent to where pesticides were being applied.[29]

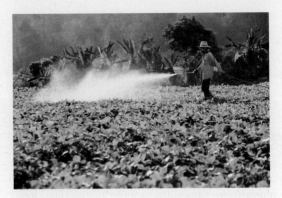

Figure 5.4 The spraying of pesticides.
© Toa55/Shutterstock.

Many agricultural workers in less-developed countries have similar vulnerabilities, sometimes compounded by the continued use of pesticides now banned in the more developed countries. Female agricultural workers in less developed countries may be particularly highly exposed because they are often casual workers doing low-skill, high-exposure jobs without protection or training.[30] (see **Figure 5.4**).

Integrated Pest Management as an Alternative to Routine Pesticide Use

Although the concept of **integrated pest management (IPM)** predates modern synthetic pesticides, it has been expanded and elaborated in response to the obvious problems stemming from the indiscriminate use of these chemicals. These problems include the development of resistance among pests, rebound effects such as target pest resurgence and secondary pest outbreaks, and widespread environmental contamination, with its health impacts on wildlife and people.

The *integrated* in integrated pest management refers to the use of multiple tactics (e.g., biological and chemical) to manage multiple pests in a manner consistent with ecological principles.[8] For example, a vertically integrated approach recognizes the problem of target pest resurgence, and a horizontally integrated approach recognizes the problem of secondary pest outbreaks. The term *management* acknowledges that the goal is to suppress pests rather than to wipe them out. Integrated pest management also incorporates the notion that populations of target pests (and their predators and competitors) should be monitored, and that pest control measures should be undertaken when some predefined threshold is met, rather than on a regular schedule.[8] IPM tactics include introducing beneficial insects (e.g., predators or parasites of the pest), using synthetic pheromones (chemicals that female insects use to attract males) to confuse male insects and reduce mating, and changing irrigation or crop rotation practices.

There is disagreement over the degree to which IPM techniques have become a part of U.S. farming. Survey data from the Department of Agriculture (USDA) suggest widespread adoption of some IPM techniques.[31] However, critics suggest that much of what passes for IPM is simply monitoring pest populations as a way to decide when to begin treatment with pesticides.[32] In fact, the challenges of integrating the flexible and nuanced IPM approach into large-scale, mechanized agriculture are substantial.

5.2 Modern Crop Production

U.S. agriculture has seen sweeping changes since the mid-20th century. Farms have become fewer and larger, and many large farms are now owned by corporate entities (including some family-held corporations). Since 1950, the number of farms in the United States fell by more than half, and the average size of a farm nearly doubled, to 418 acres.[33] On average, corporate farms are nearly four times as large as farms held by individuals or families.

It is not only the statistical picture of U.S. agriculture that has changed, but also the landscape itself. Today, there is little variety in the crops grown: A relatively small number of varieties of wheat, for example, are now planted on a very large scale. Similarly, crops are grown mostly

in monoculture: immense swaths of land planted in wheat, for example, rather than the traditional checkerboard of smaller fields planted with different crops or even with two crops interspersed in the same field. The production process relies heavily on chemical inputs, such as pesticides and fertilizers, mostly derived from petroleum. Production is further subsidized by the use of fossil fuels to power heavy machinery involved with tilling, planting, weed control, and harvesting. In 2012, U.S. agriculture used almost 800 trillion British thermal units (Btu) of energy, equivalent to the energy from 6,000 million gallons of diesel, and crop operations consumed the highest amount of this energy.[34]

Intensive Use of Fertilizers and Pesticides

Nitrogen is an essential nutrient for plants, and nitrogen-containing fertilizers are widely used in agriculture. The nitrogen in fertilizers is in the form of nitrates (NO_3), which are highly soluble in groundwater and are readily taken up by plants. However, when more fertilizer is applied than can be used by crops, the result is elevated nitrate concentrations in groundwater. This ultimately contributes to the degradation of water quality as well as global climate change (see Section 5.5); more immediately, if this groundwater is used as a source of drinking water, the elevated nitrate concentrations can have a direct human health impact.

Young infants who consume well water contaminated with nitrates may be made ill, usually when the well water is used to make infant formula. Nitrates, converted to nitrites either before or after ingestion, change hemoglobin in the bloodstream into a form that cannot carry oxygen. The resulting condition is called **methemoglobinemia**; with inadequate oxygen in the blood, the child takes on a bluish color. The condition, also called **blue baby syndrome**, can be fatal. Methemoglobinemia affects hundreds of infants in the United States each year,[35] mostly in rural areas. In some locations, nitrate contamination is more common: Researchers in Romania, for example, reported 42 to 239 cases per 100,000 live births during the years 2000–2004.[36]

Synthetic pesticides are unique among environmental health hazards in that they are developed specifically to be toxic and then are deliberately spread widely and repeatedly for agricultural purposes. In the United States in 2007, almost 450,000 tons of conventional pesticides were used, about 80% of this amount in agriculture.[2] Although pesticides are the most familiar agricultural chemicals, they are not the only ones. A number of chemicals, some of which are also used as pesticides, are used as plant growth regulators. The basic purpose of these chemicals is

Feeding a Growing Population

The goal of intensively using fertilizers and pesticides in modern agriculture is to produce more food per acre, or *yield*, to sustain an ever-increasing human population. The number of people on the planet remained under one billion until approximately 1800. Today, there are over 7 billion people on the planet and even more alarming, it only took only 12 years to add these last billion human residents. It is estimated that there could be 10 billion people alive on the planet before the next Century.[1] Will we be able to feed everyone?

Studies of other species have revealed that populations grow toward their environment's *carrying capacity* in two distinct ways. If a species' population grows exponentially until it nears the environment's capacity to provide necessary resources, that population no longer increases and remains at a level near this capacity's threshold-a manner of growth termed a S-curve growth pattern. Other species may also increase in size exponentially but not slow down even as the size of the population surpasses its environment's ability to sustain all of its members. This J-curve pattern of growth results in massive die-offs among the population until the size returns to a level that its environment may sustain.[1] Such a growth pattern is termed a *Boom and Bust cycle* and has been observed for several species in the Artic, such as wolves and hares.

Will such dramatic die-offs have to occur among humans, either from famine or other equally alarming mechanisms, such as war or pestilence, to stay within our planet's carrying capacity? Several factors must be figured out to answer this question, such as what is that capacity and also whether the human population adheres to a S-curve or J-curve growth rate. Almost 300 hundred years ago, the British political economist Thomas Malthus argued that the human population would increase, if unchecked, in a geometric progression, while the means of subsistence will increase in only an arithmetic progression (refer to graph below).

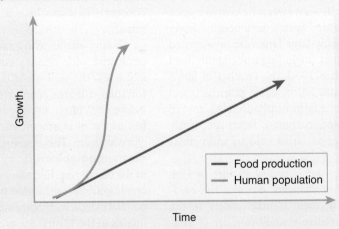

Malthusian prediction regarding the growth of human population compared to increase in food production.

Malthus pessimistically predicted that wide-spread famines would be nature's way to combat human population pressures.[1]

The exponential growth of the human population during the past 150 years may be characterized as the result of decreasing death rates brought about by the industrial-medical-scientific revolution[1]. However, associated innovations in agriculture managed to keep pace. The largest gains in the world's food supply after World War II occurred by dramatically improving the yield per acre from farms rather than by expanding the agricultural footprint. Technological improvements and innovations in irrigation, in addition to the use of fertilizers and pesticides mentioned previously, resulted in tripling and quadrupling crop yields.

Another key contributor during this time was the creation of "miracle seeds," the result of decades of research into plant breeding and hybridization. Agronomist Norman Borlaug was awarded the 1970 Nobel Peace Prize for developing miracle wheat that allowed countries from Mexico to India to more than double their wheat production. Borlaug, who came to be called the "Father of the Green Revolution," warned that his contribution might buy humankind two to three more decades of food security, but efforts to tame the *population monster* must also occur.[1]

1. Nadakavukaren, A. *Our Global Environment: A Health Perspective* (7th ed. 33-37 and 89-90). Waveland Press, Inc. 2011.

to produce a crop that is amenable to mechanical harvesting. For example, chemicals may be used to slow down or speed up growth; to dry out leaves or even defoliate plants; to open cotton bolls; or to keep the straw of a grain crop short and strong.[37, 38]

Genetically Modified Crop Plants

The stated rationale for developing **genetically modified (GM)** (or **genetically engineered**) plants is to augment the world's food supply. The global population was estimated at 6.9 billion in 2010 and is expected to increase to 9.4 billion by 2050.[39] Because most of the world's arable land is already under cultivation, the only way to increase total crop production is to increase yield per acre. Genetically modified crops are seen by many as the only plausible means to achieve this goal. For example, it would be advantageous to create plants that are not susceptible to disease, that repel pests (yet another approach to pest control), or that ripen more quickly. Crop plants might also be genetically modified to improve their nutritional value—for example, to be richer in essential vitamins. Proponents also argue that the use of GM crops can reduces the amount of fertilizer and pesticides needed.

Of course, people have been modifying plants through selective breeding for centuries, but the new technologies work at the level of DNA rather than at the level of the individual plant; in fact, such techniques are sometimes called "molecular breeding."[40] The basic approach is to first isolate a gene that codes for the desired characteristic (it might come from any species) and then transfer this DNA to the species of interest—for example, corn. Specifically, the gene being transferred (called the **transgene**, or **biotech gene**) is inserted into a simple loop of bacterial DNA, which is used to make the transfer. The processes by which the gene is integrated into the corn DNA (so that it causes the corn to take on the desired characteristic) and appears in seed are far too complex to describe here. But if these steps are successful, subsequent generations of the **transgenic** corn (the corn into whose DNA the transgene has been imported) will have the characteristic coded by the imported DNA. For example, plants of one variety of transgenic corn produce a protein that is toxic to certain insect pests, thus protecting the plants from the pests; the gene that produces this effect comes from a soil bacterium called *Bacillus thuringiensis*, and the corn is referred to as *Bt* corn. This corn has, in effect, a built-in pesticide.

The cultivation of genetically modified crop plants, and the consumption of foods made from these plants, raise two distinct public health concerns: The first arises directly from the foreign genes present in transgenic plants; the second arises from the techniques used to transfer genes from one species to another.

Allergic Reactions to Genetically Modified Foods

The core human health concern related to genetically modified foods is that they may cause allergic reactions in susceptible individuals. Allergens—the biological substances that induce allergic reactions—are proteins, and the proteins in a plant species (e.g., peanuts) have characteristic chemical structures determined by the genes of that species. As a result, if a peanut gene is transferred into a soybean plant, for example, peanut proteins will be present in the genetically modified soybeans. If any of the peanut proteins is an allergen, then a person with a peanut allergy who eats these soybeans will have an allergic reaction to it. And because the modified soybeans do not look different or taste different, the allergic individual has no way of knowing the allergen is present. Before candidate biotech genes are transferred to a different species, they are studied to see if any of the proteins they encode are considered likely to be allergenic—for example, whether a sequence of amino acids in the protein is similar to a sequence in a known allergen.[40] However, some concern remains about allergic reactions to genetically modified foods.

The safety of specific transgenic plants is a critical question because the practical challenges of limiting the spread of genetic material in the environment are truly intractable. For example, in the United States, fields planted in genetically modified corn are not physically segregated from fields of traditional corn by distance or barriers, and pollen from genetically modified corn can easily be carried on the wind to traditional corn plants. A recent assessment of 604 canola plants growing by the roadside in North Dakota, sampled over 3,000 miles of highways and county roads, found that about 80% were genetically

modified (compared with approximatley 90% of the U.S. canola crop overall).[41] Most of the genetically modified plants were one of two commercial varieties, each resistant to a specific herbicide. Two plants were found to be genetically resistant to both of these herbicides, suggesting a cross between the two engineered varieties. Findings like these suggest that the longer-term ecological impacts of planting genetically modified food plants cannot be predicted. Equally daunting is the task of keeping track of biotech ingredients as they wend their way through the labyrinth of the modern food supply, as described later.

Genetically Modified Foods and the Spread of Antibiotic Resistance

As described earlier in the context of infectious disease, bacterial populations can become resistant to an antibiotic over time, much as pests develop resistance to pesticides. Such antibiotic resistance among pathogens is a major challenge in the battle against infectious disease because it makes certain antibiotics ineffective. There has been some concern that transgenic plants could contribute to the problem of antibiotic resistance through a somewhat convoluted series of events.

When a culture of plant cells is exposed to a foreign gene in the laboratory, in hopes that the cells will take up the transgene and integrate it into their DNA, only a small percentage of the cells actually do so. As a result, it is a practical challenge to locate those cells that have been modified and can be used to start the new genetic line—for example, of transgenic corn. This has usually been done by coupling a gene for antibiotic resistance to the gene being transferred; then, when the plant cells are exposed to the appropriate antibiotic, those few that survive are identifiable as those carrying the transgene.

But these survivors, of course, also carry the antibiotic resistance gene. The concern is that, in the broader environment, such antibiotic resistance genes might somehow be transferred from transgenic plants to bacteria. The two settings

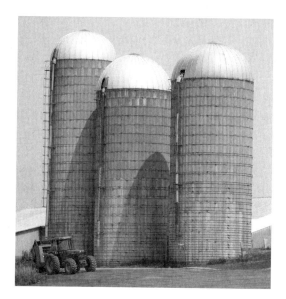

Figure 5.5 Bacteria digest crop wastes in silos like these.

in which this is most likely to occur may seem rather different, but they share an important bacterial process. One is silos on farms (see **Figure 5.5**)—storage cylinders where resident bacteria digest crop wastes, producing a moist material called silage, which is used as animal feed. The other is the gut of humans or other animals, where resident bacteria help to digest plant matter in food.[42] No one knows how likely it is that antibiotic resistance genes might be transferred from transgenic plants to bacteria in the environment; the U.S. Food and Drug Administration's (FDA) stance is that it is a remote possibility, but not all scientists agree.[43]

Use of Water for Irrigation

The irrigation of crops accounted for 42% of U.S. water consumption in 2015; more than half of water used for irrigation (52%) came from surface sources.[44] In all, about 118 billion gallons per day were used for irrigation during the year, or about 415 gallons per person per day. California alone accounted for 16% of water used for irrigation; other high-quantity users were Idaho and Arkansas, Montana, and Colorado form a second

tier of major users of water for irrigation. Depending on the method of irrigation used, water losses to evaporation can be substantial; for example, much more water is lost when large sprinkling systems are used than when water is dripped slowly into the soil.

In 1995, the U.S. Geological Survey identified the region of the Lower Colorado River as an area where the consumptive use of water exceeded its renewable water supply, and the Rio Grande region as an area of some concern.[45] In 2006, the World Health Organization identified parts of the Central Plains and the Southwest as areas whose water supplies are over-exploited or heavily exploited.[46] In the Great Plains, agriculture has increasingly been subsidized by tapping the fossil groundwater of the deep Ogallala Aquifer that underlies the region. This confined aquifer is sandwiched between impermeable layers of rock and is no longer being replenished by precipitation. During the 19th century, westward-moving settlers of European origin gradually displaced the native inhabitants of the Great Plains, and in fact an entire ecosystem, converting grassland into farms. This massive disturbance of the Plains ecosystem, in combination with a cyclical drought, led to the dustbowl conditions of the 1930s. To a great extent, it was deep wells into the Ogallala Aquifer that later converted the native plains into a breadbasket. Unfortunately, this deep groundwater is not a renewable resource on the time scale of human planning. Thus, it seems clear that current irrigation practices are not sustainable over the long term in the United States. The problem of water scarcity in the future, of course, is much broader than water use for irrigation, and it is global in scale.

Mechanical Hazards to Workers

In addition to exposures to chemicals in crop production, farmers and farmworkers face mechanical hazards. In 2017 and 2018, there were roughly 250 fatal injuries each year in crop production in the United States.[47] The great majority of these fatalities were attributable to either transportation incidents or contact with objects or equipment.[47] The average annual rate of fatal occupational injuries in crop production during a five-year period from 2005–2010 was only slightly less than that for coal mining (35.9 per 100,000 full-time-equivalent (FTE) workers) for a period that included two mining disasters (at the Sago Mine in 2005 and the Upper Big Branch Mine in 2010).[48] In 2018, the fatality rate for crop production was 20.1, much higher than the mining rate of 15 16.1 per 100,000 FTE, and twice as high as that for construction workers (9.5 per 100,000 FTE).[47] The rate for nonfatal injuries associated with crop production in 2018 was 5.6 per 100 full-time workers, and fractures were the leading type of injury, unlike the majority of all other occupations where sprains, strains and tears are the leading injury category.[49] In epidemiologic studies, farmers commonly report being struck by objects or equipment, with injuries to fingers and feet, and they cite human error and haste as frequent causes of injury.[50]

5.3 Modern Livestock Production Practices

In the past, most farmers grew crops and also kept animals, and these two aspects of farming were integrated. Crop wastes were fed to cows or pigs, for example, and the animals' manure was used as fertilizer on crops. Today, especially on larger farms, the production of crops and the production of animals are essentially segregated processes. Fields are treated with synthetic chemicals, and animals grown for meat are fed a modified diet to speed their growth and shorten the period before they can be slaughtered. For the same reason, and also for the sake of efficiency in meat production, cattle, swine, and chickens spend much of their lives in confinement at specialized facilities, sometimes called factory farms.

In energy terms, eating meat is a luxury. Only a small part of the energy stored in a plant's tissues ends up stored in the tissues of an herbivore that eats the plant. Similarly, only a small part of the energy stored in the tissues of an herbivore ends up stored in the tissues of a carnivore that eats the herbivore. This is because animals, whether herbivore or carnivore, use most of the energy they take in to stay warm, move around, reproduce, and so forth. People, of course, can be either vegetarians (herbivores) or meat eaters (carnivores). For example, people can either eat the corn grown on 100 acres of land or eat the beef from the cows supported by the 100 acres of corn, but they will derive much more energy if they simply eat the corn.

In the face of this physical reality, modern livestock production has subsidized the growing of feed crops with fossil fuels and synthetic chemicals, has emphasized mechanization and economies of scale, and has introduced new feeding and veterinary practices for livestock. This section presents key elements of modern livestock production:

- Concentrated animal feeding operations where cattle, pigs, and poultry are brought to market weight
- The processes of slaughter and meat processing, including the rendering of animal carcasses
- Dairy farming, which is rapidly becoming more consolidated

Concentrated Animal Feeding Operations

Some people in the United States (and many more worldwide) are vegetarians, either by economic necessity or by cultural or personal preference. In nature, however, human beings are omnivorous, eating both plants and animals, and animal husbandry is an integral part of traditional agriculture. In this tradition, there is a sort of contract between farmer and animal: In return for his food supply, the farmer cares for his animals so that they thrive; and the farmer's own productivity is tied to the welfare of his animals.[51]

In contrast, modern industrial agriculture in the United States is not driven by the farmer's need to survive but by the corporate objective to produce food more cheaply in order to increase profits. And on the scale of industrial agriculture, productivity no longer seems to include the welfare of individual animals. For example, "crowding hens results in less egg laying per hen, but also in high productivity for the whole operation, since hens are cheap and cages are expensive."[51] What has been lost in industrial agriculture is the element of *husbandry*: caring for animals in a way that allows them not just to survive but to thrive in a natural way, even if they will ultimately be killed and eaten.

In the United States today, most animals raised for their meat are brought to market weight in **concentrated animal feeding operations**, or **CAFOs** ("kay-foes"), after weaning. Beef cattle in CAFOs are administered steroid hormones to increase their growth rate and produce meat with less fat and more lean mass.[52] The hormones are released slowly from pellets implanted under the skin of the ear; the concentrations of the hormones in meat remain within the normal range of untreated animals.[53] Animals are transported from CAFOs to slaughtering and meatpacking facilities, from which meat enters the marketplace and carcasses become a waste stream, undergoing a process called rendering.

A Profile of CAFOs in the United States

In the United States in 2010, some 34.4 million cattle, 110 million hogs, and 8.6 billion chickens were slaughtered for meat.[54, 55] Most of these animals were raised in confinement: cattle in outdoor pens and hogs and chickens in enclosed housing. By the end of 2017, there were almost 20,000 CAFOs in the United States with an addition of 1,400 new large-scale operations since 2010.[56]

Poultry CAFOs are the most common type of CAFOs operated in the United States. Chickens raised for their eggs (layers) are produced separately from chicken raised to be eaten. Iowa is the leading egg-producing state in the United States with the greatest number of egg-laying operations estimated to contain almost 72.5 million hens.[57] Indiana and Ohio are ranked second and third in egg production. The great majority of commercially produced chickens are **broilers**—that is, chickens under 13 weeks old, for meat. The

production of broilers increased 21-fold in the United States between 1950 and 1999,[58] transforming chicken from something of a luxury into a relatively inexpensive and accessible food. As of 2010, the leading broiler-producing states, which together account for nearly 40% of production, were concentrated in the south (see **Table 5.1**).

In 2019, North Carolina and Mississippi joined Georgia, Alabama and Arkansas as the top five broiler producing states, with 9.2 billion broiler chickens.[57]

About two-thirds of U.S. beef cattle are to be found in large CAFOs (those confining 16,000 or more animals), and nearly half are in operations of 32,000 or more. In 2008, more than half of the animals were concentrated in two states, with 36% of operations in the largest category found in Texas, and 22% in Kansas.[54] As of 2018, Texas still produces the largest amount of beef, but has decreased its number of CAFOs by 59, or the equivalent of 400,000 head of cattle.[56] Kansas is still the second largest producer of beef and has increased its production by almost 10% during the last decade.[56]

Overall, swine CAFOs have fewer animals than cattle feedlots, but the profile of the industry is similar. More than three-quarters of hogs are in facilities of at least 5,000 animals, and more than half are in the largest operations. Iowa produces the greatest number of hogs and has actually

Table 5.1 **Broiler Production in Leading U.S. States, 2010**

State	Number	Percentage
Georgia	1,313,500	15%
Arkansas	1,043,500	12%
Alabama	1,033,400	12%
U.S. Total	8,625,200	100%

Data from U.S. Department of Agriculture. National Agricultural Statistics Service, Poultry—Production and Value; 2010 Summary. Statistical Bulletin Pou 3–1(11), April 2011.

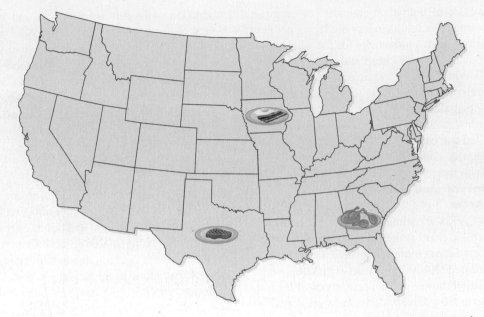

Figure 5.6 States in the U.S. with the largest CAFO production of beef, chicken, eggs or pork.

Data from U.S. Department of Agriculture. National Agricultural Statistics Service. Cattle: Final Estimates 1999–2003. 2004. Available at: http://usda.mannlib.cornell.edu/usda/reports/general/sb/sb989.pdf; U.S. Department of Agriculture, National Agricultural Statistics Service. Livestock Operations: Final Estimates 1998–2002. 2004. Available at: http://usda.mannlib.cornell.edu/usda/reports/general/sb/sb1002.pdf; U.S. Department of Agriculture, National Agricultural Statistics Service. Poultry Production and Value: Final Estimates 1998–2002. 2004. Available at: http://usda.mannlib.cornell.edu/usda/reports/general/sb/sb994.pdf. All accessed April 19, 2008.

increased the overall number of its CAFOs by 2000 farms during the past decade, making Iowa the state currently with the greatest growth rate in CAFOs.[56] Although some of the growth in these industrial livestock farms in Iowa was for poultry production, it is estimated that there are almost 23 million hogs in Iowa today. North Carolina has the second largest number of swine CAFOs with a population of roughly 9 million hogs. **Figure 5.6** shows the state in the U.S. with the largest CAFO production of beef, chicken, eggs or pork.

Conditions of Animal Confinement

The EPA has provided a description of conditions in concentrated animal feeding operations,[59] which are summarized here. Beef cattle are generally held in open feedlots (see **Figure 5.7**), which may be unpaved, paved in the areas where food and water are provided, or fully paved. Urine and manure accumulate and are removed periodically. Cattle in CAFOs are fed grain, although they are grazing animals whose natural diet is grass.

Swine are raised in enclosed housing (see **Figure 5.8**), usually with slotted floors so that urine and manure can drop into a collection area below. Beef cattle and swine produce manure equal to their own body weight about every 16 days. Wastes from feedlots are generally removed by scraping; swine houses are flushed with water to move wastes into the receptacle below the pens. In hog CAFOs like the one sketched in **Figure 5.8**, about 1,000 animals are held in pens in each of the long, narrow buildings, and their manure is collected in a man-made lagoon nearby.

The design of egg producing CAFOs are quite complex, involving systems to carefully carry eggs from the confined hens, typically in raised cages, to egg-washing stations and chillers. Broilers are also raised in enclosed housing, but usually with a solid floor and straw bedding, and they produce manure equal to their body weight about every 12.5 days. In many poultry houses, the top few inches of litter is removed five or six times a year when a new flock is brought in, and the building is fully cleaned just once a year.

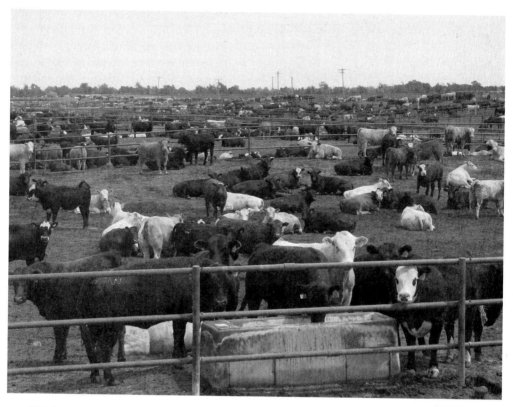

Figure 5.7 Cows study the photographer from the fringes of a mass of cattle in this CAFO.
Courtesy of Cathryn Dowd

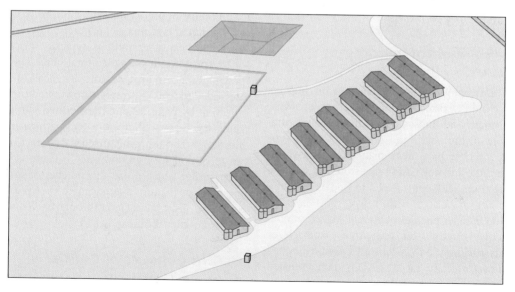

Figure 5.8 This sketch shows a typical layout for a hog CAFO, with a series of barns and an associated manure lagoon. A large operation might consist of several such units.

In all concentrated animal feeding operations, feed is ground and pelletized to increase its digestibility, and is provided in troughs or by mechanical feeding devices. Pesticides may be applied both to the buildings and directly to the animals.

Animal wastes release two toxic gases: ammonia, created as nitrogen in urine moves into the air; and hydrogen sulfide, produced as manure is broken down by bacteria in the absence of oxygen. Concentrations of particulate matter are high.[60] Mechanical ventilation systems run constantly in swine and poultry houses to reduce the risks to both workers and animals from inhaling toxic gases and dusts, but the fans cannot dispel the odors or eliminate respiratory effects.

Most beef cattle in the United States are slaughtered at age 15–18 months[61] and may change hands several times during this period. During 2010, just over 4% of cattle and calves died before slaughter; the single most common cause of death was respiratory problems.[62] Most hogs in the United States are slaughtered at about 6 months of age, and until recently were brought to slaughter weight in one location, though increasingly growers specialize in one phase of the pig's short life.[63] In 2000, the mortality rate among postnursery swine was 3%, and, as among calves, the single most common cause of death was respiratory problems.[64]

Environmental Impacts of CAFOs

The environmental and human health impacts of the industrialized rearing of beef cattle, swine, and poultry fall most heavily on poor and rural regions in the South and Midwest. CAFOs produce airborne particulate matter. Animal wastes from cattle and hog CAFOs are stored in lagoons, sprayed on fields, or released to bodies of water. Flooding associated with heavy rains contributes to broader releases of animal wastes. Several nationwide recalls on ready-to-eat spinach or salads packages have occurred because flooded wastewater from cattle CAFOs contaminated crops downstream with pathogenic bacteria, such as the potentially fatal bacterial strain *E. coli* O157:H7 that resides in in the guts of cattle.

Wastes placed on land contribute heavy nitrogen loads to soil, where bacteria convert nitrogen to nitrates. In this way, like fertilizers used on crops, animal wastes contribute highly soluble nitrates to local groundwater, with the potential to cause methemoglobinemia in infants.[65] CAFO wastes also contribute to global climate change (see Section 5.5).

When CAFO wastes are released in large quantities to surface waters, they cause a different problem: a dramatic reduction in the dissolved oxygen in the water. This decline occurs through two natural processes. First, organic wastes like manure are decomposed by bacteria in the water, a process that consumes oxygen, and when large amounts of organic waste reach a river or lake, the level of dissolved oxygen in the water can fall dramatically as the decomposers do their work. Second, the overload of the nutrients phosphorus and nitrogen to the aquatic system supports an overgrowth of algae (called **eutrophication**); and as the algae die off and are decomposed by bacteria, more dissolved oxygen is consumed. Through these processes, heavy inputs of waste may cause the receiving water to become anaerobic or nearly so, resulting in wholesale die-offs of fish and other aquatic organisms that depend on oxygen dissolved in water.

Poultry house waste, euphemistically called *chicken litter*, is a mix of manure, straw, spilled food, and carcasses, and is typically disposed of by spreading it on agricultural land. There is growing concern that organic arsenicals, which are added to feed to promote growth and prevent infection by parasites, are transformed into inorganic arsenic in soil, in waste, and perhaps in the chicken.[66] The inorganic arsenic can leach from waste or soil into groundwater.[66] There is now even greater concern that this practice of spreading chicken manure may promote the spread of antibiotic resistant bacteria through the environment and impact human health.[67]

Health Impacts of CAFOs

Routine Administration of Antibiotics to Food Animals. Antibiotics are given to livestock in CAFOs to prevent disease and promote growth, making it possible to bring animals to market weight more quickly on less feed. Antibiotics used for this purpose are administered to poultry, beef cattle, and swine at low doses through much of the animals' lifetime. An antibiotic is even injected into the eggs that will hatch into broilers.[68]

The routine use of an antibiotic shapes populations of bacteria, over time increasing the share of the population that is resistant to the drug. A number of the same antibiotics are used to treat illness in people, to treat illness in farm animals and pets, and to promote growth in food animals (see **Figure 5.9**). In the United States, annual antibiotic use in animals destined to become human food was estimated at 15 to 17 million pounds in 2002 and 29 million pounds in 2009.[69, 70] In 2015, 80% of all antibiotics produced were used for agricultural purposes.[71]

Antibiotic resistance among bacterial populations in livestock has a direct effect on human health. The practice of using manure to fertilize fields has resulted in demonstrated soil contamination with antibiotic resistant germs (ABGs) variants of both tetracycline and sulfonamide at significantly greater concentrations compared to control soil samples, placing vegetables grown in these soils at risk of contamination.[67] Runoff from these fields also introduces ABGs to local surface and groundwater supplies. During the process of slaughtering, it is not uncommon for the flesh of an animal to be contaminated by fecal matter from its intestine, in which certain bacteria are naturally present. For example, *Campylobacter* and *Salmonella* bacteria are often present on poultry products when they are purchased. If these organisms are resistant to certain antibiotics, then the antibiotics are ineffective in treating human illness resulting from eating contaminated poultry products.

However, the ineffectiveness of antibiotics in treating foodborne illness is merely the tip of the iceberg. Whether in an animal's gut or in the broader environment, bacteria routinely swap genes, including genes for antibiotic resistance. Resistant organisms that enter the environment in CAFO wastes, slaughterhouse wastes, or human sewage circulate through many ecological niches,

trading in what has been called a "global web of bacterial genetics."[72] As a result, antibiotic resistance, including multidrug resistance, poses a very broad public health challenge, and the overuse of antibiotics in livestock rearing is a key part of this problem.

CAFO Workers and Neighbors. In 2018, the fatality rate among animal production workers was 18.6 per 100,000 FTE workers, nearly eight times the rate among manufacturing workers (average 2.2 per 100,000 FTE).[47] Both neighbors and workers are regularly exposed to ammonia emanating from CAFOs; ammonia is a respiratory irritant, as is the organic dust from CAFOs, which may contain a wide range of irritants and allergens, including fecal matter, antigenic urinary proteins, animal dander, pollens, antibiotics, and pesticides.[65] Asthmatics may be particularly vulnerable to the respiratory effects of CAFO dust.[73] Workers also face the risk of death by respiratory arrest from exposure to high concentrations of hydrogen sulfide—for example, when pumping manure out of storage lagoons.[21] Concentrations of hydrogen sulfide, ammonia, carbon dioxide, and methane may rise to dangerous levels in manure pits at CAFOs, sometimes displacing oxygen.[74] Even family members may be at risk: Manure pits have repeatedly claimed multiple lives when family members jump into a pit in a vain attempt to rescue a relative.[74, 75]

The putrid odors associated with CAFOs—manure, dead fish, ammonia, the rotten-egg smell of hydrogen sulfide—are very disturbing to those who live nearby, often profoundly affecting their quality of life. At least one study suggests that residential exposure to odors from a hog CAFO is associated with increased feelings of stress, depression, fatigue, and confusion.[76]

In North Carolina, where hogs now outnumber people, poor, non-White communities bear a disproportionate burden of CAFOs and their impacts.[77] Although the state has a long history of hog farming, recent decades have seen a shift from family-owned hog farms to a new way of doing business, in which a large corporation owns the animals and provides feed and transport, and

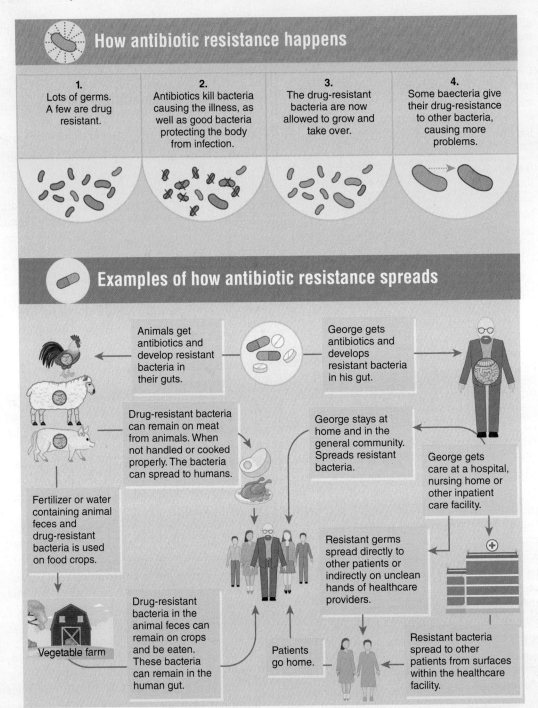

Figure 5.9 Spread of Antibiotic resistance from Livestock Production.

Centers for Disease Control and Prevention. What can I do to reduce the chance of infection with resistant bacteria from foods? Available at: https://www.cdc.gov/narms/faq.html

the local farm operator owns the land, the buildings, and the wastes.[77]

Slaughter and Meat Processing

Slaughter and meat processing are the conjoined industries that together convert animals on the hoof into meat on the table. These processes are largely invisible in many parts of the United States, but they are well known for their difficult and hazardous working conditions. In fact, the dangers faced by slaughterhouse workers were first brought to light in the early 20th century in Upton Sinclair's famous novel *The Jungle*, about Chicago's meatpacking industry. Much has changed since that time, but even today, meatpacking and poultry processing are hazardous trades.

Processing of larger animals such as cattle and swine begins with the animals being herded single file through a chute, stunned with a bolt to the brain, hung by the hind legs, and bled.[78] The carcasses then move down a production line at a set pace; they are cut open, eviscerated, cleaned, split in half, and then placed in walk-in coolers overnight. Each task on the production line is allotted about five seconds per carcass. Workers stand on elevated grated platforms (the floor is slippery) and wear protective gear. The line is noisy, and temperatures range from about 75°F to 100°F, depending on the season. Later, the refrigerated carcass is cut up in a cold room, with temperatures hovering around 40°F; these workers use power saws, power knives, and manual knives to produce chops, roasts, and so forth.[78]

Because they are much smaller animals, chickens are electrically stunned, bled, scalded to facilitate defeathering, eviscerated, cut into parts, deboned, and packed in a continuous process before being refrigerated. The division of labor in poultry processing is extreme—the Occupational Safety and Health Administration (OSHA) defines 13 steps in evisceration, nine in cutting, and 6 in deboning[79]—and the production line moves rapidly.[80]

Workers who process meat or poultry face an array of occupational hazards, with injury and illness rates higher than those for private industry overall. Acute injuries, including lacerations from knives, are common in slaughterhouses; slips, falls, strains, and sprains also occur frequently.[78] Further, meat and poultry workers suffer repetitive strain injuries, including carpal tunnel syndrome, from doing the same task over and over.[81] The incidence of respiratory illness is about twice that for private industry as a whole; incidence of hearing loss among slaughterhouse workers is almost 30 times that for private industry as a whole; among poultry-processing workers, almost 10 times.[49]

In addition, workers are potentially exposed to zoonotic diseases through contact with infected animals. Preventive measures vary; for example, prevention of brucellosis (a flu-like disease that can lead to severe infections or cause chronic symptoms) has focused on eliminating the disease in U.S. animals, whereas risks of *Salmonella* and *Campylobacter* are managed through measures to prevent workers from contacting fecal matter.[81] Respiratory irritation is common because pathogens, animal dander, or bits of feathers are likely to be present in the air of the workplace.[81] There is some evidence of elevated risk of lung cancer, oral cancer, and stomach cancer among meatpackers and butchers, but it is not known what specific exposures might be responsible.[82–84]

Finally, the origin of some foodborne illness in the general public is found in the processes of slaughter and meat processing. Given the rapid pace of production lines, meat or chicken products can easily be contaminated with an animal's fecal matter. Contamination by *Salmonella* and *Campylobacter*, two very common but rarely fatal illnesses, originates in this way. Undercooked hamburgers are the most common vehicle for exposure to the deadly bacterial strain *E. coli* O157:H7, and as few as 10 organisms can cause illness. Two features of the production of ground beef make it more susceptible to contamination than solid cuts of beef, such as steaks. First, in a major meatpacking plant, many cows contribute to a single well-mixed batch of ground beef, increasing the chance of contamination. And second, grinding the meat both aerates it and increases the surface area available for bacterial growth.

Rendering of Animal Carcasses

In industrialized livestock operations, the disposal of carcasses after the meat has been removed at slaughter is an enormous logistical challenge. In the United States at present, for example, some 34 million cattle are slaughtered commercially each year,[85] leaving the same number of carcasses to be disposed of. These animal carcasses are reprocessed into animal feed and other products through a process called rendering, as shown in **Figure 5.10**. Dead animals from feedlots, veterinary practices, shelters, and zoos also enter the rendering stream.

Rendering is essentially the heating of animal remains in a large vat. Fat is separated and removed; this rendered fat is **tallow**, used as an ingredient in various products, including candles, soap, and some cosmetics. The remaining slurry is dried and then ground, producing what is called **meat and bone meal**. This meal is fed to farm animals as a high-protein dietary supplement, shortening the time needed to bring the animals to market. It is also an ingredient in many pet foods.

The rendering cycle has been used, with variations, since the early 20th century, when growing quantities of slaughterhouse wastes became a problem. In the 1960s and 1970s, as cattle were increasingly moved from grass pastures to feedlots, meat and bone meal began to be widely used in feed. Within the livestock industry, rendering has long been seen as a form of recycling—a process that turns a waste product into something useful.

But everything changed in the 1980s and 1990s, when a novel and frightening disease of cattle morphed into a novel and frightening disease of humans—both ultimately shown to be caused by prions distributed through the rendering cycle. In the United Kingdom, where these diseases emerged, about 4 million cattle were slaughtered, most of them as a precautionary measure,[86] and 176 people have died to date from the newly identified human illness. As of early 2012, no probable or definite cases of variant Creutzfeldt-Jakob disease in the United Kingdom were still living. A total of four cases of bovine spongiform encephalopathy (BSE) have been documented in the United States.

Prion Diseases

As described previously in the context of infectious disease, abnormal prion proteins cause a set of degenerative brain diseases known as transmissible spongiform encephalopathies, which

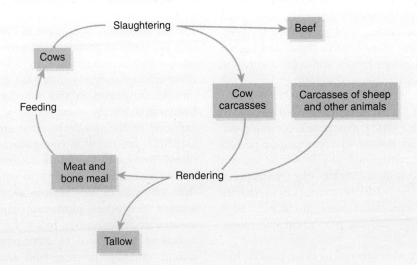

Figure 5.10 The rendering cycle.

are uniformly fatal. The prions form plaques in the brain, creating gaps that produce the sponge-like texture visible at autopsy—the hallmark of these illnesses. One such disease is **Creutzfeldt-Jakob disease (CJD)**, a rare human illness that has been known since the 1920s. It typically occurs in older people, causing neurological symptoms: dementia, loss of speech and coordination, and ultimately death. Cases of CJD occur sporadically, and no environmental risk factors are known for the disease, although iatrogenic transmission (i.e., transmission caused by medical treatment) can occur.*

Several transmissible spongiform encephalopathies affecting animals have also been known for some time, including **scrapie**, a familiar disease of sheep in the United Kingdom. Scrapie has never been known to pose a hazard to people who have contact with infected animals. Several prion diseases are known in other **ruminants** (a group of animals, including sheep and cattle, that have multichambered stomachs and that regurgitate and rechew food that they have previously swallowed). A chronic wasting disease that affects deer and elk, for example, is a prion disease.

The two prion diseases that emerged in the United Kingdom late in the 20th century were new to scientists. The disease that affected cattle was given the name **bovine spongiform encephalopathy (BSE)**, though it was commonly called **mad cow disease** in reference to the dementia suffered by the animals. Affected cows also experienced a loss of coordination, and many became downer cows—cows too ill to stand (see **Figure 5.11**). The human disease, like Creutzfeldt-Jakob disease, was a fatal degenerative neurological illness, but it affected mostly younger people and had a somewhat different

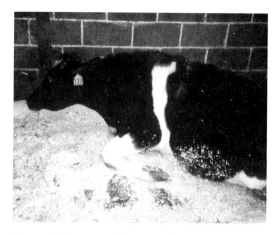

Figure 5.11 A cow afflicted with BSE struggles to stand up.

Courtesy of CDC public Health Image Library. ID# 5438. Content providers: CDC/Dr. Art Davis. Available at: http://phil.cdc.gov/phil/home.asp. Accessed October 29, 2012.

constellation of symptoms. The new illness was designated **variant Creutzfeldt-Jakob disease (vCJD)**. The first case of BSE appeared in 1986; the first case of vCJD was diagnosed in 1993. BSE cases were also reported in several other European countries in the 1990s.

In the United Kingdom, epidemiologic evidence indicated that eating beef was a risk factor for vCJD, suggesting that prions from diseased cattle were being transmitted to people. A U.K. government inquiry documented how neural matter from a cow's brain or spinal cord could in fact contaminate beef at the time of slaughter.[87] As in the United States, processing of beef in the United Kingdom was a fast-moving, partially mechanized process. The U.K. investigation documented that the carcass was split in half lengthwise using saws or cleavers, and the spinal cord was scraped out with a tool or sometimes by hand.[87] The head was removed for separate processing, and some low-quality meat was obtained from the head. All these processes created opportunities for prions to contaminate meat products intended for human consumption.

In sum, a complete transmission cycle was documented, made possible by prions' capacity to survive heat, freezing, and drying. Prions

---

*For example, CJD can be transmitted through transplants of dura mater (the membrane that sheathes the spinal cord), taken from cadavers. It is estimated that 267 cases of iatrogenic CJD may have occurred worldwide in the year 2000 (S-Juan, P., Ward, H., De Silva, R., Knight, R. & Will, R. Ophthalmic surgery and Creutzfeldt-Jakob disease. *British Journal of Ophthalmology,* 2004;88:446-449).

present in cattle carcasses survived the process of rendering, causing illness in cows that ate meat and bone meal; and prions present on beef survived the processes of food preparation, causing illness in people. The question remains: How did the first cow get BSE? The answer to this question is not known, but there are two likely possibilities. One is that a sporadic case of BSE occurred in a cow, much as sporadic CJD occurs in humans, and that this cow's remains were rendered, beginning the cycle of amplification. The other possibility is that prions from a sheep with scrapie, which were present in meat and bone meal, crossed the species boundary, becoming able to infect cattle.

In either case, the factor that transformed this rare event into an epidemic among cattle was the amplification of exposure through the rendering cycle, in which the remains of many animals are mixed together and then fed to many more animals, whose carcasses also ultimately enter the rendering cycle. In contrast, if a cow on a farm in 1930 had spontaneously developed BSE, the consequences would have been limited to the circle of people who ate parts of this animal. Thus, it seems fair to say that the epidemics of BSE and vCJD resulted from breaking another "biological taboo" by turning cows into carnivores (and, in effect, cannibals).

In fact, the only other setting in which a prion disease is known to have been transmitted and amplified in this way was in a remote tribal group in New Guinea, where transmission occurred through the ritual eating of certain body parts (including the brain) of deceased family members.[88] The disease, known locally as **kuru**, was a fatal degenerative neurological condition. By the late 1960s, it had been demonstrated that kuru was transmitted by the eating of body parts,[88] and the practice came to an end. But the infectious agent remained a mystery for more than a decade as scientists painstakingly documented the existence of infectious proteins, which came to be called prions. The kuru epidemic is believed to have begun with a case of sporadic CJD in the population.[89]

U.S. Safeguards Against BSE

To prevent an epidemic of BSE and variant Creutzfeldt-Jakob disease in the United States, there initially was a ban in 1989 ban on importing animals or animal products from any country affected by BSE. In 1997, a **ruminant feed ban** was imposed—that is, a ban on *feeding ruminant protein* (meat and bone meal from rendered ruminant mammals) to ruminants. This restriction was expanded a few years later into a full **mammalian feed ban**, banning the *feeding of any mammalian protein* to ruminants (because nonruminant mammals, such as swine and horses, might have been fed rendered ruminant protein). Nonmammalian protein (e.g., from rendered poultry) can still be fed to ruminants because birds are not believed to be susceptible to prion diseases. Regulations also address the considerable practical challenges of preventing cross-contamination between segregated rendering processes. In addition to establishing controls on rendering, BSE surveillance program was established and plans developed to respond to any U.S. outbreak. Fortunately, to date, only four cases of BSE have been diagnosed in U.S. cows, the last in 2012.

Dairy Farming

Like the production of food crops and meat, the production of dairy goods is being consolidated into larger operations in the United States. From 2001 to 2009, the proportion of U.S. dairy cows found in operations of more than 2,000 animals more than doubled, as did the share of dairy production represented by these large operations (to almost one-third). These large operations are less likely than small ones to be family-owned or to be integrated into a broader farming operation, and thus they are more likely to purchase feed and young cows rather than grow their own feed and raise their own heifers.[90] Like CAFOs for beef cattle, large dairy operations produce large quantities of manure, with similar environmental and human health impacts.

The overall number of licensed dairy operations has been declining since 2003 when there were 70,375, with the largest annual decline occurring in 2019, with only 34,187 operations now in the U.S.[91] However, annual milk production in the U.S. has grown every year over the past decade, with 218.4 billion pounds of milk produced in 2019, California being the largest milk-producing state, followed by Wisconsin.[91] The ever-increasing productivity per cow over the past decade has actually hurt dairy farmers with large supplies outweighing demand, and only the larger dairy operations being able to compensate for lower demand and still make a profit. The reasons for lower milk prices are because there are fewer opportunities to export milk combined with a decrease in demand domestically.[91]

One reason for reduced demand for U.S. milk internationally was the introduction in the early 1990s of synthetic hormones used in dairy cows to improve productivity. **Bovine growth hormone** (also called **bovine somatotropin**) is a natural hormone in cows that, among other things, regulates milk production. A genetically engineered version of this hormone, **recombinant bovine growth hormone (rBGH)**, has been developed by Monsanto Corporation under the name Posilac. Regular injection of slow-release rBGH to dairy cows (every 2 to 4 weeks) increases their milk production substantially and makes them convert feed to milk more efficiently.[92] The economics of using rBGH favor larger dairy operations. Farmers not using rBGH most often cited its cost and their animals' health, but some cited personal beliefs or the wish to maintain their organic status. There has been some concern that rBGH may increase the frequency of udder infections and may cause stress in cows. Although potential human health concerns have been raised related to possible antibiotic residues in milk from treatment of udder infections, no human health effects have been documented.

rBGH was approved in 1994 for use in the United States, though it has been banned in the European Union and in Canada. Several large grocery store chains in the United States have also refused to sell milk produced using rBGH. The reasons for these bans relate to consumer concerns about growth hormone in milk causing premature reproductive development in children and obesity.[93] Recent research also suggests a link between the presence of steroid hormones in dairy products as a risk factor for various cancers.[93]

5.4 Modern Fishing

Fish and seafood provide an alternative source of protein to land-based livestock meat and modern fishing has changed dramatically, too. In recent decades, human capacity to catch marine fish has increased dramatically as a result of mechanized methods to take fish from the water, as well as the use of high-tech means, such as sonar, to locate fish. Large nets dragged across the sea floor—a sort of mechanized underwater harvest—disrupt or even destroy ecosystems. A substantial share of the catch is now processed on factory ships at sea. Like farming, fishing is powered by fossil fuels (about 500 liters of diesel fuel are expended for every metric ton of deep-sea fish caught[94]) and is a high-risk occupation.

Occupational Hazards of Fishing

Fishing is one of the most dangerous of occupations for U.S. workers, second only to logging in terms of fatal accidents by occupation during 2018.[47] For the period 2006–2010, the average annual fatality rate among U.S. fishermen averaged 149 per 100,000 FTE workers, a rate four times that for coal miners and 62 times that for manufacturing workers.[48] An analysis of deaths in the Alaskan commercial fishing fleet over an earlier 8-year period (1991–1998), during which a total of 167 fishermen of the Alaskan fleet died on the job, gives a more detailed picture.*,[95] Nearly all those who died were males, ranging in age from 10 to 67 years. Of the fatalities, 107 were caused

---

*Even more than for farming, national data on deaths and injuries among fishermen are incomplete because many fishermen are self-employed and the number of workers on individual vessels is small. For this reason, regional research data are presented here.

by the sinking or capsizing of a vessel; of the 60 deaths not caused by the loss of the vessel, 42 were nevertheless caused by drowning or hypothermia, mostly because a man went overboard. More than half of these fishermen were washed overboard by a wave or dragged overboard after becoming entangled in equipment; more than 20% of man-overboard events were unobserved. Other than being washed overboard, the most frequent cause of death among Alaskan fishermen was crushing by machinery or equipment. More recent data on the U.S. East Coast commercial fishing fleet over a 9-year period (2000–2009) show a similar pattern: Of 165 total fatalities, 98 (59%) were attributed to the capsizing of a vessel, and 36 (22%) occurred because a man was washed overboard.[96]

Declining Wild Stocks and Growth of Fish Farms

For a given fishery (the population of a species of fish in a particular location), the volume caught follows a typical time course, increasing to a peak level of production and then falling off. Marine scientists define a fishery as *fully exploited* during the period around its peak production, when yearly production is more than 50% of the peak year's production. This fully exploited period is bracketed by periods defined as *developing* and *overfished* (during which production is at 10% to 50% of peak production); and these periods in turn are bracketed by periods labeled *undeveloped* and *collapsed* or *closed* (during which production is at less than 10% of the peak).[97]

In 1950, more than 90% of the world's fisheries were classified as either undeveloped or developing. By 2000, fewer than 10% were classified as undeveloped or developing, and nearly 20% had collapsed.[97] To date, the challenges of protecting this resource—from gaining the compliance of fishing crews to ceding some national authority to international commissions—have largely stymied efforts to do so.[98]

In the context of declining stocks of wild fish, along with the current recommendation to eat fish as a healthy alternative to red meat, **aquaculture**, the farming of fish, has become widespread and now accounts for 40% of the world's fish food.[99] Although the term is not generally used in this context, fish farms are essentially concentrated animal feeding operations. Some use simple mesh enclosures placed in natural waters; others are similar in concept, but much larger and more durable, with large mesh tanks arrayed on a floating metal platform, not unlike an oil rig. Still others are buildings on land that house fish in large, fully enclosed tanks.

The most commonly farmed species is salmon; the global production of farmed salmon has increased more than 40-fold over the past 2 decades.[100] Farmed fish are fed an intensive diet consisting mainly of fish meal and oils derived from small ocean fish. Although the public perception is that farmed fish is cleaner,[99] research has shown that concentrations of PCBs and dioxins, as well as DDT and other organochlorine pesticides, are higher (sometimes up to 10 times higher) in farmed salmon than in wild-caught salmon.[100] Aquaculture is also not as environmentally friendly as the public perceives, contributing to the eutrophication of natural waterways as well as to the spread of antibiotic resistance into the ecosystem from farm wastewater discharges.[99] Aquaculture also further contributes to the decline in wild stocks of fish since a large quantity of wild-caught fish is used as feeds for aquaculture.[99]

5.5 Impacts of Modern Agriculture on Global Resources

Modern agricultural practices have managed so far to keep pace with supplying adequate calories to the world's growing human population.[101] However, in doing so, agriculture has also become the planet's dominant environmental threat, consuming a large portion of the earth's land surface and destroying habitats, using up freshwater, polluting oceans and emitting greenhouse gases.[102] Agriculture already uses about 40% of the earth's land surface, not including Greenland or Antarctica, covering much of the *best* land.

Furthermore, agricultural practices since the last ice age have disrupted ecosystems dramatically, transforming 70% of grasslands, half of the savannas, and more than a quarter of tropical forests. Currently, agriculture's footprint on the earth's surface is 60 times that of urban pavements and buildings.[102]

Agricultural irrigation uses 70% of freshwater withdrawals, and much of is consumptive meaning that the water is not returned to the world's water supply cycle, compared with other major water consumers, such as thermoelectric power generation. Not only does agriculture use up freshwater, it also pollutes both fresh and marine water supplies. Fertilizer runoff and CAFO wastes both contribute to eutrophication that results in enormous hypoxic *dead zones* at the mouths of several of the world's major rivers,[102] including where the Mississippi meats the Gulf (refer to **Figure 5.12**).

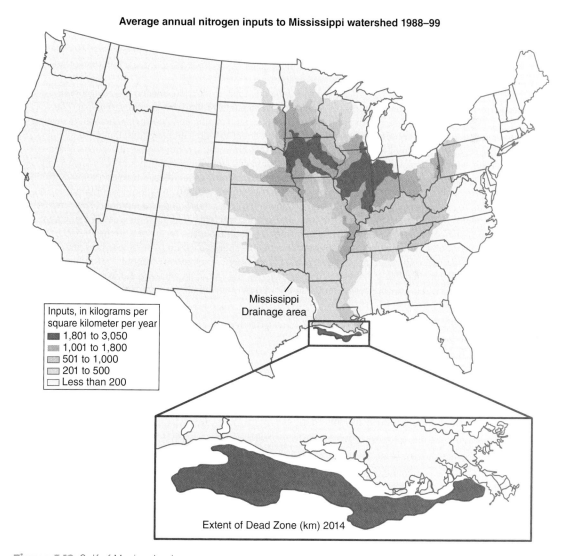

Average annual nitrogen inputs to Mississippi watershed 1988–99

Inputs, in kilograms per square kilometer per year
- 1,801 to 3,050
- 1,001 to 1,800
- 501 to 1,000
- 201 to 500
- Less than 200

Mississippi Drainage area

Extent of Dead Zone (km) 2014

Figure 5.12 Gulf of Mexico dead zone.

The Great Food Transformation

Modern agricultural practices are generating more food calories than ever before, yet almost one billion people on the planet are hungry and almost two billion are eating too much unhealthy food.[1] Globally, the prevalence of malnutrition, obesity and being overweight has increased and unhealthy diets currently pose a greater risk to human wellbeing than unsafe sex, and alcohol, drug and tobacco use combined.[2] The modern diet based on high intakes of red meat, processed sugar and saturated fats with too few vegetables and whole grains is estimated to account for up to 11 million avoidable, premature deaths globally each year.[1]

Modern agriculture is also not environmentally sustainable. To quote Lucas and Horton's editorial in *The Lancet*, "For the first time in 200,000 years of human history, we are severely out of synchronization with the planet and nature."[1] Our global food production system is one of the largest contributors to climate change, biodiversity loss associated with land-system transformations, and water pollution. Globally, scientists and researchers have joined forces to sound the alarm. After more than two years of collaboration, the EAT-Lancet Commission of almost forty experts in health, nutrition, environmental sustainability, food systems, and economic and political governance from 16 countries published their recommendations for how to fix our broken food system.

Recognizing that dietary demand is inextricably linked to food production, solving the environmental problems associated with agriculture will require a great transformation in how many of us eat. The EAT-Lancet Commission diet strives to be a win-win diet (i.e., sustainable and healthy), adaptable to diverse regional food cultures and production systems, with the potential to feed a global population of 10 billion people.[2] The recommended diet will be a big change for most Americans, requiring large portions of vegetables, fruits, whole grains, legumes, nuts, and unsaturated oils, with moderate amounts of seafood and poultry, and no to very low portions of red or processed meats, starchy vegetables, sugar, and refined grains.

To achieve such a transformation, the Commission recognizes that international and national commitments to an unprecedented global collaboration will be necessary and challenging.[2] Their report describes specific mitigation strategies for addressing factors, such as yield gaps between regions and countries and the need to redistribute the use of nitrogen and phosphorus fertilizers. In the United States, perhaps the best motivation to support such dramatic dietary changes would be to stress how personal health can be improved with reduction in obesity, also highlighting the economic benefits of reducing costly medical care for modifiable diseases such as diabetes. By changing what we eat, we can achieve a win-win situation not only for ourselves, but also our planet upon which our future generations will depend.

1. Lucas T, Horton R. The 21st-century great food transformation. *Lancet*. 2019. Comment Section. http://dx.doi.org/10.1016/50140-6736(18)33179-9
2. Willett W, Rockstrom J, Loken B. et al. Food in the Anthropocene: the EAT-Lancet Commission on healthy diets from sustainable food systems. *Lancet*, 2019;393:447-92.

Agriculture also makes a substantial contribution to global climate change. Both nitrous oxide and methane are greenhouse gases. Nitrous oxide is estimated to account for about 5%, and methane about 16%, of the Earth's net gain in radiation energy from the five major anthropogenic greenhouse gases. In fact, both nitrous oxide and methane are more potent greenhouse gases, molecule for molecule, than the gas with the greatest overall impact, carbon dioxide. As explained earlier, both wastes from CAFOs and the intensive use of fertilizers on crops contribute to contamination of groundwater with nitrates. Bacteria in soil convert nitrates to either nitrogen gas (N_2) or nitrous oxide (N_2O), which are released into the atmosphere. In 2009, nitrate fertilizers accounted for more than two-thirds (69%) of U.S. nitrous oxide emissions.[103]

Methane (CH_4) is produced by agricultural activities in which organic matter is digested or decomposes under anaerobic conditions. For example, a single cow releases 250 to 500 liters of methane per day, mainly by belching.[104] If manure from CAFOs is allowed to accumulate in lagoons, it produces methane as it decomposes. And the cultivation of rice in paddies also releases methane as crop residues decompose under flooded conditions. Belching by livestock, manure disposal, and rice cultivation together are estimated to account for almost one-third (28%) of U.S. emissions of methane.

Agriculture's reliance on fossil fuel also contributes significantly to the global climate change. In addition to the enormous amount of fuel consumed for crop production, discussed previously, modern agriculture is a global affair with foods processed, packaged, and shipped while refrigerated from all far-flung corners of the planet. To quote the environmental writer, Barbara Kingsolver,[105] the "global grocery store is a stunning energy boondoggle, transporting five calories' worth of strawberry from California to New York using 435 calories of fossil fuel."

5.6 From Source to Table

Previous sections of this chapter describe methods used to cultivate crops, to raise and slaughter food animals, and to capture or farm fish. Although some of these activities produce items ready for the table, more often they produce inputs to a complex web of manufacturing processes. This section first touches on a few specific issues related to the quality of food as it is processed, and then takes up a broader issue: the capacity to trace foods backward through the systems of distribution and production.

Food Defects

Food products may become contaminated—on the farm or during storage or processing—by foreign substances such as insect fragments or rodent hairs. Although these things are unappetizing, at low levels they do not make people sick, and they are unavoidable at acceptable levels of pesticide use. The regulatory term for such contaminants is **food defects**, and acceptable levels of these

substances in food have been established. Foreign substances present in food at or below these levels are considered to present no health hazard to people. Food defects include insects (e.g., no more than 30 aphids and/or thrips per 100 grams of frozen Brussels sprouts), insect larvae (e.g., no more than 5% of maraschino cherries are rejects due to maggots), insect fragments (e.g., no more than 25 per 50 grams of cornmeal), rodent hairs, rodent filth, grit, rot, mold, glass fragments, and so on.[106]

Food Additives

In contrast to these accidental additions to food products, various substances are deliberately added to foods during processing to achieve specific purposes. Such **food additives** are used as preservatives (e.g., butylated hydroxyanisole [BHA]), sweeteners (e.g., aspartame), flavor enhancers (e.g., monosodium glutamate [MSG]), fat replacers (e.g., Olestra), nutrients (e.g., vitamin C), thickeners, leavening agents, anticaking agents, and so forth. The additives that can be used are regulated, as are the amounts that can be present in food.

Since 1958, the Food and Drug Administration must approve any new additive to be used in food, set limits on its use, and set labeling requirements. Two groups of substances are exempted: one set that the FDA had determined to be safe before the 1958 amendment, and another set that are *generally regarded as safe* (GRAS; "grass") by experts. This term has a regulatory meaning: Several hundred substances are on the GRAS list, which is subject to modification. Finally, the FDA cannot approve any additive that is found to cause cancer in either humans or animals—a restriction known as the Delaney Clause.[107] However, pesticides were removed from the scope of the Delaney Clause in 1996.

Rather than use a preservative, foods can be irradiated during processing to kill microbes and prevent foodborne illness. Irradiation of food, though not widely used in the United States, has been technically feasible for decades. Food is irradiated relatively late in the production process to minimize the opportunity for later microbial contamination—for example, a piece of beef might be irradiated after being wrapped for sale. Typically, cobalt-60 is used as a source of gamma radiation. Food is irradiated by passing it through a machine on a conveyor belt; the speed of the conveyor belt determines the dose. This technique kills by fragmenting DNA; it is effective against insects, parasites, and bacteria, but it is not effective against viruses, prions, bacterial spores, or toxins previously produced by bacteria.[108] Similar techniques are used to sterilize instruments and materials in medical settings.

Irradiation does *not* leave food radioactive. Rather, the immediate health concerns revolve mainly around the destruction of vitamins and micronutrients in food and the potential toxicity of chemicals created by irradiation (called **radiolytic chemicals**).[108, 109] Taking a broader view, irradiation substitutes a late process for preventive strategies farther upstream—for example, changes in feedlots to reduce the prevalence of *E. coli* in cattle; in addition, there is some concern over the use of nuclear technologies in a large number of local food-processing facilities.[110] Radiation is not unique in creating new chemicals in food; other types of food processing (e.g., broiling steak) also do so.

The symbol shown in **Figure 5.13** is known as the **radura** and signifies on a food label when that food has been irradiated. Under U.S. law, irradiated food must bear the radura symbol on its label, along with the words "treated with radiation" or "treated by irradiation."[111] In regulatory terms, irradiating food without complying with these requirements amounts to using an unapproved additive.

"Traceability" in the Modern Food Supply System

The modern food system is marked by complex, large-scale operations and the rapid distribution of foods. Taken together, these features make it challenging to trace food products backward through the system, but events have shown that this can be important. For example, tracing meat to its origins has been critical in containing outbreaks of illness from the virulent pathogen

Figure 5.13 The radura logo, indicating irradiated food.

Morehouse K. Food irradiation: The treatment of foods with ionizing radiation. Food Testing Anal. 1998;4(3): 9, 32, 35.

E. coli O157:H7. A small number of large companies now slaughter most U.S. cattle, and the slaughtering industry is also concentrated geographically. Facilities that produce half of U.S. meatpacking shipments by value (not including poultry) are in just four states—Nebraska, Kansas, Texas, and Iowa.[112] Ground beef from such facilities—some in the form of ready-made hamburger patties—is promptly shipped to locations around the country. For reasons detailed elsewhere, ground beef is particularly susceptible to contamination with *E. coli* O157:H7.

Fast-food restaurants further promote the rapid distribution of pathogens. In 1993, more than 200 people were made ill, and 4 died, from an *E. coli* O157:H7 outbreak traced to hamburgers served by the Jack in the Box fast-food chain.[113] Although recalls of meat can prevent some illness, their effectiveness is limited in the context of a rapid-distribution food system. For example, the source of an *E. coli* O157:H7 outbreak in Colorado in 1997 was traced to ground beef, sold as hamburger patties in grocery stores, from a large meatpacking plant in Nebraska. The company voluntarily recalled about 35 million pounds of ground beef, but 25 million pounds had already been eaten.[113]

Although corn is not transformed into grain products as rapidly as livestock is transformed into meat, it has proved extremely difficult to trace or recall grain from genetically modified crop plants. This became clear in 1998, when the EPA took the highly unusual step of restricting the use of a specific genetically engineered corn to animal feed. A *Bt* corn named StarLink was not to be used in foods for human consumption because proteins of this transgenic corn had been found to be similar to known human allergens.[43]

However, it soon became clear that corn bound for human consumption was not necessarily segregated from corn bound for animal consumption. And because corn is processed and transported en masse, some mixing is likely to occur in grain elevators or elsewhere. Testing of corn products from supermarket shelves documented the presence of StarLink corn in taco shells made by Taco Bell. Ultimately, StarLink corn was found in various other products, including non-genetically modified seed corn and corn shipped to Japan.[43] Unlike cattle, kernels of corn cannot be tagged and tracked, and it does not appear realistic to segregate genetically modified grains from other grains. The StarLink saga ultimately involved about 2500 farmers and 350 grain elevators, as well as 17 corporate entities that produced or sold seed or flour or taco shells.[43]

The globalization of the food supply also makes it difficult to trace the origins of food contamination back to its source. An increasing number of foodborne disease outbreaks have occurred during the past 40 years in the United States associated with imported fresh produce. For example, Mexican cantaloupes were responsible for nine *Salmonella* outbreaks where the contamination was traced back to unsanitary condition for the Mexican agricultural workers either during harvesting or packaging.[114] In addition to different standards regarding occupation hygiene, other countries often have different rules pertaining to the use of agricultural pesticides and other chemicals. Recent concerns with orange juice samples containing elevated levels of lead and the organophosphate Chlorpyrifos, a substance banned in the United States for fruit production, demonstrate the challenges of keeping track of all the global inputs into our morning breakfast.[115] Orange juice manufactured in the U.S. may combine oranges imported from several different countries, and federal food inspectors are tasked with monitoring millions of tons of imported food annually. In sum, the broad-scale industrial systems that make it possible to produce and distribute foods rapidly also make it difficult to manage certain hazards of the food supply.

5.7 Locally Grown Foods and Organic Farming

Since the 1950s, the U.S. food industry has succeeded in making varied and nutritional foods, including high-protein meat, poultry, and fish products, available to a much broader segment of the population. These achievements are attributable mainly to economies gained through large-scale, mechanized processes, along with the use of synthetic chemicals and other technical innovations and globalization.

Of course, these changes bring costs as well as benefits. As detailed earlier, various practices of modern agriculture may leave residues in foods, including low levels of pesticides, hormones, or antibiotics; and genetically modified foods can cause unexpected allergic reactions. Microbial contamination continues to be a risk associated with a global food supply chain and its fossil fuel consumption contributes greatly to greenhouse gas emissions. In addition to these concerns, some people are simply uncomfortable with the extent to which we have manipulated nature, or contaminated the environment, or treated animals as mere inputs to industrial processes. Others are disturbed by the homogenizing effect (not to mention the empty calories) of many fast foods and convenience foods. These concerns are evidenced in a renewed interest in locally grown foods bought at farmers' markets or grown in community gardens (see **Figure 5.14**).

In addition to trying to eat locally and *in season* with what is naturally available in the region, there is also strong interest in trying to eat foods grown more naturally, or *organically*. The organic

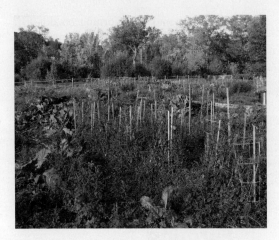

Figure 5.14 This urban community garden, seen here in early autumn, provided homegrown vegetables for city dwellers through the summer months.

Courtesy of Keith J. Maxwell

approach to farming is roughly the antithesis of the modern approach described in the introduction to this chapter, which characterizes most U.S. agriculture. **Organic farming** is, at a minimum, sustainable; its practices do not degrade the soil but rather maintain and even build it, because good soil is the foundation of successful agriculture.[116] A second defining characteristic of organic farming is that it rejects the use of synthetic pesticides and commercial fertilizers.[116]

Together, these principles yield the typical features of organic farming—for example, raising both crops and animals, feeding crops to animals, and using manure to fertilize crops. Similarly, organic farmers may grow two crops together or in rotation. For example, grains may be alternated with legumes such as peas or beans, whose roots have nodules containing nitrogen-fixing bacteria. These bacteria convert organic nitrogen compounds to nitrates, which are water-soluble nutrients easily taken up by plants. Organic farming shares some features with traditional farming—that is, farming in the era before gasoline-powered tractors and synthetic organic chemicals. Although organic farming does not have to be small in scale, it usually is.

It was only in 1990 that organically grown produce and meats gained official regulatory standing at the federal level, though various private and regional entities had offered organic certification for some time. Between 1992 and 2008, organic pasture acreage in the United States increased threefold and organic crop acreage more than five-fold.[117] Organic beef cattle and swine increased 6- to 8-fold, organic milk cows 100-fold, and broilers 500-fold. A few crops also stand out: Organic cropland planted in vegetables has increased 9-fold and land area in apple orchards 5-fold. Yet, the overall percentage of cropland that is organic remains very low at about 0.5%,[118] and although environmentally sustainable, organic farming does not produce nearly enough food, and the food produced tends to be more expensive.

5.8 Food Quality Regulations

Agencies and Laws Specific to Aspects of Food Quality

The regulation of food, agriculture, and fisheries in the United States is complex, involving numerous laws implemented by several agencies. It also has very deep roots. The federal Meat Inspection Act was passed in 1906 and later amended as the Wholesome Meat Act (1967); the Poultry Products Inspection Act was passed in 1957. The Pure Food and Drug Act was also passed in 1906; it has been amended several times and is known today as the Federal Food, Drug, and Cosmetic Act (FFDCA). Two other laws are central to food regulation: the Federal Insecticide, Fungicide, and Rodenticide Act (FIFRA; "fif-ra") of 1972, and the Food Quality Protection Act (FQPA) of 1996, which amended some sections of both FIFRA and the FFDCA.

Three federal agencies are most involved in the regulation of food and agriculture[119]:

- The Department of Agriculture regulates the safety and labeling of most meat and poultry.
- The Environmental Protection Agency is responsible for controlling the effects of pesticides on human health.

- The Food and Drug Administration is responsible for the safety, nutritional value, and labeling of most foods other than meat and poultry, and related to concerns other than pesticides.

Key elements of the U.S. regulatory framework for food and agriculture also appear in **Table A-1 (see appendix).**

Pesticides

Before a pesticide can be sold or distributed in the United States, it must be registered with (licensed by) the EPA. Pesticides are registered for a specific use or set of uses. Registration is intended to ensure that if the pesticide is used as instructed on its label, there is a "reasonable certainty of no harm to human health" (i.e., to workers or others at hand when it is applied) and the pesticide will not pose "unreasonable risks to the environment."[120] For pesticides used on crops consumed by people or by food animals, the EPA also sets a **pesticide tolerance**, which is the maximum pesticide residue level allowed in human food. Pesticide tolerances are to be set low enough to protect infants and children. Pesticide tolerances were originally set under authority of the Federal Food, Drug, and Cosmetic Act, but with the passage of the Food Quality Protection Act in 1996, an effort to reassess all pesticide tolerances over a 10-year period was begun, and was successfully completed in 2007.

Genetically Modified Food Plants

There is no single federal law governing genetically modified foods, or **biotechnology** more generally. (The term *biotechnology* is often used synonymously with **genetic engineering**, but also refers more broadly to applied biological science.) This fact reflects a 1986 policy judgment that biotechnology does not pose any unique risks and that its products can be regulated in the same way as conventional products, using laws that predate biotechnology.[121] As a result, at least three federal agencies are involved in the regulation of genetically modified food plants—the USDA, EPA, and FDA—and their responsibilities in this area are closely intertwined.[121, 122]

The USDA regulates plant pests, and therefore also evaluates whether genetically modified plants in the field could harm other plants; for example, a plant that incorporates a pesticide might harm insects that are beneficial to other plants. There are three regulatory routes to commercialization of a genetically modified crop plant[123]: permitting (obtaining a permit ahead of conducting a field test); notification (notifying the USDA 30 days before a field test begins); or petitioning for nonregulated status, which obviates the requirement for a field test. Petitioning for nonregulated status has been the most commonly used path to commercialization.[123]

The EPA registers pesticides and sets food tolerances for pesticides, and therefore does the same for pesticides produced by genetically engineered plants (e.g., *Bt* corn).

The FDA has responsibility for food safety and therefore has this same responsibility for foods derived from transgenic plants. The FDA recommends that developers of transgenic plants consult early with the agency and that they follow certain procedures to evaluate potential harm (e.g., the potential allergenicity of new proteins), but these steps are not required. The FDA also does not require that transgenic foods be labeled as such.

Humane Slaughter of Food Animals

In keeping with the 1978 Humane Methods of Slaughter Act, the USDA employs a veterinarian and slaughter line inspectors at each of the more than 900 federally inspected slaughterhouses.[124] Mandated methods for humane slaughter are incorporated into the Hazard Analysis and Critical Control Point systems (described later in this chapter) in use at these plants. The law does not cover chickens or other birds.

Inspection and Grading of Meat

In keeping with requirements of the Wholesome Meat Act, carcasses are inspected for wholesomeness in meat processing plants and approval is stamped on the carcass.[125] For the most part, consumers do not see this stamp because they see only individual cuts of meat in the grocery store.

However, customers typically do know the *grade* of the meat they buy in the grocery or eat in a restaurant. Most familiar to consumers is the Department of Agriculture's traditional grading of beef (e.g., USDA Prime and USDA Choice steaks). This voluntary grading is based on the marbling of the meat; that is, higher-grade beef has more fat streaks running through the meat, making it juicier and more flavorful.[125]

In general, beef from grain-fed cattle is fattier than beef from grass-fed cattle, and the two types of beef also taste somewhat different. The USDA recently established a voluntary certification process for labeling beef as grass-fed. To be labeled as grass-fed, beef must come from cows that were not fed grain, but rather ate only grass (or forage) and had ready access to pasture.[126]

Conservation and Management of Fisheries

The Magnuson-Stevens Fishery Conservation and Management Act, reauthorized most recently in 2006, includes provisions to address three critical issues: overfishing of the regional fisheries in ocean waters surrounding the United States; environmental degradation in these fisheries; and the incidental catching of fish other than the species being sought, often resulting in the death of these fish.[127] Regional fishery management councils are required to define what constitutes overfishing of a given fishery and to establish plans to rebuild fish stocks.

Organic Foods

The Organic Foods Production Act of 1990 set national standards for producing and handling of foods given the organic label. It also created the National Organic Standards Board, an advisory body that includes organic farmers and retailers, scientists, and environmental and consumer advocates. The law sets criteria that qualify crops and livestock as organically grown and certifies organic growers and handlers that conform to these criteria.[128] For example, organically raised cattle must have access to pasture and fresh air and be able to exercise. Their feed must be organically produced and cannot include products from rendering. Products from certified growers can carry the organic seal shown in **Figure 5.15**. Unlike the term *organic*, the term *natural* has no regulatory meaning under U.S. law.

Food Safety

Individuals can do much to prevent foodborne illness by using appropriate practices at home. In reality, microbial contamination of food is a fact of life. However, many hazards can be prevented or controlled by following some general practices for safe food handling. As the term *food safety* is typically used in environmental health, it focuses on procedures to prevent food-borne illness at the point where food is prepared by controlling the environment in which pathogens find themselves.

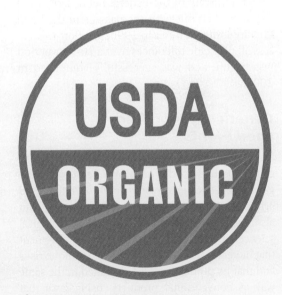

Figure 5.15 The USDA organic seal.
© cash1994/Shutterstock

If pathogenic bacteria are to survive and prosper in food, their basic needs must be met. Most human pathogens (which are adapted to live in the human body and also to survive a passage through the ambient environment) survive and multiply at temperatures from 40°F to 140°F—a temperature range known in food safety as the **danger zone**. Bacteria also require water and nutrients, and individual species have other requirements (such as an aerobic environment or an anaerobic environment) or tolerances (e.g., for a high-salt environment). In favorable conditions, the growth of a population of bacteria follows a typical pattern (see **Figure 5.16**). During the first 1 to 4 hours in a new environment, bacteria multiply only slowly. This early period is known as the **lag phase**. The lag phase is followed by a period of logarithmic growth (the **log phase**), followed in turn by a plateau as the bacterial population exhausts the resources of its environment.

Some foodborne pathogens form spores that can survive inhospitable conditions. Of course, cleanliness of hands, work surfaces, and implements is also a key to controlling foodborne illness.

Thus, two basic levers for the control of bacterial contamination of food are time and temperature, and a general rule of thumb in food safety is "keep it hot, or keep it cold, or don't keep it." That is, although the lag phase offers a sort of grace period, the key to food safety is to limit the time that food spends in the danger zone.

Food should be stored cold and cooked to a high enough temperature to kill pathogens. (Instructions for specific foods should be followed; the recommended temperatures for broiled meat and poultry, for example, are higher than 140°F.)

Upstream controls are also important; however, using institutional controls to ensure food safety is a difficult challenge because many individuals and entities may be involved in a long line of processes in food production and food service (refer to **Figure 5.17**). Inspection of food products and processes has long been at the heart of regulating food safety, as evidenced in the early laws requiring inspection of meat and poultry. Traditionally, federal food safety efforts rested on inspectors who made a physical examination of foods, such as carcasses in a meatpacking facility. Although this approach (sometimes referred to as the "poke and sniff" method) was not fully scientific, it was a direct inspection of the food itself.

Since the 1990s, the USDA and FDA have increasingly implemented a different approach to food safety, known as the **Hazard Analysis and Critical Control Point (HACCP**; "hassip") system, which has broad international acceptance. The HACCP approach rests on seven key actions:[129]

- Identify the hazards that may be associated with a food (e.g., microbial contamination)
- Identify **critical control points** in the production of the food (i.e., points at which the hazard could be controlled or eliminated, such as cooking); and for each critical control point establish:

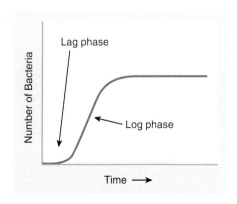

Figure 5.16 A schematic bacterial growth curve under favorable conditions.

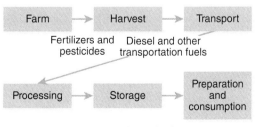

Figure 5.17 Farm to table system.

- Specific measures to prevent the hazard (e.g., requirements for cooking time and temperature)
- Procedures to monitor the preventive measures (e.g., how cooking time will be monitored)
- Corrective actions to be taken when monitoring shows a failure in preventive measures (e.g., disposing of inadequately cooked food)
- Establish procedures to ensure that pieces of the system are in good working order (e.g., that a cooking unit is working properly)
- Establish recordkeeping systems to document each of the preceding steps

Because HACCP systems incorporate both scientific and practical understanding of food safety, they offer the possibility of much more effective control of foodborne illness than "poke and sniff" inspections. On the other hand, HACCP systems rely on food industries, such as meatpackers and poultry processors, to police themselves. Federal inspectors no longer inspect food directly, but rather evaluate the HACCP systems that industry has created to monitor itself, a change that is of concern to some food inspectors.[69]

The USDA and FDA have concluded that on balance the modernization offered by HACCP is an improvement over traditional food inspections. The USDA has required the meat and poultry industries to implement HACCP.

Specifically, each meat or poultry establishment must develop a HACCP system and then demonstrate that the system can and does work in practice.[130] The FDA has also implemented HACCP requirements for producers of dairy products and juice, producers of fish and seafood, processors of seafood and seafood products, and processors of fruit and vegetable juice and juice products. In conjunction with the FDA and the food service industry, the USDA offers guidance in the form of standard operating procedures (based on HACCP principles) for food service operations[131]; however, state and local governments regulate food safety in food service and retail food establishments.

In addition to international, federal and regional governmental oversight, ensuring that the food you eat is safe *for you* is a personal responsibility bigger than just adhering to safe food handling practices. Knowing what is in the food you eat and where it comes from is also important, especially if you have unique food intolerances or allergies. Food labels play an important role in providing consumers with the information they need to eat well and safely. Labels also have the ability to keep us informed about the food production processes bringing us our meal. Public health practitioners must to be vigilant about modern agricultural practices and continue to advocate for truly informative food labeling laws.

Study Questions

1. Contrast chemical pesticides with industrial chemical pollutants as environmental health hazards.
2. Contrast the perspective of most of the world's more developed countries with the perspective of sub-Saharan African nations on the use of DDT to control mosquitoes.
3. Why do you think integrated pest management is not more widely used in the United States?
4. Describe three major human health concerns associated with modern food production practices.
5. Explain the global environmental health impacts of modern food production.
6. Do you think current food quality regulations and agencies are adequate to ensure food safety? Explain.

References

1. Nadakavukaren A. *Our Global Environment: A Health Perspective* (7th edition). Waveland Press, Inc. 2011

2. Atwood D, Paisley-Jones, C. (2017). Pesticides Industry Sales and Usage: 2008 – 2012 Market Estimates. United States Environmental Protection Agency. https://www.epa.gov/sites/production/files/2017-01/documents/pesticides-industry-sales-usage-2016_0.pdf.

3. Geisz, HN, Dickhut RM, Cochran MA, Fraser WR, Ducklow HW. Melting glaciers: a probable source of DDT to the Antarctic marine ecosystem. *Environ Sci Technol.* 2008;42(11):3958-3962.

4. Encyclopedia Britannica. Paul Hermann Müller. 2007. www.britannica.com/eb/article-9054225/Paul-Hermann-Muller

5. World Health Organization. WHO and DDT for Malaria Control—June 2009.

6. World Health Organization. (2011). WHO Assessment: DDT use for malaria a concern for human health [press release].

7. Encyclopedia Britannica Bhopal disaster. Retrieved June 30, 2020 from https://www.britannica.com/event/Bhopal-disaster

8. Ehler L. Integrated pest management (IPM): definition, historical development and implementation, and the other IPM. *Pest Manag Sci.* 2006;62:787–789.

9. Kamel F, Hoppin JA. Association of pesticide exposure with neurologic dysfunction and disease. *Environ Health Perspect.* 2004;112(9):950-958.

10. Alavanja M, Hoppin J, Kamel F. Health effects of chronic pesticide exposure: cancer and neurotoxicity. *Ann Rev Public Health.* 2004;25:155-197.

11. World Health Organization. Pesticides are a leading suicide method. 2006. www.who.int/mediacentre/news/notes/2006/np24/en/index.html

12. Clapp RW, Jacobs MM, Loechler EL. Environmental and occupational causes of cancer: new evidence, 2005–2007. *Rev Environ Health,* 2008;23(1):1-37.

13. Blair A, Zahm S. Cancer among farmers. *Occup Med,* 1991;3: 335-354.

14. Blair A, Zahm S. Patterns of pesticide use among farmers: implications for epidemiologic research. *Epidemiology,* 1993;4(1):55-62.

15. Blair A, Zahm SH. Agricultural exposures and cancer. *Environ Health Perspect.* 1995;103(suppl 8):205-208.

16. Blair A, Zahm SH, Pearce NE, Heineman EF, Fraumeni JF. Clues to cancer etiology from studies of farmers. *Scand J Work Environ Health.* 1992;18(4):209-215.

17. Blair A, Freeman LB. Epidemiologic studies in agricultural populations: observations and future directions. *J Agromed.* 2009;14(2):125-131.

18. Weichenthal S, Moase C, Chan P. A review of pesticide exposure and cancer incidence in the Agricultural Health Cohort Study. *Environ Health Perspect.* 2010; 118(8):1117-1125.

19. Cohn BA, Wolff MS, Cirillo PM, Sholtz RI. DDT and breast cancer in young women: new data on the significance of age at exposure. *Environ Health Perspect.* 2007;115(10):1406-1414.

20. Garcia A. Occupational exposure to pesticides and congenital malformations: a review of mechanisms, methods, and results. *Am J Indust Med.* 1998;33(3):232-240.

21. Kirkhorn SR, Schenker MB. Current health effects of agricultural work: respiratory disease, cancer, reproductive effects, musculoskeletal injuries, and pesticide-related illnesses. *J Agri Safety Health.* 2002;8(2):199-214.

22. Perry MJ. Effects of environmental and occupational pesticide exposure on human sperm; a systematic review. *Human Reprod Update,* 2008;14(3):233-242.

23. Garry VF. Pesticides and children. *Toxicol Appl Pharmacol.* 2004;198(2):152-163.

24. Infante-Rivard C, Weichenthal S. Pesticides and childhood cancer: an update of Zahm and Ward's 1998 review. *J Toxicol Environ Health Part B.* 2007;10(1-2):81-99.

25. Van Maele-Fabry G, Lantin AC, Hoet P, Liston D. Childhood leukaemia and parental occupational exposure to pesticides: a systematic review and meta-analysis. *Cancer Causes Control.* 2010;21:787-809.

26. Wigle DT, Turner MC, Krewski D. A systematic review and meta-analysis of childhood leukemia and parental occupational pesticide exposure. *Environ Health Perspect.* 2009;117(10):1505.

27. Economic Research Service. Rural Labor and Education: Farm Labor. U.S. Department of Agriculture. April, 2012.

28. McCauley LA, Lasarev MR, Higgins G, Rothlein JE, Muniz J, Ebbert C. Work characteristics and pesticide exposures among migrant agricultural families: a community-based research approach. *Environ Health Perspect,* 2001;109:533-538.

29. Robinson E, Nguyen HT, Isom S, et al. Wages, wage violations, and pesticide safety experienced by migrant farmworkers in North Carolina. *New Solutions,* 2011;21(2), 251-268.

30. London L. Occupational epidemiology in agriculture: a case study in the Southern African context. *Int J Occup Environ Health,* 1998;4(4): 245-256.

31. Brower V. Growing greener: the impact of integrated pest management. *EMBO Reports,* 2002;3(5):403-406.

32. Ehler L, Bottrell DG. The illusion of integrated pest management. *Issues in Science and Technology.* 2000; 16(3):61-64.

33. U.S. Department of Agriculture. 2007 Census of Agriculture/Summary and State Data/Volume 1, Geographic Area Series, Part 51, AC-07-A-51. 2009. www.agcensus.usda.gov/Publications/2007/Full_Report/usv1.pdf

34. U.S. Energy Information Administration. Today in energy – energy for growing and harvesting crops is a large component of farm operating costs. 2014. https://www.eia.gov/todayinenergy/detail.php?id=18431

35. Knobeloch L, Proctor M. Eight blue babies. *Wisconsin Med J.* 2001;100(8), 43-47.

36. Curseu D, Sirbu D, Popa M, Ionutas A. The relationship between infant methemoglobinemia and environmental exposure to nitrates. In: Gokcekus H, Turker U, Lamoreaux JW, eds. *Survival and Sustainability*, Springer. 2011:635.

37. Sørensen M, Danielsen V. Effects of the plant growth regulator, chlormequat, on mammalian fertility. *Intl J Androl.* 2006;29(1):129-133.

38. Ball S, Glover C. *Defoliants, Desiccants, and Growth Regulators Used on New Mexico Cotton.* New Mexico State University Press. 1999.

39. U.S. Census Bureau. International programs. Retrieved April 21, 2010 from https://www.census.gov/data-tools/demo/idb/informationGateway.php

40. Lehrer SB, Bannon GA. Risks of allergic reactions to biotech proteins in foods: perception and reality. *Allergy.* 2005;60(5):559-564.

41. Pollack, A. *Roadside Invader: Engineered Canola. New York Times.* (2010, August 6).

42. Heritage J. Transgenes for tea? *Trends in Biotechnology,* 2005;23(1):17-21.

43. Nestle, M. *Safe Food: Bacteria, Biotechnology, and Bioterrorism.* University of California Press. 2003.

44. Dieter CA, Maupin MA, Caldwell RR, et al. *Estimated use of water in the United States in 2015: U.S. Geological Survey Circular* 2018;1441:65.

45. U.S. Geological Survey. Comparisons of Average Consumptive use and Renewable Water Supply for the 21 Water-Resources Regions of the United States, Puerto Rico, and U.S. Virgin Islands (Updated using 1995 Estimates of Water use); 2002. Retrieved October 30, 2012

46. United Nations Development Programme. Human Development Reports 2006. 2006. Available at: http://hdr.undp.org/en/media/HDR06-complete.pdf

47. Bureau of Labor Statistics. National census of fatal occupational injuries in 2018. 2019. Retrieved July 4, 2020 from: https://www.bls.gov/news.release/pdf/cfoi.pdf

48. Bureau of Labor Statistics. Injuries, Illnesses, and Fatalities/Census of Fatal Occupational Injuries (CFOI)—current and revised data. Retrieved April 23, 2012 from www.bls.gov/iif/oshcfoi1.htm

49. Bureau of Labor Statistics. Injuries, Illnesses, and Fatalities/Industry Injury and Illness Data. Retrieved July 9, 2012 from: www.bls.gov/iif/oshsum.htm

50. Rautiainen RH, Lange JL, Hodne CJ, Schneiders S, Donham KJ. Injuries in the Iowa certified safe farm study. *J Agri Saf Health,* 2004;10(1):51-63.

51. Rollin BE. Animal agriculture and emerging social ethics for animals. *Journal Animal Science,* 200482: 955-964.

52. Lone K. Natural sex steroids and their xenobiotic analogs in animal production: growth, carcass quality, pharmacokinetics, metabolism, mode of action, residues, methods, and epidemiology. *Crit Rev Food Sci.* 1997;37(2)93-209.

53. U.S. Food and Drug Administration. Steroid hormone implants used for growth in food-producing animals. 2002. Retrieved October 30, 2012 from https://www.fda.gov/animal-veterinary/product-safety-information/steroid-hormone-implants-used-growth-food-producing-animals

54. U.S. Department of Agriculture, National Agricultural Statistics Service. Livestock Slaughter: 2010 Summary. 2011. Retrieved June 20, 2012 from https://downloads.usda.library.cornell.edu/usda-esmis/files/r207tp32d/7p88ck085/1v53k090s/LiveSlauSu-04-25-2011.pdf

55. U.S. Department of Agriculture. Poultry—Production and Value: 2012 Summary. 2013. Retrieved October 2, 2020 from https://downloads.usda.library.cornell.edu/usda-esmis/files/m039k491c/1z40kw41x/2z10ws53c/PoulProdVa-04-29-2013.pdf

56. Walljasper, C. Several states see shifts in animal production since 2011. 2018. *Agribusiness Report.* Retrieved July 1, 2020 from https://investigatemidwest.org/2018/06/07/large-animal-feeding-operations-on-the-rise/

57. National Chicken Council.. Broiler Chicken Industry Key Facts 2019. Retrieved July 4, 2020 from: https://www.nationalchickencouncil.org/about-the-industry/statistics/broiler-chicken-industry-key-facts/

58. U.S. Department of Agriculture, National Agricultural Statistics Service. Trends in U.S. agriculture. 2018. Retrieved October 30, 2012 from: www.nass.usda.gov/Publications/Trends_in_U.S._Agriculture/

59. U.S. Environmental Protection Agency. Profile of the agricultural livestock production industry. EPA 310-R-00-002. 2000. Retrieved April 19, 2008 from: www.epa.gov/compliance/resources/publications/assistance/sectors/notebooks/aglivestock.pdf

60. Cambra-López, M, Aarnink, AJ, Zhao Y, Calvet S, Torres AG. Airborne particulate matter from livestock production systems: a review of an air pollution problem. *Environ Pollution,* 2010;158(1):1-17.

61. U.S. Food and Drug Administration. Overall reproductive efficiency and health statistics for U.S. animal agriculture, Appendix B: a risk-based approach to evaluate animal clones and their progeny (draft). 2007. Retrieved March 10, 2007

62. U.S. Department of Agriculture, National Agricultural Statistics Service. Cattle Death Loss. 2011. Retrieved June 20, 2012 from www.nass.usda.gov/Statistics_by_State/Florida/Publications/Livestock_and_Poultry/catloss2010.pdf

63. 2012 Census of Agriculture. (2014). Hog and pig farming. Retrieved October 2, 2020 from https://www.nass.usda.gov/Publications/Highlights/2014/Hog_and_Pig_Farming/Highlights_Hog_and_Pig_Farming.pdf

64. U.S. Department of Agriculture, Animal and Plant Health Inspection Service. Swine 2000. 2005. Retrieved October 30, 2012 from: www.aphis.usda.gov/animal_health

/nahms/swine/downloads/swine2000/Swine2000_dr
_PartII.pdf

65. Cole D, Todd L, Wing S. Concentrated swine feeding operations and public health: a review of occupational and community health effects. *Environ Health Perspect.* 2000;108:685-699.

66. Nachman K, Graham JP, Price LB, Silbergeld EK. Arsenic: a roadblock to potential animal waste management solutions. *Environ Health Perspect,* 2005;113(9):1123-1124.

67. Zhao X, Wang J, Zhu L, Ge W, Wang J. Environmental analysis of typical antibiotic-resistant bacteria and ARGs in farmland soil chronically fertilized with chicken manure. *Science of the Total Environment,* 2017;593-594: 10–17.

68. Marano N, Stamey K, Barrett T, Angulo F. High prevalence of gentamicin resistance among selected *Salmonella* serotypes in the United States: associated with heavy use of gentamicin in poultry. Infectious Disease Society of America 37th Annual Meeting; Philadelphia, PA. 1999.

69. PBS Frontline. Modern meat/antibiotic debate overview. 2002. Retrieved September, 19, 2012 from: www.pbs .org/wgbh/pages/frontline/shows/meat/safe/overview .html

70. U.S. Food and Drug Administration. 2009 Summary report on antimicrobials sold or distributed for use in food-producing animals. 2010. Retrieved June 20, 2012 from: www.fda.gov/downloads/ForIndustry/UserFees /AnimalDrugUserFeeActADUFA/UCM231851.pdf

71. Center for Veterinary Medicine. Summary report on antimicrobials sold or distributed for use in food-producing animals. 2015. Food and Drug Administration Department of Health and Human Services. Retrieved January 13, 2017 from http://www.fda.gov/downloads /ForIndustry/UserFees/AnimalDrugUserFeeActADUFA /UCM476258.pdf

72. Sørum H, L'Abée-Lund TM. Antibiotic resistance in food-related bacteria—a result of interfering with the global web of bacterial genetics. *Int J Food Microbiol.* 2002; 78(1-2):43-56.

73. Sigurdarson S, O'Shaughnessy PT, Watt JA, Kline JN. Experimental human exposure to inhaled grain dust and ammonia: towards a model of concentrated animal feeding operations. *A J Indust Med.* 2004;46(4): 345–348.

74. National Institute of Occupational Safety and Health (NIOSH). NIOSH Warns: Manure Pits Continue to Claim Lives. 1993. Retrieved October 30, 2012 from www.cdc.gov/Niosh/updates/93-114.html

75. Brubaker B. (2007, July 4). Four family members, farm-hand killed by gas fumes in manure pit. *Washington Post.*

76. Schiffman SS. Livestock odors: implications for human health and well-being. *American Society of Animal Science,* 1998;76(5):1343–1355.

77. Wing S, Cole D, Grant G. Environmental injustice in North Carolina's hog industry. *Environ Health Perspect.* 2000;108, 225-231.

78. Cai C, Perry MJ, Sorock GS, Hauser R, Spanjer KJ, Mittleman MA, Stentz TL. Laceration injuries among workers at meat packing plants. *Am J Indust Med.* 2005;47(5):403-410.

79. U.S. Occupational Safety and Health Administration. Poultry processing industry eTool. Retrieved October 30, 2012 from www.osha.gov/SLTC/etools/poultry/index .html

80. Quandt SA, Grzywacz JG, Marin A, et al. Illnesses and injuries reported by Latino poultry workers in western North Carolina. *Am J Indust Med.* 2006;49(5):343-351.

81. Campbell D. Health hazards in the meatpacking industry. *Occup Med.* 1999;14(2):351-372.

82. Besson H, Banks R, Boffetta P. Cancer mortality among butchers: a 24-state death certificate study. *J Occup Environ Med.* 2006;48(3):289-293.

83. McLean D, Pearce N. Cancer among meat industry workers. *Scand J Work Environ Health.* 2004;30(6): 425–437.

84. Boffetta P, Gridley G, Gustavsson P, et al. Employment as butcher and cancer risk in a record-linkage study from Sweden. *Cancer Causes & Control,* 2000;11:627–633.

85. U.S. Department of Agriculture, National Agricultural Statistics Service. QuickStats: Agricultural Statistics Database. 2019. Retrieved October 2, 2020 from https:// www.nass.usda.gov/Quick_Stats/index.php

86. BBC News. Why mad cow disease lingers on. Retrieved March 23, 2007 from http://news.bbc.co.uk/2/hi/uk _news/493435.stm. 1999.

87. U.K. Ministry of Agriculture, Fisheries and Food. The BSE inquiry report. *BSE Inquiry.* 2000. Retrieved February 7, 2008 from http://www.fao.org/livestock /agap/frg/feedsafety/uk-bse.htm

88. Rhodes R. *Deadly Feasts.* 1997. Simon & Schuster.

89. Doyle E. Bovine spongiform encephalopathy: an updated scientific literature review. 2004. University of Wisconsin, Food Research Institute, Retrieved October 30, 2012 from https://www.semanticscholar.org/paper /Bovine-Spongiform-Encephalopathy-An-Updated -Review-Briefings-Doyle/248099c60e6d430c13019b92 0e0f3a0f112c63d3

90. MacDonald JM, McBride WD, O'Donoghue E, Nehring RF, Sandretto C, Mosheim R. Profits, costs, and the changing structure of dairy farming: USDA economic research report number 47. 2007. Retrieved December 7, 2012 from www.ers.usda.gov/media/188030/err47_1_.pdf

91. National Agricultural Statistics Service, United States Department of Agriculture. Largest decline in U.S. dairy farms in 15-plus years in 2019. *Market Intel Milk Production Report.* 2020. Retrieved July 5, 2020 from https://www.fb.org/market-intel/largest-decline-in-u.s. -dairy-farms-in15-plus-years-in-2019

92. Keown JF, Kononoff PJ. Can you afford to use bovine somatotrophin (bovine growth hormone)? *University of Nebraska-Lincoln Extension, Institute of Agriculture and Natural Resources.* 2007. Retrieved February 7, 2008 from www.ianrpubs.unl.edu/epublic/live/g1664/build /g1664.pdf

93. Malekinejad H, Rezabakhsh A. Hormones in dairy foods and their impact on public health – a narrative review article. *Iran J Public Health*. 2015;44(6), 742-758.

94. Tyedmers P. Fisheries and energy use. In: Cleveland C, ed. *Encyclopedia of Energy*, 2, Elsevier. 2004;2:683-693.

95. Thomas TK, Lincoln JM, Husberg BJ, Conway GA. Is it safe on deck? Fatal and non-fatal workplace injuries among Alaskan commercial fishermen. *A J Indust Med*, 2001;40(6),693-702.

96. National Institute for Occupational Safety and Health. Fatal occupational injuries in the U.S. Commercial fishing industry: Risk factors and recommendations, East Coast region. 2010. NIOSH 2011-105. Retrieved July 9, 2012 from www.cdc.gov/niosh/docs/2011-105/pdfs/EC_CFID_Summary_EV.pdf

97. Froese R, Kesner-Reyes K. Impact of fishing on the abundance of marine species. International Council for the Exploration of the Sea Annual Science Conference; Copenhagen. 2002.

98. Grainger R. Global trends in fisheries and aquaculture (National Oceanic and Atmospheric Administration's National Dialogues on Coastal Stewardship). Retrieved April 19, 2008 from https://biotech.law.lsu.edu/cphl/noaa/ctrends-proceed-1999.pdf

99. Cole DW, Cole R, Gaydos SJ, Gray J, et al. Aquaculture: environmental, toxicological, and health issues. *Int J Hygiene Environ Health*. 2009;212(4):369-377.

100. Hites RA, Foran JA, Carpenter DO, Hamilton MC, Knuth BA, Schwager SJ. Global assessment of organic contaminants in farmed salmon. *Science*. 2004;303(5655):226-229.

101. Willett W, Rockström J, Loken B, et al. Food in the Anthropocene: the EAT-Lancet Commission on healthy diets from sustainable food systems. *Lancet*, 2019;393(10170):447-492.

102. Foley JA. Can we feed the world and sustain the planet? *Scientific American*, 2015;60-65.

103. U.S. Environmental Protection Agency. Inventory of U.S. greenhouse gas emissions and sinks: 1990–2010. 2012. Retrieved June 20, 2012 from https://www.epa.gov/ghgemissions/inventory-us-greenhouse-gas-emissions-and-sinks-1990-2010

104. Johnson K, Johnson DE. Methane emissions from cattle. *Journal of Animal Science*. 1995;73(8):2483-2492.

105. Kingsolver B. (2002). Lily's Chickens. *Small Wonder*. Harper Collins.

106. U.S. Food and Drug Administration. (n.d.). Defect Levels Handbook. Retrieved April 24, 2012.

107. U.S. Food and Drug Administration. (n.d.). Food Additives. Retrieved October 30, 2012.

108. Shea KM. Technical report: irradiation of food. *Pediatrics*. 2000;106(6):1505-1510.

109. Louria D. Counterpoint on food irradiation. *Int J Infect Dis*. 2000;4(2):67-69.

110. Epstein SS, Hauter W. Preventing pathogenic food poisoning: sanitation, not irradiation. *Intern J Health Services*. 2001;31(1):187-192.

111. U.S. Food and Drug Administration. Food irradiation: The treatment of foods with ionizing radiation. Retrieved March 22, 2007.

112. U.S. Department of Agriculture, National Agricultural Statistics Service. Livestock Slaughter: 2011 Summary. 2012. Retrieved July 11, 2012.

113. Schlosser E. *Fast Food Nation*. 2002. Perennial.

114. Walsh KA, Bennett SD, Mahovic M, Gould LH. Outbreaks associated with cantaloupe, watermelon, and honeydew in the United States, 1973-2011. *Foodborne Pathogens and Disease*. 2014;11(12):945-952.

115. Shende C, Inscore F, Sengupta A, Stuart J, Farquharson S. Rapid extraction and detection of trace Chlorpyrifos-methyl in orange juice by surface-enhanced Raman spectroscopy. *Sensing and Instrumentation for Food Quality and Safety*, 2010;4:101-107.

116. Kuepper G, Gegner L. Organic crop production overview. 2004. U.S. Department of Agriculture, National Center for Appropriate Technology. Retrieved April 19, 2008 from https://pdfs.semanticscholar.org/04e8/54028ad338dfe0470c2ced6aed1644f1b028.pdf

117. U.S. Department of Agriculture, Economic Research Service. Data sets/organic production, Table 2 [data]. Retrieved April 23, 2012 from https://www.ers.usda.gov/data-products/organic-production/documentation.aspx

118. U.S. Department of Agriculture, Economic Research Service. Data sets/organic production, Table 3 [data]. Retrieved April 23, 2012 from https://www.ers.usda.gov/data-products/organic-production/documentation.aspx

119. University Libraries: UNT Digital Library. Food biotechnology in the United States: science, regulation, and issues. Library of Congress. 2001. Retrieved October 30, 2012 from: http://digital.library.unt.edu/ark:/67531/metacrs1376/

120. U.S. Environmental Protection Agency. Pesticides: regulating pesticides. Retrieved March 22, 2007 from www.epa.gov/pesticides/regulating

121. Pew Initiative on Food and Biotechnology. Guide to U.S. Regulation of Genetically Modified Food and Agricultural Biotechnology Products. 2001. Retrieved February 7, 2008 from: https://www.pewtrusts.org/en/research-and-analysis/reports/2001/09/03/guide-to-us-regulation-of-genetically-modified-food-and-agricultural-biotechnology-products

122. Rawson JM, Vogt DU. Congressional Research Service. Food Safety Agencies and Authorities: A Primer. *Library of Congress*, 1998;98-91 ENR.

123. National Research Council. *Environmental Effects of Transgenic Plants*. National Academies Press. 2002.

124. U.S. Department of Agriculture, Food Safety and Inspection Service. *Key Facts: Humane Slaughter*. Retrieved March 22, 2007.

125. U.S. Department of Agriculture, Agricultural Marketing Service. How to Buy Meat. *Home and Garden Bulletin* [serial online], 1995;265. Retrieved December 10, 2007.

126. U.S. Department of Agriculture. Grass Fed Marketing Claim Standards. Retrieved April 30, 2012 from www .ams.usda.gov/AMSv1.0/ams.fetchTemplateData.do ?template=TemplateN&navID=GrassFed MarketingClaimStandards&rightNav1=GrassFed MarketingClaimStandards&topNav =&leftNav=Grading CertificationandVerfication&page=GrassFedMarketing Claims&resultType=

127. National Oceanic and Atmospheric Administration. *Sustainable Fisheries.* Retrieved March 14, 2007 from https://www.fisheries.noaa.gov/topic/sustainable -fisheries

128. U.S. Department of Agriculture, Agricultural Marketing Service. The National Organic Program: Production and Handling–Preamble. Retrieved December 12, 2007 from www.ams.usda.gov/nop/NOP/standards/DefinePre .html

129. U.S. Food and Drug Administration. HACCP: A State-of the-Art Approach to Food Safety. Retrieved February 7, 2008 from: www.ams.usda.gov/nop/NOP/standards /DefinePre.html

130. U.S. Department of Agriculture. HACCP Validation. Retrieved April 30, 2012 from https://www.fsis.usda .gov/wps/portal/fsis/topics/regulatory-compliance /haccp/resources-and-information/haccp-validation /Validation

131. U.S. Department of Agriculture, National Food Services Management Institute. Food safety standard operating procedures (SOPs). Retrieved April 30, 2012 from https://professionalstandards.fns.usda.gov/content/food -safety-standard-operating-procedures-sops

CHAPTER 6

Producing Manufactured Goods

LEARNING OBJECTIVES

After studying this chapter, the reader will be able to:

- Define or explain the key terms introduced throughout the chapter
- Characterize the uses, common sources of environmental exposure, and toxicity of these groups of synthetic organic chemicals: organic solvents, phthalate plasticizers and bisphenol A, PCBs, dioxins and furans, PBDEs, and PFCs
- Describe in simple terms the effect of chlorofluorocarbons in the stratosphere and the implications for human health
- Appreciate the toxicity of certain metals to workers and the general population, especially children
- Summarize briefly the current status of nanotechnology and what is known about its risks to human health
- Describe the field of occupational health and the major causes of worker mortality and morbidity
- Discuss the physical occupational exposures associated with respiratory health effects and hearing loss
- Appreciate that certain occupational exposures cause cancer or pose reproductive hazards
- Characterize the disparity in hazardous exposures among national and international workers
- Describe key approaches and the U.S. regulatory framework for managing the public health risks associated with producing manufactured goods

In the prosperous decades that followed World War II, many people in the more developed countries were able to acquire more material goods. Especially in the United States, this period saw a rapid change from an ethic based on thrift and self-denial to expectations of convenience and instant gratification. Whereas an earlier generation's motto had been "use it up, wear it out, make it do," a new generation yearned for "the good life." In the 1950s, the symbols of the good life were a house, a car, a washing machine, and a television. By the start of the 21st century, consumerism had reached new heights, and "the good life" had become "lifestyles" that encompassed large suburban homes, sport utility vehicles, luxury housewares, and an astounding array of electronic devices for computing, communications, and entertainment.

Of course, these products do not spring magically into existence. Each one has a history: Raw materials are obtained and then transformed through manufacturing. Nothing ever really goes away, and so industrial processes create wastes or byproducts—resulting in exposures to workers, to neighboring communities, and sometimes even to consumers. In the mid-20th century, smokestack industries and air pollution dominated the landscape of many U.S. cities and towns (see **Figure 6.1**). By the end of the century, the icon of industrial pollution had become the 55-gallon drum of chemical waste (see **Figure 6.2**).

Modern consumers are increasingly insulated from the realities of industrial pollution. For example, in 2019, more than five times as many Americans were employed in service industries as in manufacturing[1]; at the same time, more and more manufacturing has moved, and continues to move, to less-developed countries. To many residents of an industrialized country who purchase and use a product, that product's footprint—in environmental destruction or pollution, in consumption of nonrenewable energy resources, and in workers' illnesses and injuries—may be largely invisible.

This chapter describes the environmental health issues associated with the manufactured products of modern society, specifically the associated major chemical and physical risks. The uses and health effects of several groups of synthetic organic chemicals are discussed in Section 6.1 as are a number of toxic metals in Section 6.2. The chapter then describes the origins of occupational health and the hazards that especially affect workers (Section 6.3). Section 6.4 concludes the chapter with a discussion of the management and

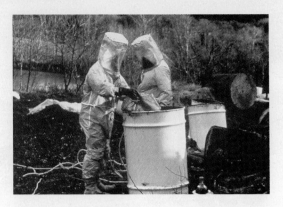

Figure 6.2 Workers wear protective gear as they handle hazardous wastes.

Courtesy of CDC Public Health Image Library. ID# 1530. Content provider: CDC. Available at: http://phil.cdc.gov/phil/home.asp. Accessed October 15, 2012.

disposal challenges associated with the hazardous materials used in modern production as well as their inadvertent byproducts.

6.1 Synthetic Organic Chemicals

In the United States today, thousands of **organic chemicals** are in use. The great majority of these chemicals are manmade and are produced from petroleum. The capacity to make such **synthetic organic chemicals** from oil, a hydrocarbon resource, rests on carbon's unique flexibility in forming stable bonds.

In an oil refinery, the constituents of crude oil are separated into lighter and heavier fractions, which are then used to make many products, including various fuels (e.g., gasoline, diesel fuel, jet fuel, kerosene), nonfuel products (e.g., lubricating oils, greases, petroleum jelly, asphalt), and chemicals that become the raw materials for the production of other chemicals in the chemical industry. Thus, some of what we think of as chemical manufacturing takes place at oil refineries and some at separate chemical plants.

Synthetic organic compounds have been designed and produced for many uses. Among these are many products so familiar that we might not even think of them as chemicals: soaps and detergents; cosmetics and toiletries; plastics and

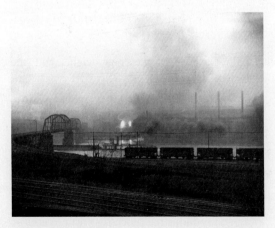

Figure 6.1 Polluted air blankets a U.S. city in 1946.

Courtesy of CDC Public Health Image Library. ID# 8998. Content provider CDC/Roy Perry. Available at: http://phil.cdc.gov/phil/home.asp. Accessed October 15, 2012.

synthetic rubbers; inks and dyes; paints, coatings, polishes, and adhesives; pharmaceuticals; and even explosives. Because there are far too many synthetic organic chemicals to consider individually, this discussion focuses on some groups that are both widespread and pose a risk to human health:

- Organic solvents
- Chemicals used in the production of plastics
- A set of environmentally persistent toxic substances
- Chemicals that deplete the stratospheric ozone layer

Another important group of toxic chemicals, pesticides, were already discussed in the context of agriculture and food production.

Organic Solvents

Organic solvents, often referred to simply as **solvents**, are chemicals that dissolve other substances. They are used as intermediaries in synthesizing chemicals, and they are useful in many cleaning applications in industry; for example, solvents are used in "degreasing" metals in the manufacture of electronic components, which today are found in products ranging from airplane navigation systems to coffeemakers and cell phones.

Although solvents have a broad range of chemical structures, many widely used solvents fall into one of two groups, both of which are low-molecular-weight, volatile chemicals (see **Table 6.1**).

One group is simple hydrocarbons, in which the carbon atoms are arranged in a ring. Four common solvents in this group—benzene, toluene, ethylbenzene, and xylene, commonly referred to together as BTEX ("bee-tex")—are often derived from petroleum at the refinery and are used as feedstocks in the production of other chemicals. In the other group of widely used solvents, the carbon atoms are arranged in a chain rather than in a ring, and one or more of the hydrogen atoms has been replaced with a chlorine atom. This group of chlorinated (chlorine-containing) solvents includes trichloroethylene (TCE) and other

Table 6.1 Some Widely Used Organic Solvents

Nonchlorinated Solvents	Chlorinated Solvents
Benzene	Trichloroethylene (TCE)
Toluene	Tetrachloroethylene (PCE)
Ethylbenzene	1,1,1-Trichloroethane (TCA)
Xylene	

compounds that have environmental breakdown products similar to TCEs, including tetrachloroethylene (commonly known as perchloroethylene, or PCE) and 1,1,1-trichloroethane (TCA; also known as methyl chloroform), among others.

Industrial solvents are released into the environment mainly by the industries that produce them and the industries that use them. In 2010, some 56 million pounds of BTEX were released or disposed of, on- or offsite, by U.S. industries, and smaller quantities of the chlorinated solvents TCE, PCE, and TCA were released.[2] The industries with the largest BTEX releases are the chemical, printing and publishing, and petroleum industries, which together account for about half of the annual total releases; the transportation equipment, paper, and hazardous waste/solvent recovery industries together account for another quarter. For both BTEX and the three chlorinated solvents named above, most of the quantity released was disposed of onsite—for example, in surface impoundments, landfills, or underground injection wells. Solvents are common contaminants of U.S. groundwater, which is an important source of drinking water in many areas. Many solvents are moderately soluble in water and can be transported over long distances, making cleanup a difficult challenge.

In the textile industry, solvents are widely used in dyeing, and their use in dry cleaning results in occupational exposures at a large number of small businesses. At one time, highly toxic benzene was used as a dry cleaning agent (see **Figure 6.3**). Over time, benzene was largely

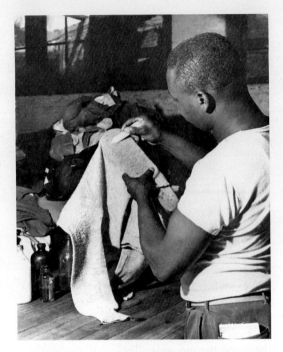

Figure 6.3 In 1950, this dry cleaning worker used benzene to spot-clean a garment.

Courtesy of CDC Public Health Image Library. ID# 9453. Content provider CDC/Barbara Jenkins, NIOSH. Available at: http://phil.cdc.gov/phil/home.asp. Accessed October 15, 2012.

replaced by trichloroethylene, and TCE in turn has been largely replaced by PCE, now used by approximately 28,000 U.S. dry cleaners.[3] Some cleaners also offer water-based cleaning methods that do not damage fabrics that cannot be washed in a home washing machine.

Most solvents affect the central nervous system. Acute high-level exposures cause symptoms such as dizziness, loss of coordination, confusion, and unconsciousness; and chronic lower-level exposures can lead to memory loss or other intellectual impairment.[4] Long-term exposure to many solvents damages the liver, kidneys, or both; benzene also causes anemia.[4] Among the seven solvents mentioned here, the World Health Organization's (WHO) International Agency for Research on Cancer (IARC) lists benzene in Group 1 (carcinogenic to humans); benzene is well known to cause leukemia in people.[5] IARC places TCE and PCE in

Group 2A (probably carcinogenic to humans), ethylbenzene in Group 2B (possibly carcinogenic to humans), and toluene, xylene, and trichloroethane in Group 3 (not classifiable as to carcinogenicity to humans). A further cancer concern associated with the chlorinated solvent TCE, is that vinyl chloride, a known human carcinogen listed in IARC's Group 1, is generated during TCE's decay in the environment.[6]

Phthalate Plasticizers and Bisphenol A

Plastics are a set of synthetic organic chemicals familiar in items we use every day. The word *plastic* means flexible or malleable, and **plasticizers** are the chemicals used in the manufacturing process to make plastics flexible. As a result, the chemicals used as plasticizers, called **phthalates**, are present in plastic products. Even plastics that seem fairly hard need some flexibility so that they can sustain an impact without shattering. Another chemical, **bisphenol A (BPA)**, is used widely during the production of certain plastics to stiffen or harden the product. Bisphenol A has also been used in the linings of food and aluminum drink cans to provide stability. A polycarbonate plastic bottle may contain small amounts of both phthalates and bisphenol A.

Phthalates and bisphenol A are classed as semivolatile compounds; they slowly move from a plastic product into the air. Similarly, although these chemicals are not highly water-soluble, they slowly mobilize from a plastic container into a liquid held in the container, particularly if that liquid is carbonated. Phthalates are somewhat lipophilic and bioaccumulate in fish; however, they do not biomagnify across higher levels in ecosystems, because higher animals metabolize and excrete them.[7]

Different chemicals in the phthalate family are used for different purposes.[7] The most widely used phthalate plasticizer is di(2-ethylhexyl) phthalate (DEHP): The United States, for example, produces approximately 240 million pounds of this higher-molecular-weight phthalate annually.[8] DEHP is present in polyvinyl chloride (PVC) plastic. This very common plastic material is used in many products, including water pipes, flooring, upholstery, credit cards, and plastic shower curtains. Phthalates have been measured in many consumer products purchased in stores, including air fresheners, dryer sheets, and various products for hair and skin care.[9] In a study that sampled dust and indoor air in 120 homes, DEHP was found in every home.[10] PVC plastic is also used in food packaging and intravenous bags used for blood or other medical products. Intravenous exposures to DEHP are of particular concern for three reasons[11]: The plastic may be as much as 30%–40% DEHP by weight; the DEHP is not bound to the plastic material and thus moves freely into the contents of a plastic bag; and the intravenous exposure route bypasses normal metabolic processes. The earliest reports of contamination of stored blood by its plastic container came more than 40 years ago.[12,13]

Until recently, di-isononyl phthalate (DiNP) was used in many plastic toys in the United States. Other, lower–molecular-weight plasticizers— dibutyl phthalate (DBP), diethyl phthalate (DEP), and dimethyl phthalate (DMP)—are used mostly in household or cosmetic products that are spreadable or sprayable. For example, these phthalates are used in hair spray and nail polish, lotions and perfumes, glue and insect repellent, insecticides, and coatings on pharmaceuticals. As a result of their large-scale production and use over time, phthalates are ubiquitous in the environment, and due to the wide use of phthalates in products, people living in more developed countries are routinely exposed to these chemicals at low levels.

Phthalates and bisphenol A are considered **endocrine disruptors**, or **endocrine-disrupting compounds**—that is, chemicals that interfere in some way with the body's hormonal signaling. Endocrine disruptors can mimic the effect of a hormone, or block its effect, or even influence the body's production of the hormone. The term **environmental hormone** is also sometimes used to refer to endocrine-disrupting chemicals in the environment, and the term **xenoestrogen**

refers to environmental chemicals with effects similar to those of the female hormone estrogen.*

In laboratory studies, DEHP, DINP, and di-n-hexyl phthalate have been shown to cause developmental toxicity in animals, and the body system most sensitive to their effects is the immature male reproductive system.[7] In male rats exposed perinatally, phthalate exposure has been linked to increased risk of cryptorchidism (undescended testis), hypospadias (wrongly placed opening of the urethra), low sperm counts, and reduced anogenital distance.[14,15] (A reduction in the distance between the anus and the genitals is considered a marker of feminization because anogenital distance is typically shorter in females than in males.) Data from animals also show clearly that phthalates both cross the placenta and are present in breastmilk,[7] indicating the potential for high exposure in utero and in infancy. A case-control study has found a roughly twofold risk of hypospadias associated with the mother's self-reported occupational exposure to hair spray during pregnancy.[16] An earlier epidemiologic study documented a link between higher maternal phthalate exposure during pregnancy and a smaller anogenital distance in the newborn male infant.[17]

Mechanistic evidence is emerging of a link between exposure to environmental chemicals and obesity, and there is limited evidence of such a link from studies in rodents and humans. Prenatal exposure to bisphenol A has been linked to early weight gain and adult obesity in rodents.[18] Exposure to tributyl tin, an organic tin compound used in PVC plastics and fungicides, has been linked to increased lipid accumulation in rodents.[19] In humans, a national cross-sectional study showed that obese men (as measured by

---

*The pharmaceutical diethylstilbestrol (DES), administered to pregnant women from the late 1940s through the 1960s (because it was believed to prevent miscarriage), was an early endocrine disruptor. Among other effects, it has been linked to reproductive abnormalities in the sons, daughters, and even granddaughters of the women who took the drug.

waist circumference) were more likely to have high concentrations of phthalate metabolites in their urine,[20] after controlling for potential confounding variables. Findings like these await confirmation in long-term epidemiologic studies (and diet, exercise, and genetics remain important predictors of obesity), but scientists are now using the term **obesogen** to refer to a chemical that causes weight gain. The obesogen hypothesis specifically links environmental endocrine-disrupting chemicals to obesity promoting mechanisms such as increasing the commitment, differentiation and size of adipocytes (fat cells) in the body or altering the body's regulatory signaling of hormones associated with appetite and satiety.[21]

Determining the true extent of hazard posed by plasticizers and BPA is challenging health researchers due to their ubiquitous presence now in the environment and our bodies. Some of these challenges include trying to adequately characterize exposure, such as characterizing the amount of BPA ingested from drinking carbonated sodas or beer packaged in aluminum cans. Other challenges include trying to locate similar populations to study, but where one may serve as a nonexposed or control group with little exposure. Also, many of the suspected risks are nebulous and hard to diagnose, which makes conducting clinical-based studies difficult.

Despite the limited scientific data available at the time, consumers became outraged about 20 years ago over the quantity of detectable plasticizers and BPA to which they were being exposed. Parents of infants were particularly alarmed to learn about BPA exposure from baby milk bottles and phthalate exposure from pacifiers (**Figure 6.4**). The fact that any amount of these substances was detectable caused significant controversy and a mass migration of the public from polycarbonate to steel or BPA-free bottles, even though much research remains to be done to translate these exposure amounts into their specific health risks. The Consumer Product Safety Improvement Act of 2008 included a ban on the sale of toys and children's products containing any of six phthalates, including all those mentioned earlier in this chapter. No regulatory action

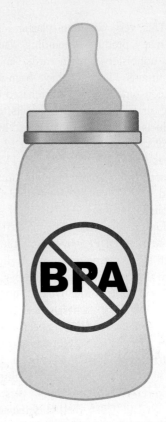

Figure 6.4 Toxic BPA found in plastic bottles.

has been taken yet to ban products that contain bisphenol A; however, significant consumer pressure has resulted in a great variety of BPA-free products now widely available.[22] Unfortunately, there is accumulating evidence that the substances replacing BPA pose equal or potentially greater risk.[23]

Reducing the use of plasticizers and BPA appears to be working as demonstrated by comparing older data with the most recent exposure data available from the National Health and Nutrition Examination Survey (NHANES), a nationwide, cross-sectional, representative sample of approximately 10,000 individuals in the U.S. population. The NHANES survey cycle occurs every two years since its initiation in 1999 and includes physical examinations, physiological measurements, and laboratory tests of blood and urine samples, including biomarkers of phthalate exposure (phthalate metabolites) in the urine of males and females of all ages and ethnic groups.[24] In 2000, children ages 6 through 11 years had a significantly higher average (geometric mean) urinary concentration of a DEHP metabolite, measured at 5.12 µg/L, than 10 years later, when measured at 1.64 µg/L. Among those aged 20 and older, the average concentration of the same metabolite dropped from 3.21 µg/l to 1.55 µg/L. The most recent cross-sectional assessment of bisphenol A concentrations in urine, using NHANES data from 2009-2010, found the same decline in urinary BPA levels from a peak in 2003-2004 of 3.55 µg/L for children ages 6 to 11 years down to 1.81 µg/L, and adults 20 years or older declined from 2.41 µg/L down to 1.79 µg/L.[24] Non-Hispanic Blacks have demonstrated the highest mean levels for BPA during every sample period, also indicating that low-income children have borne a heavier burden of exposure.[25] However, reducing exposures may occur much more quickly than the national sampling studies can reveal. An analysis of a "fresh foods intervention"—a three-day period during which study subjects consumed no packaged foods—documented a 66% reduction in average (geometric mean) concentration of urinary metabolites of BPA during the intervention and a 53% to 56% reduction in average concentration of urinary metabolites of DEHP.[26]

Persistent Toxic Substances

At the opposite end of the physical–chemical spectrum from volatile solvents is a set of organic compounds known for their persistence in soil and sediment. Most originate as manmade chemicals, created for specific purposes, but some are unanticipated byproducts of industrial chemical processes. These persistent compounds bioaccumulate in animal tissues and biomagnify through an ecosystem's food chain. As a result of these traits, these chemicals have become ubiquitous in the global environment: They have spread throughout the world in soil carried by wind and water and also in the bodies of birds and aquatic animals that are long-distance travelers.

Several groups of persistent chemicals are now known to be toxic to people, and these are the chemicals of concern here. The descriptive term **persistent toxic substances** is used in this text; other labels, some of which have regulatory meaning, have been used to refer to overlapping sets of chemicals.* The persistent toxic substances described here are halogenated compounds; that is, they contain an element from the group known as **halogens**, which includes chlorine, fluorine, bromine, and iodine. As a group, the halogens are highly reactive, which accounts for both their usefulness in organic chemistry and their potential to cause harm in the body. In fact, chlorine does not occur naturally in organic compounds in mammals, and it has been argued that the chemical industry violated a "biological taboo" in introducing synthetic chlorinated compounds into ecosystems.[27]

The first generation of synthetic halogenated hydrocarbons were high–molecular-weight chlorinated compounds. Within this group, polychlorinated biphenyls (PCBs) are a set of chemicals that were used mainly to insulate electrical devices. Dioxins and furans,** a large group of structurally related chlorinated compounds, were never manufactured but have been created as byproducts of various chemical processes. More recently, two other groups of persistent toxic substances have emerged as causes of concern.

---

*The term *persistent organic pollutants* (POPs) originates with the Stockholm Convention (see text). Another term, *persistent, bioaccumulative,* and *toxic* (PBT) *chemicals,* has been used more recently by the Environmental Protection Agency (EPA) to designate a set of chemicals of regulatory concern. This list has some overlap with the POPs list but includes other organic chemicals as well as the heavy metals lead and mercury. Both terms are often used more loosely as descriptive rather than regulatory names. A more recent coinage, *ubiquitous bioaccumulative toxins,* captures the implications of persistence; however, the term *toxin* typically refers to a substance produced naturally by a plant or animal.

**The term *dioxins and furans* is shorthand for polychlorinated dibenzo-p-dioxins (PCDDs) and polychlorinated dibenzofurans (PCDFs).

These halogenated chemicals are not chlorinated, but rather contain bromine or fluorine. Polybrominated diphenyl ethers (PBDEs) have been used mostly as flame retardants in fabrics, electronic devices, and furniture; and perfluorochemicals (PFCs) have been widely used in nonstick coatings.

Polychlorinated Biphenyls, Dioxins, and Furans

Polychlorinated biphenyls (PCBs) are a large family of related manmade compounds; there are 209 distinct PCBs, which were produced by the Monsanto Corporation and sold mainly as seven different mixtures, under the trade name Aroclor. These compounds have high molecular weights and are oily liquids or solid waxy substances at room temperature. As a group, PCBs are chemically stable and nonflammable, and have low electrical conductivity. Because of these properties, they were widely used as insulating fluids in electrical equipment, such as transformers; General Electric (GE) was Monsanto's main customer for PCBs. PCBs were manufactured in the United States from 1930 through 1977.[28] Globally, about 1.5 million metric tons of PCBs were produced, and perhaps 20% to 30% of this amount ultimately found its way into the environment.[29]

Although PCBs were used in closed systems, they entered the wider environment in large quantities as industrial wastes and several of these now abandoned PCB-contaminated waste sites are federal Superfund sites. For example, two GE manufacturing plants in New York released up to 1.3 million pounds of PCBs into the Hudson River between 1947 and 1977.[30] In 2002, the EPA issued a detailed plan (a Record of Decision, ROD) justifying its intended remedial actions over a 40-mile stretch of the river; Phase 1 of the remedial work was completed in 2009, and Phase 2 is expected to be a five- to seven-year effort. The sediments of many rivers and lakes, including the Great Lakes on the U.S.–Canadian border, are contaminated with PCBs from industrial releases. Further south, the Sangamo capacitor manufacturing plant is estimated to have dumped 400,000 pounds of waste PCBs during operations from 1955 to 1977 into Lake Hartwell,

a 56,000 acre lake between South Carolina and Georgia, with significant sediment deposition occurring along a seven-mile stretch of Twelve-Mile Creek downstream of the plant.[31] The ROD for Lake Hartwell stipulates ongoing monitoring and public fish advisories restricting consumption of predator fish throughout the lake and all species nearer Twelve Mile Creek. Although modern regulations have curtailed these industrial releases of waste PCBs, accidental releases still occur from time to time when aging PCB-laden equipment fails or burns in a fire, releasing PCBs into the atmosphere.

The manufacture of PCBs also created a family of chemicals called dioxins as byproducts. *Dioxins* are a group of structurally related compounds, as are the *furans*, which are chemically similar to dioxins and often occur with them. The most toxic of the **dioxins and furans** is 2,3,7,8-tetrachlorodibenzo-*p*-dioxin, or TCDD. Dioxins, furans, and PCBs behave similarly in the environment and have been found to have mostly similar health effects.

Dioxins not only occur as byproducts in the production of PCBs but also of various other chemical processes involving chlorinated organic compounds. For example, dioxins were chemical byproducts in the manufacture of an herbicide—a chemical used to kill unwanted plants—known as 2,4,5-trichlorophenoxyacetic acid (2,4,5-T). As a result, dioxins were present as contaminants in 2,4,5-T. This herbicide in turn was one of two major ingredients in a defoliant (dubbed "Agent Orange" after its color-coded container) used by the U.S. military during the Vietnam War. A defoliant is a substance that causes the leaves to fall off plants; defoliants are sometimes used in war to deny cover to enemy combatants. The U.S. military sprayed Agent Orange widely in Vietnam from 1962 to 1971.[32] As a result, both U.S. soldiers and many Vietnamese were exposed to the dioxin that contaminated this defoliant.

Dioxins also appear in the waste streams of the pulp and paper industry whenever chlorine is used in the production processes, and dioxins can be produced when chlorinated plastic materials are burned. In a modern waste incinerator, temperatures are usually kept high enough to minimize the production of dioxin. However, any uncontrolled burning of ordinary household waste—or, for that matter, any fire in a home or office building—produces dioxins.

Dioxins have also been released into the environment through accidents. In 1972 and 1973, for example, waste oil, later found to be contaminated with dioxin, was spread on dirt roads to control dust in the town of Times Beach, Missouri, mysteriously sickening children and animals. The town was evacuated a decade later when soil samples taken in 1982 showed high concentrations of dioxin.[33] In 1999, elevated concentrations of PCBs in chicken feed, ultimately traced to recycled fat used by the feed manufacturer, sickened birds at several poultry farms in Belgium; for a short time, contaminated meat reached the food supply.[34]

Acute exposure to PCBs or dioxins causes **chloracne**, a painful and disfiguring skin condition that can last for a few months or for more than 15 years.[35] Chloracne has been documented in accident victims: for example, those who consumed rice oil contaminated by PCBs in a Japanese factory in 1968[36]; and those who lived near a chemical plant in Seveso, Italy, in 1976, when an explosion released a cloud containing dioxins and their chemical precursors.[35] Chloracne came to public attention in a political context with the dioxin poisoning in 2004 of the Ukrainian political leader Viktor Yushchenko.[37]

Today, the general population has ongoing low-level exposure to PCBs and dioxins, mostly from eating fish, meat, and dairy products, because these chemicals are persistent in sediments and soil and become magnified in animal tissues. Indeed, studies in more developed countries have documented that everyone carries low levels of dioxins and furans in his or her tissues.[29] Although PCBs are no longer in production, workers can be exposed when handling older electrical equipment. PCBs, dioxins, and furans are controlled, along with DDT and other organochlorine pesticides, under the Stockholm Convention on Persistent Organic Pollutants.

In humans and other mammals, PCBs, TCDD, and many other dioxins and furans have several health effects in common because these effects are mediated through a single biological mechanism with wide-ranging impacts.* Effects of TCDD documented in animals include liver damage, immunotoxicity, birth defects, reduced fertility, endometriosis, and cancer.[29] In studies of nonhuman primates, chronic PCB exposure has been shown to lower birthweight, affect memory and learning, and affect the immune and endocrine systems.[38] IARC classifies PCBs in Group 2A (probably carcinogenic to humans) and TCDD in Group 1 (carcinogenic to humans).[5]

Epidemiologic study of everyday exposures to PCBs and dioxins is challenging because these exposures are relatively low and are likely to occur along with exposures to other chemicals. However, several studies in the United States and Europe provide some evidence that these compounds affect human neurologic development, especially with in utero exposure.[29] Studies of cancer mortality among workers have linked PCB exposure to death from melanoma of the skin, lymphoma, brain cancer, and liver and biliary tract cancers.[39]

Polybrominated Diphenyl Ethers

Polybrominated diphenyl ethers (PBDEs) are a large group of related compounds with structures somewhat similar to those of PCBs and dioxins. However, in contrast to PCBs (whose use was industrial) and dioxins (which are accidental byproducts), PBDEs have been manufactured and sold in flame-retardant products. Flame retardants, which slow the ignition and spread of fire with the goal of reducing deaths and injuries, came into wide use in the 1970s. In a PBDE molecule, bromine atoms are substituted for

---

*Chemicals in this group exert their effects by binding to the aryl hydrocarbon (Ah) receptor protein; on the basis of this shared biological mechanism, these chemicals are sometimes referred to together as dioxin and dioxin-like compounds (Webster, T.F. & Commoner, B. Overview: the dioxin debate. In Schechter A, Gasiewicz T, eds. *Dioxins and Health*, [2nd edition], John Wiley and Sons. 2003:1-53.)

hydrogen atoms. PBDE compounds are named according to the number of bromine substitutions; most commercially produced PBDEs are penta-, octa-, or deca-BDEs (5, 8, or 10 bromine substitutions). On the whole, PBDEs are relatively high–molecular-weight compounds; they are generally not volatile, instead accumulating in dust or sediment; and they are lipophilic.[40] The large-scale synthesis of these chemicals was a relatively recent phenomenon, yet approximately 200,000 metric tons of brominated flame retardants were produced annually during the peak years of their production.[41]

PBDEs are used mostly in consumer products—penta-BDEs, phased out in 2004, were used mostly in fabrics (e.g., in children's pajamas) and foams (e.g., in mattresses). A different flame retardant, tris(1,3-dichloroisopropyl) phosphate (known as Tris), was in common use in foam products.[42] The octa- and deca-BDEs are used in plastics, both in consumer products (e.g., the plastic housings of televisions, computers, and other electronic devices) and in building materials.[43] PBDEs are not chemically bound to these plastic or textile materials, and thus they can move out of products,[40] entering the indoor environment from consumer products in use and entering the ambient environment when products are discarded.

PBDEs are now widespread in the environment. They have been measured in fish, shellfish, and fish-eating birds in the Baltic Sea, North Sea, Arctic Ocean, and Pacific Ocean,[44] and in seals and beluga whales in North American waters.[45] They have also been measured in humans. Indeed, a 1999 study found that the concentration of a set of PBDEs in the breastmilk of Swedish women had doubled every 5 years over the preceding 25 years.[46]

The human health risks of PBDEs at the low doses that most people experience are not well known. PBDEs have been shown to disrupt the thyroid hormone system; this is not surprising, given that their chemical structure is similar to that of thyroid hormones.[41,47] It has been suggested that because thyroid hormones play an important role in aspects of brain development

that are important to autism risk, PBDE exposure might be a risk factor for autism.[47] Mice exposed to PBDEs show learning and motor deficits.[45] As yet, the evidence on the carcinogenicity of these chemicals is too limited to make any judgment of their possible cancer risk.[45]

Neither penta- nor octa-PBDEs are still produced in the United States, and the EPA has disallowed resumption of production, although these chemicals can still be imported. Although there is no federal restriction on the use of deca-PBDEs, the EPA strongly recommends alternative compounds be considered and a number of states have enacted bans. In 1977, the Consumer Product Safety Commission banned the sale of children's garments made of fabric treated with Tris[48]; such fabric had been widely used in children's pajamas. Critics note that in addition to being hazardous, halogenated flame retardants shift the focus away from preventing fires and fire-related injuries through other means (e.g., fire-safe candles, child-resistant cigarette lighters, sprinklers, smoke detectors) and also that most deaths and injuries from fire are not due to flame, but to inhalation of carbon monoxide, other gases, and soot.[49]

Perfluorochemicals

A set of fluorine-containing chemicals called **perfluorochemicals** or **perfluorinated compounds (PFCs)** has been widely used since the 1950s in the production of coatings for carpets and fabrics, packaging materials for fast foods, and many other commercial applications and consumer products.[50] For example, PFCs have been used in the manufacture of some familiar brand-name products designed to repel water or stains or sticky food—Scotchgard (made by 3M), Stainmaster and Teflon (made by DuPont), and Gore-Tex (made by W. L. Gore and Associates). Perfluorooctanoic acid (PFOA) was the primary PFC used at the 3M facility, although other PFCs, such as perfluorooctane sulfonate (PFOS) were also produced.[51] Even though these chemicals have been used for over 60 years, concern about their associated health effects only emerged recently because the use of PFCs was not subject to toxicologic testing associated with the federal Toxic Substances Control Act in the late 1970s; PFCs had received blanket approval since they were already in commerce when the law was passed.[51]

Perfluorochemicals are now widely distributed in the natural environment and these compounds are perhaps the most persistent toxic substance yet created. Neither PFOS nor PFOA biodegrade in the environment by any known mechanism.[52] Perfluorochemicals bioaccumulate in individuals and biomagnify in ecosystems. Perfluorooctane sulfonic acid has been detected at low levels in the tissues of fish, fish-eating birds (including bald eagles), and marine mammals (including dolphins and seals) at locations in North America, Europe, and the Arctic and Pacific Oceans,[53,54] with higher concentrations reported in animals in more industrialized areas. More than a decade ago, when 3M scientists discovered PFOS in the livers of *unexposed* laboratory rats, they traced the source to fish meal that was an ingredient in the commercial rat food fed to the animals.[55] In contrast to BPA, cross-sectional analysis of 2003–2006 NHANES data found that higher exposure to perfluorochemicals was associated with *higher* family income.[25]

In an early study of nine retired 3M chemical workers, the mean half-life of PFOS in the body was estimated to be about 8.7 years.[55] PFOS and PFOA tend to bind to protein in the blood and circulate through the body. In fact, they may be repeatedly removed by the liver, excreted into the intestine in bile, and then reabsorbed from the intestine. (This is a well-known toxicokinetic process called enterohepatic cycling.) Fortunately, the human body appears to be more successful than the environment at eventually removing PFOA and PFOS substances, based on the most recent NHANES 2015-2016 data. The geometric mean serum PFOS level for the total population has decreased from 30.4 µg/L observed during the 1999-2000 survey to 4.72 µg/L with the 2016 data, and serum PFOA measurements from 5.21 µg/L then, to 1.56 µg/L in 2016.[24]

Ingestion of food and water is believed to be the major route of exposure today. The dietary sources of particular concern are fish and meat (because the chemicals bioaccumulate and biomagnify) and packaged foods (because the chemicals may migrate into food from packaging materials).[56] Drinking water supplies sampled near manufacturing and industrial sites and disposal areas have been found to contain elevated levels of both PFOS and PFOA. Another route of exposure involves inhalation of either particulate matter containing PFAS from soils or in dust or vapor phase PFC precursors.[57] The chemicals are also known to pass through the placenta and have been measured in breastmilk.[56]

Recent epidemiologic studies (refer to **Case Study The C8 Science Panel**) have found associations between exposure to PFOS and high cholesterol. Exposure to PFOA has been associated with decreased vaccine response, pregnancy-induced hypertension, thyroid disorders, high cholesterol, and testicular and kidney cancer, and assigned an IARC Group 2B classification.[57]

Initial efforts at the federal level to protect the public from exposure to PFCs involved the EPA adding PFOA and PFOS compounds to its list of unregulated contaminants of concern in drinking water in 2009 and setting preliminary drinking water health standards of 400 parts per trillion (ppt) for PFOA and 200 ppt for PFOS.[51] In 2016, the EPA reduced its advisory to a lifetime level for PFOA and PFOS in drinking water of 70 parts per trillion (ppt) separately or combined,[57] although no official national standard has been promulgated as of July of 2020.

Chemical companies also curtailed their use of PFOA and PFOS, partially in response to pending litigation as well as part of a voluntary agreement with the EPA to eliminate production of these compounds worldwide by 2015.[52] Unfortunately, the attempts by these companies to find a substitute fluorinated compound may still be a source for the release of PFOA into the environment since they often degrade and transform into PFOA over time. The alternatives, however, have been shown to be less bioaccumulative in the human body.[52]

The C8 Science Panel

The majority of the human health effects information reflected in the recent EPA technical documents concerning PFOS and PFOA came about in a rather unique way—as part of the settlement agreement from a large class-action lawsuit against DuPont, one of the original manufacturers of PFCs. The lawsuit spearheaded by environmental attorney Robert Bilott alleged that farmers and residents near DuPont's Washington Works plant in Parkersburg, West Virginia, were unknowingly exposed to PFOA released from the plant for years. The story of this lawsuit is the subject of the movie *Dark Waters*, released in 2019, starring Mark Ruffalo as Bilott. Part of the settlement required the formation of the C8 Science Panel, consisting of a team of well-respected epidemiologic researchers. (*C8* was the name for PFOA used by DuPont workers, referring to the number of carbons in its chemical make-up.).

Beginning in 2005, the C8 Science Panel conducted exposure and health effect investigations in the communities near the Parkersburg plant. The settlement stipulated that the Panel submit "Probable Link" reports to the court summarizing whether they found or did not find a link between exposure and disease. By the end of 2012, 17 Probable Link reports were filed, six of which concluded the probability of a link between exposure to C8 to: diagnosed high cholesterol, ulcerative colitis, thyroid disease, testicular cancer, kidney cancer, and pregnancy-induced hypertension.[1] Detailed descriptions of the epidemiologic studies conducted by the Panel have been published in peer-reviewed scientific journals that may be accessed from the C8 Science Panel website, http://www.c8sciencepanel.org/index.html.

1.   Data from C8 Science Panel. (n.d.). Retrieved July 10, 2020 from: http://www.c8sciencepanel.org /index.html

Ozone-Depleting Chemicals

Another group of synthetic organic chemicals can affect human health indirectly by depleting the Earth's stratospheric ozone layer. This layer of more concentrated ozone in the stratosphere absorbs some of the ultraviolet radiation in sunlight, protecting people and other animals from extreme exposure. The less effective screening out of UV-A and UV-B radiation, due to stratospheric ozone depletion, results in an increased risk of skin cancer. Fortunately, the ionizing UV-C radiation in sunlight is most effectively screened out by the stratospheric ozone layer, even in its depleted state.

In the stratosphere, all three forms of oxygen— the single atom (O), the familiar oxygen molecule (O_2) that animals use for respiration, and ozone (O_3)—are present in a state of dynamic equilibrium, such that ozone is constantly being created and destroyed. Certain chemicals, including chlorine (naturally present in the stratosphere at low concentrations), are involved on the destruction side of the equation.

In the era of synthetic organic chemicals, human beings have created large quantities of synthetic chemicals containing chlorine. When long-lasting, chlorine-containing gases are released into the air, they accumulate in the troposphere and over time are transported by air movements to the stratosphere, where they take on a more chemically reactive form.[58] This infusion of reactive chlorine upsets the natural balance in stratospheric chlorine chemistry, and the result is a net loss of ozone. The loss of stratospheric ozone has been more extreme over the South Pole (creating the "ozone hole") because of its unique weather conditions. Eventually, reactive chlorine gases are transported back to the troposphere, where they are removed from the atmosphere by precipitation.[58]

The predominant cause of stratospheric ozone depletion has been a family of chemicals called **chlorofluorocarbons (CFCs)**, a subgroup of halocarbons that contain chlorine, fluorine, and carbon in different combinations. These chemicals have been used mainly as refrigerants in air conditioners, as blowing agents in the creation of foam products, and as propellants in aerosol spray products. For a time, CFCs seemed the perfect chemicals: They have many uses; they are nontoxic and odorless; they are not flammable or corrosive; and they are chemically stable, producing no toxic breakdown products. Yet, precisely because CFCs are chemically stable, they last for many years in the lower atmosphere, with some eventually moving into the stratosphere. Two chlorinated solvents, carbon tetrachloride and 1,1,1-trichloroethane, play a lesser role in ozone depletion, as do some brominated compounds. The ozone-depleting halocarbons also act as minor greenhouse gases.

During the 1970s, springtime ozone concentrations in the stratosphere over Antarctica began to decrease slowly; in the 1980s, the decline sped up, and ozone concentrations reached their lowest point in the mid-1990s. The "ozone hole" is not quite a literal hole in the ozone layer but a region in which ozone concentrations are dramatically lower than elsewhere. Its areal extent is largest in late summer and early fall. From the mid-1990s, stratospheric ozone concentrations and the size of the ozone hole have changed little.[59] However, with controls in place from the Montreal Protocol, substantial recovery of stratospheric ozone is anticipated by about the middle of the 21st century.

The Montreal Protocol on Substances that Deplete the Ozone Layer, an international agreement, was opened for signatures in 1987 and went into force in 1989. Subsequent modifications, most recently in 1999, have made controls more stringent. A total of 197 nations, including the United States and other more developed countries as well as less-developed countries, have ratified the agreement.[60] The Montreal Protocol sets country-specific limits on the production and consumption of specific chemicals in terms of their ozone-depleting potential. For example, the U.S. no longer allows the use of the CFC-containing refrigerant freon in home and car air-conditioning systems. Despite the long timeline for success, the Montreal Protocol is a working example of international cooperation on an environmental health problem of global scale.

The preceding text has described several sets of synthetic organic chemicals that raise serious public health concerns—two developed for specific uses in industry (solvents, plasticizers/BPA),

and others that have had large-scale unanticipated impacts, either through their persistence in the environment (PCBs, PBDEs, PFCs) or through their depletion of stratospheric ozone (CFCs). Many of these chemicals appear near the top of the Agency for Toxic Substances and Disease Registry's (ATSDR) Substance Priority List (refer to **Table 6.2**). As described earlier, part of the federal Superfund law established the ATSDR as the lead agency to evaluate and rank hazardous

Table 6.2 Leading Chemicals and Metals on the ATSDR's 2019 Substance Priority List

2019 Rank	Substance Name
1	Arsenic
2	Lead
3	Mercury
4	Vinyl Chloride
5	Polychlorinated Biphenyls (PCBs)
6	Benzene
7	Cadmium
8-10, 15	Polycyclic Aromatic Hydrocarbons (PAHs)*
11	Chloroform
12	Aroclor 1260
13	DDT, P,P'-
14	Aroclor 1254
16	Trichloroethylene (TCE)
17	Chromium, Hexavalent
18	Dieldrin
19	Phosphorus, White
20	Hexachlorobutadiene

*Polycyclic Aromatic Hydrocarbons are discussed later in the context of fossil fuel combustion.
Data from Agency for Toxic Substances and Disease Registry. (2019). The ATSDR 2019 Substance Priority List. Retrieved from: https://www.atsdr.cdc.gov/spl/index.html#2019spl

waste sites for listing on the National Priority List. Part of this evaluation involves the creation of a list of substances that are most commonly found at sites on the NPL and which are determined to pose the most significant potential threat to human health due to their known, or suspected, toxicity and potential for human exposure.[61] Several other chemicals near the top of this list are the pesticides discussed in the last chapter. Most of the remaining substances are toxic metals with arsenic, lead, and mercury topping the list.

6.2 Toxic Metals

As a group, **metals**—elements that are shiny, are solid at room temperature (mercury is an exception), can be melted or formed using heat, and conduct electricity and heat—have proven extremely useful to human beings. Among the 30 or more metals that are routinely used in modern industry, six are described here (lead, mercury, arsenic, cadmium, chromium, beryllium), chosen for their substantial public health impacts. All but beryllium have high atomic weights and are commonly known as **heavy metals**.

Health Effects of Lead

Lead has long been known as a neurotoxicant, and it has both acute and chronic effects. Lead from leaded gasoline, and also from lead paint, is widespread in the environment, especially in soil and dust. Young children, of course, have greater incidental ingestion exposures to soil and dust than adults, primarily through hand-to-mouth behavior. Infants in utero and young children are especially vulnerable to lead's neurotoxic effects. This is partly because their nervous systems are still developing. Children also absorb a much higher percentage of ingested lead than adults, and absorption is further increased if a child's diet is deficient in iron and calcium. Lead is distributed throughout the body, causing a range of effects including kidney toxicity, anemia, hypertension, and reproductive effects. Because lead binds chemically at sites ordinarily occupied by calcium, it accumulates in bone and teeth, especially in children whose diets are low in calcium. A landmark 1979 health study[62] assessed

exposure by measuring lead in baby teeth that children had shed.

Today, the most common biomarker used to assess children's exposure to lead is the concentration in blood, usually referred to as **blood lead level (BLL)**, measured in micrograms of lead per deciliter of blood ($\mu g/dL$). It is generally recommended that children with BLLs greater than 45 $\mu g/dL$ undergo **chelation**, a painful treatment that increases the excretion of circulating lead. Because such a reduction in blood lead can mobilize lead stored in bone, multiple rounds of chelation are often required to bring down a child's blood lead level. Blood lead levels well below 45 $\mu g/dL$ can cause neurotoxic effects in children. In the United States, the Centers for Disease Control and Prevention (CDC) designates a **blood lead action level**, the blood lead level at which action should be taken to reduce a child's exposure; any concentration greater than 10 $\mu g/dL$ is considered an elevated blood lead level. The action level has dropped steadily through recent decades as lead's effects have been discerned at ever-lower levels. In the 1960s, the action level was 60 $\mu g/dL$, and it has been lowered several times since then:

1971: 40 $\mu g/dL$
1975: 35 $\mu g/dL$
1985: 25 $\mu g/dL$
1991: 10 $\mu g/dL$

Today, there is good evidence of harm below the current action level of 10 $\mu g/dL$. Indeed, the neurotoxicity of lead is the only noncancer effect that is generally considered to have no threshold. The EPA has declined to set a reference dose for lead, because any reference dose would depend on the assumption that a threshold exists.[63]

The health impact of lead exposure is often evidenced by a lower score on an intelligence test—a lower intelligence quotient, or IQ—an effect that has been documented in many studies. A 2006 review, for example, found that each 1-mg/dL increment in blood lead level is associated with an average decrement in IQ of 0.87 points.[64] More recent evidence suggests that the IQ decrement per $\mu g/dL$ of blood lead may actually be greater at lower blood lead levels.[65]

Of course, cognitive ability is more than just IQ, and lead's detrimental effects in several domains, such as memory, learning, and spatial ability, are well documented.[65] But even the simple deficit of a few IQ points becomes a sobering loss if we think at the population level rather than the individual level. An individual with an IQ of 130 or higher is usually considered gifted; and an individual with an IQ of 70 or lower is usually considered to be intellectually impaired to a degree that limits his or her independence and places demands upon the resources of society. Of course, these are not bright lines, and similarly, people cannot discern five-point differences in IQ in their acquaintances. But in principle, if the BLL of everyone in a population were increased so that everyone's IQ decreased by five points, the entire bell curve for IQ would shift five points downward. In a population of 100 million, such a shift would substantially reduce the gifted subgroup in the population (from 6 million to fewer than 3 million) while increasing the cognitively impaired subgroup (from 6 million to more than 9 million).[64] This effect is shown schematically in **Figure 6.5**.

Furthermore, lead's neurological impacts reach beyond the cognitive domain.[65] In various studies, lead exposure has been linked to reduced postural balance, increased risk of amyotrophic lateral sclerosis (ALS, also known as Lou Gehrig's disease), and changes in brain structure and function in adults. Chronic exposure can also damage peripheral nerves, causing symptoms known as "wrist drop" and "foot drop."[66,67] In children, exposure has been linked to greater risk of failure on a reading test at the end of the fourth grade, attention-deficit/hyperactivity disorder, and delinquent or violent behavior.

And finally, lead's impacts are more than neurological.[65] Higher blood lead levels have been linked to higher overall mortality, driven mainly by mortality from cardiovascular causes. The International Agency for Research on Cancer (IARC) has placed inorganic lead compounds in the category of probable human carcinogen; lead exposure has been linked to higher overall cancer mortality and lung cancer mortality using data from the ongoing NHANES series of studies. Lead damages the kidneys and causes high blood pressure. High lead exposure impairs fertility in men and has been linked, at least tentatively, to delayed sexual maturation in both girls and boys. Exposure has also

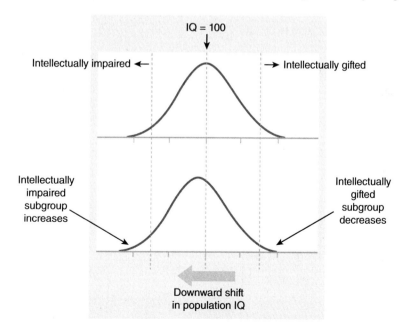

Figure 6.5 Decrease in intellectually gifted subgroup, and increase in intellectually impaired subgroup, with a small downward shift in population IQ.

Flint Water Crisis*

The Flint water crisis began as a simple cost-saving exercise. In 2012 to 2013, Flint officials began to investigate whether the city could save money by switching from its current water provider, the Detroit Water and Sewerage Department (DWSD) to a new source. Ultimately, they decided that Flint could build its own pipeline to connect to the Karegnondi Water Authority (KWA), with the goal of saving the region $200 million over the course of 25 years.[1]

In April of 2014, the city of Flint switched its water supply from the DWSD to the Flint River as an interim source while it's pipeline to KWA was being built. The Flint River had served as the water source for the city up until the 1960s. Within one month of the switch, citizens began to complain that water from their taps looked, smelled, and tasted foul. Despite complaints, city officials assured citizens that the water was safe. Unfortunately, it was not until a year later that a study by a team of researchers from Virginia Tech proved otherwise. The city's water had very high levels of lead. Water samples collected from 252 homes through a resident-organized effort indicated that citywide lead levels had spiked, with nearly 17% of samples registering above the federal "action level" of 15 parts per billion (ppb), the level at which corrective action must be taken. More than 40% measured above 5 ppb of lead, which the researchers considered an indication of a "very serious" problem.

The problems ultimately stemmed from the Flint water treatment plant, where officials failed to apply corrosion inhibitors to the water. The Flint River water that was treated improperly caused lead from aging pipes to leach into the water supply, leading to extremely elevated levels of the heavy metal neurotoxin.[1] The consequences from the Flint water crisis were devastating. It is estimated that between 6,000 and 12,000 children had been exposed to drinking water with high levels of lead. Due to the change in water source, the percentage of Flint children with elevated BLLs may have risen from about 2.5% in 2013 to as much as 5% in 2015.[2]

The water disaster called attention to the problem of aging and seriously neglected water infrastructure nationwide. But additionally, civil rights advocates characterized the crisis as a result of environmental racism (Flint's population is 56.6% African American per the 2010 census). Columnist Shaun King, for example, wrote that the crisis was "a horrific clash of race, class, politics and public health."[2]

1.   Denchak, M. (2018, November 8). *Flint Water Crisis: Everything You Need to Know*. Natural Resources Defense Council. Retrieved November 9, 2019 from: www.nrdc.org/stories/flint-water-crisis -everything-you-need-know

2.   Kennedy M. (2016, April 20). *Lead-Laced Water in Flint: A Step-By-Step Look at the Makings of a Crisis*. National Public Radio. Retrieved November 9, 2019 from www.npr.org/sections/thetwo-way/2016/04 /20/465545378/lead-laced-water-in-flint-a-step-by-step-look-at-the-makings-of-a-crisis

*Many thanks to Katie Van Valkinburgh for her assistance with this case study.

been linked to miscarriages and still birth.[67] Higher lead exposure also appears to be linked to greater risk of both tooth loss and periodontitis in adults.

The burden of lead exposure is not evenly distributed across U.S. society but rather falls more heavily on disenfranchised groups,[68] including the poor and African Americans. For example, NHANES data for 1999 to 2004 show that larger percentages of Black children and children on Medicaid fell into the higher exposure strata compared with percentages of White children and children not on Medicaid, respectively.[69] Disenfranchised populations are more likely to live near high-traffic roadways, to live in older housing, and to lack the resources to abate a lead hazard, as was demonstrated recently and dramatically in Flint, Michigan, (refer to **case study**). In addition, they are less likely to have access to information about lead's hazards and how to reduce their exposures.

Such social inequities in exposure and effect can be magnified over time, in a cycle of intergenerational effects.[70] Children in lower socioeconomic groups are likely to be more exposed to lead and are also less likely to have a diet high in iron and calcium. Thus, as a group, they bear a heavier burden of lead's cognitive, physical, and

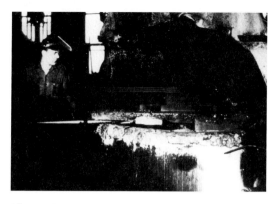

Figure 6.6 A laborer works with molten metal in a lead smelting plant in Cincinnati, Ohio, at mid-20th century.

Courtesy of CDC public Health Image Library. ID# 9527. Content providers CDC/Barbara Jenkins. Available at: http://phil.cdc.gov/phil/home.asp. Accessed October 15, 2012.

behavioral impacts. These burdens make it harder for them, as adolescents and young adults, to get a good education, acquire job skills, and stay out of trouble. And without these advantages, they are more likely to have pregnancies and rear children in settings where the risk of lead exposure is high. In contrast, children in higher socioeconomic groups generally continue to encounter conditions that insulate them, and ultimately their children, from lead's impacts.

In the more developed countries today, most adult exposure to lead, typically inorganic lead, occurs in occupational settings. For example, lead smelter workers are exposed to inorganic lead, although the acute awareness of lead's toxicity has led to generally effective controls on exposure in the United States and other more developed countries today. (**Figure 6.6** shows the type of uncontrolled exposure that was common in years past.) Workers in demolition activities, on the other hand, may have uncontrolled exposures to lead without knowing it.[62]

Health Effects of Methylmercury

Like lead, mercury is strongly neurotoxic. Mercury is also an unusual metal—liquid at room temperature and easily volatilized at warmer temperatures. This means that elemental mercury vaporizes and moves into the atmosphere. In the atmosphere, elemental mercury (also called metallic mercury) can be carried with air currents for some time, but eventually it settles out or is deposited with rain or snow. Once the elemental mercury reaches the Earth's surface, certain species of bacteria convert the mercury from its elemental form to a different form: an organic compound called **methylmercury**. This conversion occurs mostly in the sediments of oceans, lakes, and rivers (refer to **Figure 6.7**). Methylmercury is taken up by algae, the first link in an aquatic food chain that leads through zooplankton, small invertebrates, and fish of increasing size. Although methylmercury is not highly lipophilic, it does become concentrated in the muscle of fish, which in turn are eaten by people. Today, this pathway accounts for most of the general population's exposure to mercury from ambient environmental sources.* Methylmercury is found at highest concentrations in large predator fish, such as tuna or swordfish (in saltwater) and bass or pike (in freshwater). Infants in utero can be exposed to methylmercury consumed by the mother.

The neurological impacts of high prenatal exposure to methylmercury include mental retardation, cerebral palsy, deafness, and blindness.[71] These effects were made tragically clear in the 1960s in the area around Minamata Bay, Japan, where a local chemical company was using inorganic mercury as a catalyst in the manufacture of acetaldehyde. Unknown to the plant's operators, the process converted some of the inorganic mercury into methylmercury, which was then released with a waste stream into Minamata Bay.[72] The result was high levels of methylmercury in the sediments of the bay, and consequently high exposures to residents of the area, for whom fish was a dietary staple. Over a period of years, an entire cohort of children exposed in utero or after birth suffered the effects of this exposure. Exposure to methylmercury as an adult can also cause sensory and motor impairments,[71] but fetal and childhood exposures are much more damaging.

---

*In the past, a methylmercury fungicide was used to treat food grains, with tragic consequences in some populations, but this practice ceased in the 1970s.

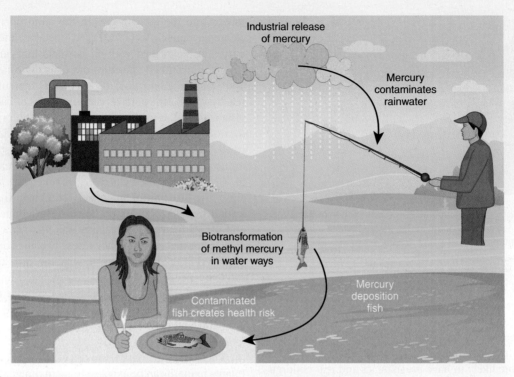

Figure 6.7 Methylmercury exposure.

Courtesy of CDC public Health Image Library. ID# 9527. Content providers CDC/Barbara Jenkins. Available at: http://phil.cdc.gov/phil/home.asp. Accessed October 15, 2012.

More recent epidemiologic research has documented subtle effects on neurological development of much lower exposures to methylmercury than those that occurred at Minamata. For example, one major study has been conducted in the Faroe Islands (located in the North Atlantic between Iceland and Norway), where the traditional diet includes whale meat and blubber. The range of exposures to methylmercury in the Faroe Islands overlaps with that in the United States but includes higher exposures. Using neuropsychological testing, researchers have measured subtle impacts of prenatal methylmercury exposure in Faroese children up to age 14 years, including effects on language, attention, and memory, and to a lesser extent on fine motor function.[73-75]

Findings like these raise concern for low-level exposure to all pregnant women and young children. But women and children in some demographic groups are at even greater risk because of their dietary habits. Canned tuna, an inexpensive

source of protein, is a staple in many households. Certain Native American groups depend heavily on fish that they catch themselves, sometimes from badly polluted waters—an unfortunate intersection of environmental pollution and traditional culture, often reinforced by poverty.[76] The EPA and the U.S. Food and Drug Administration (FDA) have jointly issued recommendations on fish consumption for women who are pregnant or might become pregnant. Public health advisories are also directed at recreational fishermen to inform them of health risks associated with mercury-contaminated game fish. Research is ongoing on the complex question of how best to balance the dietary benefits of polyunsaturated fatty acids found in fish against the risk of exposure to methylmercury.[77]

In contrast, most manufacturing workers' exposures are to either elemental mercury or inorganic mercury compounds (in which elemental mercury is combined with elements other than carbon). High-level inhalation exposure to mercury causes characteristic effects including excitability, delirium, and hallucinations.[78] In the 19th and early 20th centuries, this set of symptoms was familiar in hatters—makers of gentlemen's felt hats—who used inorganic mercury (specifically, mercuric nitrate) in processing the felt. This syndrome was brought vividly to life in the Mad Hatter of Lewis Carroll's *Alice's Adventures in Wonderland*.

The NHANES biomarker data pertaining to mercury reports blood mercury levels reflective of exposure to inorganic, ethyl, and methylmercury species. Total population averages for blood total mercury concentrations have not varied greatly during the past three NHANES sampling cycles from 2011 through 2016, with the most recent national average equal to 0.678 µg/L.[24] However, ethnicity trends show a remarkable variability, with Mexican Americans averaging the lowest levels, whereas Asians consistently exhibit levels more than twice the national average, with a blood total mercury level equal to 1.73 µg/L from the 2015 to 2016 data.[24]

A recent analysis of NHANES data has also identified another concern related to mercury, its potentially synergistic effect with PFAS substances. Researchers using NHANES data from 2009 to 2014 found high correlations between mercury and PFAS concentrations, meaning that these substances occurred within the same samples frequently. Since both PFAS and mercury have been associated with neurological development concerns, and exposure to both occurs primarily through the consumption of seafood, more epidemiologic research is encouraged that carefully considers this intertwined relationship.[79]

Arsenic, Cadmium, Chromium, and Beryllium*

Arsenic

Although arsenic may be most familiar as an acute poison, in fact, it is widespread in the Earth's crust. Its local abundance in the Earth varies widely, and in some areas, it is great enough to contaminate groundwater to a level that affects health. In

some areas of Northern New England, for example, groundwater is naturally high in arsenic. In Bangladesh, where there has been an effort in recent decades to reduce people's consumption of sewage-tainted surface waters by switching to deep groundwater, it has become clear that some groundwater contains arsenic at concentrations high enough to cause acute health effects. For a time, arsenic was used in the United States in a preservative (copper chrominated arsenic) for pressure-treated wood (e.g., in decks and play structures), but this practice has been phased out for residential uses.

Arsenic is released into the ambient environment mostly by metal smelters (especially copper smelters), by the burning of coal, and in tannery wastes. Arsenic is also an ingredient in pesticides that were widely used in the past, although much less common today. Workers in smelters and tanneries are exposed to arsenic, and neighbors of industrial facilities or hazardous waste sites may also be exposed. Arsenic has neurotoxic effects, and chronic exposure to arsenic is associated with skin cancer (basal and squamous cell carcinoma) and cancers of the lung, liver, bladder, kidney, and prostate. IARC classifies arsenic in Group 1 (carcinogenic to humans).

Cadmium

Cadmium, which often occurs with zinc or lead in the Earth's crust, is widespread in the environment, largely as a result of air pollution from the mining and smelting of these metals. Cadmium is

*Information about arsenic, cadmium, chromium, and beryllium comes mostly from three sources, which provide many of the same specifics: (1) Grandjean P. Health significance of metal exposures. In Wallace RB, Kohatsu, N., eds. *Maxcy-Rosenau-Last Public Health and Preventive Medicine* (15th ed.). New York: McGraw-Hill Medical; 2008. (2) Goyer RA. Toxic effects of metals. In Klaasen CD, ed. *Casarett and Doull's Toxicology: The Basic Science of Poisons*. New York: McGraw-Hill; 1996. (3) U.S. Agency for Toxic Substance and Disease Registry. *ToxFAQs for Arsenic, ToxFAQs for Cadmium, ToxFAQs for Chromium*, and *ToxFAQs for Beryllium*; all available at: www.atsdr.cdc.gov/toxfaqs/index.asp (accessed April 18, 2012).

used in metal plating and is present in the wastes of this industry. Workers in the mining, smelting, or metal-plating industries, among others, can be exposed to cadmium, as can those who live near industrial facilities or hazardous waste sites.

Exposure to cadmium is associated with chronic obstructive pulmonary disease and chronic kidney disease; the latter may cause skeletal changes, causing extreme bone pain, an unusual condition known by its Japanese name, *itai-itai* ("ouch-ouch"), because of an outbreak in Japan during the 1940s. Cadmium exposure has been clearly associated in epidemiologic studies with lung cancer. IARC classifies cadmium and cadmium compounds in Group 1 (carcinogenic to humans).

Chromium

Chromium occurs in several different forms. Chromium-III (trivalent chromium) is a common form and an essential trace nutrient; chromium-VI (hexavalent chromium) is rare in nature but is more often used in industry and is highly toxic. Chromium-VI is produced in industrial processes, including chrome plating, leather tanning, and the preserving of wood (in copper chrominated arsenic, as noted earlier). Workers in these facilities, as well as people living near hazardous waste sites, can be exposed. Hexavalent chromium damages the skin and has been linked to asthma and lung cancer. IARC classifies chromium-III in Group 3 (not classifiable as to carcinogenicity to humans) and chromium-VI in Group 1 (carcinogenic to humans).

Beryllium

Most exposure to beryllium occurs in the workplace; unlike the other metals described here, beryllium is not a common metal. It is extremely strong and lightweight and is used mainly in high-tech industries. Beryllium has been used to make fluorescent light bulbs; today, it is used mainly in the space and aircraft industries. Occupational exposure to beryllium can lead to acute or chronic lung disease and lung cancer. Chronic beryllium disease is a debilitating lung condition that bears some resemblance to lung diseases caused by dust and fibers, with scarring of lung tissue and severely impaired breathing. IARC classifies beryllium and beryllium compounds in Group 1 (carcinogenic to humans).

Nano-Scale Materials

Nanoparticles (or **nanomaterials**) are engineered particles less than 100 nanometers in diameter. That is, nanoparticles are in the same size range as the air pollutants known as ultrafine particulates (0.1 micron = 100 nanometers). **Nanotechnology** takes advantage of the fact that the physical and chemical properties of a given material are often different on a nanoscale, opening the door to a new world of products made from many different substances, including carbon-based materials and various metals. These technologies are being developed for industrial processes and a range of medical applications, including imaging methods and drug delivery systems.[80] The use of nanotechnology in consumer products is increasing rapidly and being marketed enthusiastically. In particular, nano-silver has been advertised as an antibacterial in a broad range of consumer products, including cosmetics, socks, undergarments, bedding, refrigerators, air purifiers, paint, flooring, hair straightening devices, toothbrushes, baby bottles, and water bowls for pets. A recent survey of products using silver nanoparticles found that 14% of them could release silver particles to the air when they were being used.[81]

Nanotechnology is still new, and so the health effects of nanoparticles have not yet been extensively studied, but there is reason for concern. Exposures can occur by all three major routes. Because of the large surface-area-to-volume ratio of these tiny particles, they are considered highly reactive and thus likely to induce an inflammatory response.[82] Like ultrafine particulates produced by combustion, nanoparticles penetrate deep into the lungs and can pass through the alveolar wall into the general circulation, perhaps making normal host defenses ineffective.[80,82] Animal studies have shown that nanoparticles can cross the blood–brain barrier and may be carried into sensory nerves.[80]

Some commercial nanoparticles are long, thin nano*tubes* which, like asbestos fibers, can cause toxicity specifically because of their shape.[80,82] As a result of their shape, carbon nanotubes cause inflammation through multiple mechanisms, activating an "inflammatory cascade."[80] In a study of surviving first responders in the World Trade Center disaster, carbon nanotubes were documented in the lung tissue of three of seven individuals and also in four of seven dust samples.[83] Given that carbon nanotubes would not have been common in commercial materials manufactured before 2001, it is posited that they were generated in the high-temperature combustion of airplane fuel. A great deal is yet to be learned about the health effects of nanoparticles, but what is known about exposures and systemic health effects suggests that some caution is warranted in adopting this new technology.

6.3 Hazards in the Workplace

Much of what we have learned about the health effects associated with exposure to chemicals and metals came at the expense of occupational workers. And this has been true for a long time. As far back as 400 BC, Hippocrates observed health effects among his patients associated with occupational exposure to metal working, and during the early centuries AD, Galen, Paracelsus, and Agricola recorded their concerns with the respiratory effects suffered by miners.[84] Ramazzini, considered the *father of occupational medicine*, investigated musculoskeletal hazards associated with the physical demands of various jobs, and was an early advocate for altering the job to better ensure the well-being of workers.[84] The health risks associated with exposure to specific substances emerged during the 1700s and 1800s, such as Pott's observation regarding soot as the cause of scrotal cancer among chimney sweeps or the identification of Mad Hatter's disease from exposure to mercury fumes. In the early 1900s, Hamilton published her concerns with both the health effects that would emerge with adding tetraethyl lead as an antiknock agent to gasoline, and the cases of jaw bone necroses among matchstick makers she observed associated with exposure to phosphorus, subsequently named *phossy jaw*.[84]

Like Ramazzini, Hamilton was a strong advocate for protecting workers' health and she was also a harsh critic of the manner in which industrial occupations went about business at the expense of their workers. In the case of phossy jaw, she argued that the matchstick industry had known of the risks for over 50 years but showed a callous disregard for their workers, primarily immigrants who should be happy to have the job and assume any risks associated with it.[84]

Passage of the Occupational Health and Safety Act (OSHA) in 1970 was a federal response that attempted to change this attitude that industrial productivity trumps workers' health. The aim of the law was to assure safe and healthful working conditions for men and women by providing resources for information, education, and training in the field of occupational health, including the establishment of the National Institute for Occupational Safety and Health (NIOSH) to conduct occupational-related research into safety standards. The Toxic Substances Control Act of 1976 was another federal effort to reduce hazardous exposures in the workplace but unfortunately did not retroactively address existing industrial substances such as the case with PFCs mentioned earlier. With occupational research and preventive efforts coming along only after the introduction of hundreds of potentially toxic substances, the result of this "business as usual" attitude is that occupational workers have often served as guinea pigs with known and elevated levels of exposure to many of the substances we now address as environmental hazards to the general population.

Occupational Fatalities

Dying on the job is obviously an extreme and distressing occupational hazard. There were 5,250 occupational fatalities reported in the United States in 2018, a rate of 3.5 deaths per 100,000 workers.[85] Jobs associated with the transportation and material moving occupations accounted for almost 30% of these fatalities in 2018, followed by jobs in construction and extraction. Half of all deaths involved a vehicle incident as the primary cause. Violence and other injuries by persons or animals caused 16% of all of the fatalities in 2018, a proportion equal to deaths caused by falls, slips, and trips among workers.[85] Wyoming, North Dakota, and Alaska had fatality rates three times greater than average, and occupational fatalities depict a clear geographic pattern with rates lower in the Northeast and West coast (refer to **Figure 6.8**).

Although these occupational statistics provide important information regarding worker mortality risks, they do not adequately capture the impact of exposures on the job that result in deaths from diseases common in the general population, such as cardiovascular disease or cancers. Medical records and death certificates rarely provide detailed occupational exposure information, and many of the exposures to plausible etiologic

agents may have occurred years prior to the development of the disease. Furthermore, in the United States, occupational records are infrequently linked to health records, especially among retired workers (with perhaps the exception of those who served in the Armed Forces).

In 1981, Doll and Peto published a study that characterized occupational cancer mortality risks showing that work exposures caused 4% of all cancer deaths and 12.5% of lung cancer deaths.[86] Almost 40 years later, these estimates are thought to woefully underestimate the true extent of risk from occupational exposure to carcinogens given that the IARC now lists almost 500 occupational agents (chemicals or exposure circumstances, such as second-hand smoke or exposure to diesel exhaust) as known or possible human carcinogens. More recent estimates have focused on the occurrence of occupationally associated cancers, rather than on mortality. In the United States in 2012, the most recent year

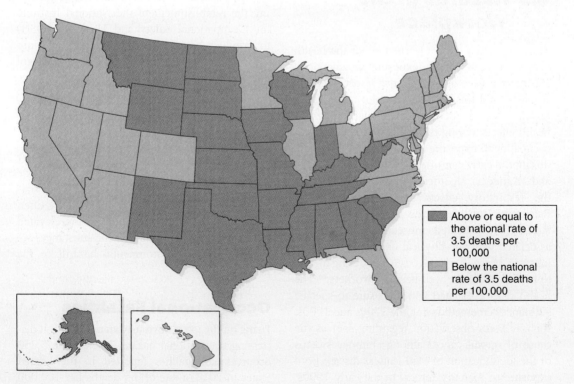

Above or equal to the national rate of 3.5 deaths per 100,000

Below the national rate of 3.5 deaths per 100,000

Figure 6.8 Map of U.S. 2018 fatality rates.

Data from Centers for Disease Control and Prevention. Fatal Injuries Charts. Retrieved from: https://wwwn.cdc.gov/NIOSH-WHC/chart/bls-fw?T=ZY&V=C&S=N00

available, between 45,000 to almost 92,000 new cancer cases were thought to be caused by past occupational exposures.[87]

An international assessment of work-related cancers, published in 2015, estimated that 666,000 fatal work-related cancers occur yearly, based on information from 2010 and 2011. This global occupational cancer assessment also suggests that a fifth of all lung cancers among men is associated with occupational exposures, and lung cancers account for more than half of all occupational cancers.[86] Radon as a major occupational cause of lung cancer among miners was observed hundreds of years ago and is discussed later in the context of coal and uranium mining. Today, asbestos is thought to be responsible for 55% to 85% of occupational lung cancers.[86]

Asbestos Fibers

In environmental health, the term *particulate* not only refers to irregularly shaped particles or dusts (classified by size as idealized spheres) but also to long, thin fibers; and *fibrosis* is a general term for scarring of the lungs in response to a physical irritant, with the formation of excessive fibrous tissue and a loss of flexibility that impairs breathing. It is workers who have typically sustained the highest exposures to particles and fibers. All miners are commonly exposed to naturally occurring silica (quartz) dust in the Earth's crust, and coal miners are also exposed to coal dust. Asbestos fibers (and cotton dust described next) are also important respiratory hazards to workers, and the public has some exposure to asbestos in building materials and various products.

Asbestos is a mineral fiber that is insulating, durable, and noncombustible. As a result, it has been widely used in building insulation and in products, such as brake linings, in which resistance to combustion is essential. Asbestos has been known for centuries, but it was only in the 20th century that it began to be mined on a large scale. There are three major types of asbestos (chrysotile, amosite, and crocidolite asbestos) as well as other minor types. Large deposits of

asbestos are located in South Africa, Canada, and elsewhere around the world.

Exposure to asbestos became widespread during the 20th century, and its effects have been experienced in an ever-widening circle that begins with miners who extract asbestos from the Earth. Workers have been exposed in industries that manufacture asbestos products, making brake linings or insulation products to be used in buildings, for example. Other workers have been exposed by using asbestos products on the job: auto repair workers, construction workers, and shipyard workers, among others. In the past, it was common for workers to carry fibers home on their clothing and bodies, exposing their families.

It was known by the late 1800s that exposure to asbestos damaged the lungs, and by 1930, the term **asbestosis** was being used in medical journals to describe a debilitating fibrotic lung disease.[88] By the 1940s and 1950s, asbestosis was well known to the Johns-Manville Company and other companies that manufactured asbestos, although they concealed this information from their workers and the government.[88] This deception culminated in a tangle of litigation and bankruptcies in the 1960s and 1970s.

Today, asbestos is well documented as a cause not only of asbestosis but also of lung cancer and mesothelioma. The lung cancer risks of asbestos exposure and cigarette smoking are synergistic; that is, the risk of exposure to both together is greater than the sum of their individual risks.[89] Long, thin asbestos fibers penetrate deep into the lungs, reaching the alveoli, and some even pass through lung cells to penetrate the chest cavity. Similarly, ingested fibers can ultimately reach the abdominal cavity. Asbestos fibers that escape the lungs or gastrointestinal tract can cause **mesothelioma**, a cancer of the pleura (the membranes that coat the outsides of the chest organs and the inside of the chest cavity) or the peritoneum (a similar membrane in the abdominal cavity). Mesothelioma is caused almost exclusively by asbestos,[90] and for this reason, it is essentially a marker of exposure to asbestos—in public health terms, a **sentinel illness**.

Mesothelioma is considered uniformly fatal, and death usually occurs within a relatively short time after diagnosis.

Over the 40 years from 1968 through 2007, U.S. deaths with asbestosis as the underlying cause rose steadily and then plateaued (see **Figure 6.9**). Nationwide data on deaths from mesothelioma as the underlying cause are available through 2015, and mesothelioma deaths consistently outnumber asbestosis deaths five to one. Deaths from asbestos-related lung cancer do not appear in the graph.

Although the regulation of asbestos lagged behind the medical understanding of its hazards, workplace controls have been in place since the 1970s in the United States, as well as in other more developed countries. Sadly, the manufacture of asbestos products has shifted to less-developed countries; although a movement to ban asbestos has gained a toehold in India, researchers project that more than 1 million asbestos-related deaths may occur there.[91,92] It is estimated that approximately 7 million metric tons of asbestos have been used in building materials in India since 1960.[93] Asbestos fibers can be released through wear and tear, demolition, or earthquakes. In New York, asbestos was found at concentrations of up to 4% in dust samples after the collapse of the World Trade Center.[93]

Various manmade mineral fibers—of aluminum silicate, ceramic, or glass—have replaced asbestos in most uses since the health hazards of asbestos became clear. IARC has categorized such fibers in Group 2B (possibly carcinogenic to humans) or Group 3 (not classifiable as to carcinogenicity to humans).[5]

Cotton Dust

Historically, cotton mill workers in the more developed countries were exposed to high concentrations of airborne cotton dust, resulting in a fibrotic lung disease called **byssinosis**, also known as **brown lung**. Despite its name, cotton dust may contain not only cotton but also bacteria or fungi, soil, pesticides, and other contaminants. Byssinosis was well known to workers in the 1940s, but U.S. industry resisted regulation for many years; exposures declined dramatically after a federal standard was promulgated in 1978.

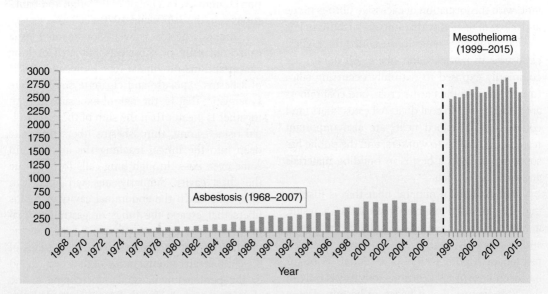

Figure 6.9 Deaths with asbestosis or mesothelioma as underlying cause.

Data from Mortality multiple cause-of-death data from National Center for Health Statistics, National Vital Statistics System. Population estimates from U.S. Census Bureau; see Appendix (www2a.cdc.gov/drds/WorldReportData /Appendix.asp) for information about data sources, methods, ICD codes, and limitations for general caution regarding inferences based on small numbers of deaths. Reference Number: 2012F01-01.

Byssinosis is a disabling disease but is not highly fatal. In 1995, for example, the Occupational Safety and Health Administration (OSHA) estimated that 35,000 individuals alive at that time were disabled by byssinosis,[94] yet the Centers for Disease Control and Prevention (CDC) has estimated that byssinosis was the underlying cause of only about seven deaths a year during the mid-1990s.[95]

In less-developed countries undergoing rapid industrialization, byssinosis is a common occupational disease. In China, for example, a cumulative incidence of byssinosis of 24% over a 15-year period (1981-1996) was documented among textile workers.[96] In India, the prevalence of byssinosis was estimated at 30% and 38% in two different groups of textile mill workers around the turn of the 21st century.[97]

Asthma-Causing Agents in the Workplace

Certain hazards from organic compounds, metals, and physical agents such as dusts or fibers—are known as causes of **occupational asthma** (asthma caused by an exposure at work) among industrial workers. One common cause of occupational asthma among industrial workers is a set of chemicals called isocyanates. They are used as paint-hardening agents, with the result that paint sprayers are exposed in various work settings and also as the raw materials for polyurethane foam and various adhesives and coatings.[98-100] Other substances found in the workplace that are known to cause or aggravate asthma include flour and wood dust; organic compounds used as cleaning agents; metal-working fluids, iron welding fumes, and solder flux (the substance used to promote joining); aluminum (e.g., in solder); chromium and nickel (used in electroplating); latex in gloves; and gluteraldehyde (in sterilizing agents).[99,100] Working as a printer, baker, sawmill worker, metal processing plant worker, spray painter, hairdresser, welder, or farmer is associated with increased asthma risk.[101,102]

Nonrespiratory Occupational Hazards

The physical demands of many jobs are responsible for a majority of the nonfatal, but severe occupational injuries that occur in the U.S. workplace. In 2018, more than 40% of all reported severe injuries involved overexertion and bodily reaction, or falls, trips, and slips, resulting in serious sprains, strains, tears, soreness, pain, bruising, or contusions. Other severe injuries include fractures, cuts, and lacerations. Overall, in 2018, the rate for severe injury or illness was 89.7 per 10,000 workers.[85]

Less dramatic than these acute outcomes are the chronic impacts of exposures to vibration or repetitive work. A worker who uses a jackhammer experiences vibration throughout his or her body, but especially in the hands and arms. Over time, such vibration can damage nerves and blood vessels in the fingers, with a loss of strength in the grip.[103] Workers who do repetitive tasks (e.g., on a production line or keyboard) may experience musculoskeletal disorders, including tendinitis or carpal tunnel syndrome, in which inflamed tissues press on nerves, causing pain and weakness in the hands.[104] Back pain, which can be related to many different activities, is a common concern among workers. Hearing loss is also one of the main less severe, nonfatal conditions associated with the physical demands of the workplace.

Noise

Noise is sometimes defined as unwanted sound (see the following sidebar titled, "About Sound"), but from the public health perspective, it is more useful to define noise as sound that can damage hearing or otherwise harm health. The full complexities of the human ear are beyond the scope of this text, but in simple terms, when sound waves in the air strike the eardrum, they are translated first into vibrations in a series of three tiny bones and then into vibrations in the fluid inside a snail-shaped structure called the *cochlea*. The cochlea is lined with special cells, which are called *hair cells*, because each one is topped by a cluster of tiny hair-like structures (a *hair bundle*). When vibrations in the cochlear fluid cause a hair bundle to move, it translates this physical energy into a signal to the hair cell, which in turn sends a nerve impulse to the brain, which interprets the sound (e.g., identifying it as a barking dog). Most hearing loss due to excessive noise exposure occurs through damage to the tiny hair bundles in the cochlea. The "hairs" in a healthy hair bundle stand upright in neat rows; in contrast, those in a hair bundle damaged by excessive noise are splayed and flattened. Such damage to a hair bundle is permanent—it cannot be repaired—and if enough hair bundles are damaged, hearing loss becomes noticeable.

The **volume threshold** (measured in decibels) at which sound can be perceived is different at each frequency; hearing loss appears as an upward shift in the threshold at which sound of a certain frequency can be perceived (**threshold shift**). It has been known for some time that hearing loss can be caused by noise exposure—not only a long-term exposure, such as working for 20 years in a canning factory, but also a brief exposure to a very loud noise, such as an exchange of gunfire at close range—and that such hearing loss can be permanent. Excessive noise exposure can also cause **tinnitus**, a continuous ringing, roaring, or other sound in the ears, which can be very distressing. Like threshold shift, tinnitus can be permanent.

Those who work in noisy environments (e.g., factory workers, ground crews at airports, farmers using tractors, or other machinery) are at risk of noise-induced hearing loss. In the 1999 to 2004 NHANES, respondents were asked whether the noise in their workplaces was loud enough that they "had to speak in a raised voice to be heard." In several industrial sectors—rubber/plastics/leather, lumber/wood products, metal, and repair and maintenance—a large share of respondents (45% or more) answered yes.[105] Industrial noise and cigarette smoking have synergistic effects in inducing hearing loss.[106] Rock musicians create their own noisy work environment: Mick Jagger (of the Rolling Stones), Mark Knopfler (of Dire Straits), and

About Sound

Sound is a form of physical energy, like vibration or radiation. Sound energy radiates outward from a source in waves, much as waves spread out when a rock is dropped into water. Sound has two important characteristics—frequency and intensity—and what we perceive as "loudness" has to do with both of these traits. *Frequency* is the number of complete wave cycles per unit of time, and higher frequency corresponds to higher pitch. Frequency is measured in Hertz (Hz; cycles per second). *Intensity* corresponds to the amplitude of the waves (the distance between trough and peak), and greater amplitude corresponds to greater pressure. Intensity is measured in **decibels (dB)**. The decibel scale is logarithmic: A 1-decibel increase in sound represents a tenfold increase in the intensity of the sound. Because most environmental sounds are made up of many different sound frequencies, composite decibel scales, which weight frequencies in different ways, are used to assess them. The scale most often used in assessing human perception of environmental noise is known as the A-weighted decibel (dBA) scale. The decibel scale measures sound relative to the hearing threshold of a healthy young person.

other rock stars have spoken out about their noise-induced hearing loss.[107,108]

The CDC estimates that the proportion of hearing difficulty among currently employed workers between 2004 to 2013 was 11.4%, with agricultural, forestry, and fishing workers having the highest rate of 18.5% of employed workers. The mining industries had the second-highest proportion during these years, with 16.6 percent of their workforce. About 14% of both construction and manufacturing workers had hearing difficulties.[85] Based on data for the four-year period from 2004 to 2007, the average annual incidence of noise-inducing hearing loss was 2.8 per 10,000 full-time workers, and this study identified animal slaughtering (excluding poultry) with a strikingly elevated annual incidence rate of 82 per 10,000 workers.[109] Annual incidence of hearing loss in the range of about 50 to 65 per 10,000 was noted in other types of foundries and also in fiber, yarn, and thread mills.

In occupational settings, it is sometimes possible to enclose or muffle sources of noise. However, in many situations, the only feasible way to reduce noise exposure and conserve hearing is by individual use of personal protective equipment, such as noise-blocking earplugs or earmuffs. NIOSH has set a recommended exposure limit for noise in the occupational setting—representing a time-weighted, 8-hour average—at 85 dbA.[110]

Military service has been linked to risk of hearing loss: Among U.S. adults 20 to 69 years of age, the prevalence of noise-induced threshold shift is about twice as great among those who have served in the armed forces (22.2%) as among those with no history of service (11.5%).[111] Similarly, the prevalence of tinnitus among adult men who are veterans of the Iraq and Afghanistan conflicts is higher (11.7% overall) than among nonveterans (5.4%).[112]

Occupational noise affects more than just hearing. In the workplace, noise that leads to ringing in the ears has been linked to higher frequency not only of accidents and injuries but also of ordinary lapses in memory, attention, or perception that are sometimes referred to as cognitive failures.[113] And, using the very large NHANES dataset from 1999 to 2004, chronic exposure to occupational noise has been linked to coronary heart disease, angina (chest pain caused by inadequate blood supply to the heart), and heart attack; these links are particularly strong in people under 50 years of age, in men, and in smokers.[114]

Light During the "Biological Night"

One more feature of modern life—extending the light hours each day through the use of artificial lighting, thereby reducing the number of dark hours each day—is now understood to have negative impacts on health. Throughout the world, but especially in the more developed countries, the hours after sunset are well lit, and one result is that many people work evening or night shifts. In 2004, among U.S. workers, alternate-shift

workers made up 51% of 16- to 19-year-old workers, and 16% of those 20 years of age and older.[115] Most alternate-shift workers worked either an evening or night shift, but smaller subgroups worked rotating or split shifts or had irregular schedules arranged by their employers. Alternate-shift work was more prevalent among men than women and among part-time workers than full-time workers, and was common in industries ranging from durable-goods manufacturing to finance to real estate to food services.[115]

IARC has designated "shift-work that involves circadian disruption" as a Group 2A carcinogen (probably carcinogenic to humans).[116] The term **circadian** refers to the cycles of roughly 24 hours that occur in various physiological processes, reflecting organisms' adaptations to the fundamental cycle of day and night. Taken as a whole, research in humans and lab animals links exposure to light at night with suppressed production of the hormone melatonin (which modulates sleep/wake patterns and whose production normally peaks during nighttime sleep), leading to increased risk of, and promotion of, tumors.[116,117] In addition, lower breast cancer risk has been linked to longer sleep time in prospective, individual-level epidemiologic studies; and an ecologic study of countries worldwide has found higher breast cancer incidence where there are higher levels of light at night.[118]

Finally, experiments in rodents have demonstrated that exposure to light during the normal dark period—analogous to the experience of nurses and other night shift workers—is associated with eating an increased proportion of calories during the normal dark period and also with an increase in body mass index.[119]

Reproductive Occupational Hazards

Shift-work has also been identified as a reproductive hazard associated with the work-place, as circadian dysregulation is linked to irregular menstrual cycles, endometriosis, infertility, miscarriage, low birth weight or preterm delivery.[120] Radiation exposure is another physical hazard known to cause miscarriage or act as a **teratogenic agent** (causing birth defects) that occurs in occupational settings, such as among X-ray technicians, dental hygienists, and imaging laboratory workers.[121] In addition to these physical hazards, the occupational setting may expose workers to other infectious or chemical types of teratogenic agents or substances that harm the reproductive system. For example, maternal infection with rubella is linked to several birth defects including cataracts, deafness, and heart defects. Spermatogenesis can be impaired by serious infections. Several healthcare occupations involve exposure to infectious agents, although social workers, teachers, butchers, and animal handlers also face exposure to infectious agents.[121]

The reproductive risks associated with the occupational chemical exposures discussed previously are highlighted in the following section. Virtually all organic solvents are known to harm the reproductive system.[121] The NIOSH warns employees that solvents increase the chances of having a miscarriage, stillbirth, preterm birth, a low–birth-weight baby, or a baby born with a birth defect. Many organic solvents are also known to pass into breast milk.[122] Similarly, chemicals that function as endocrine disruptors are associated with adverse reproductive outcomes. For example, phthalate plasticizers have been shown to disrupt ovarian function in mice at doses equivalent to human exposure related to phthalate coatings on certain medications.[121]

Reproductive risk was one of the first worries regarding persistent chemicals, when Carson described the thinning of eagle egg shells associated with DDT. Although pesticides were discussed elsewhere, it is worth noting here that agricultural workers, both males and females, face a variety of reproductive risks associated with their exposures not only to persistent pesticides such as DDT but also to dioxins from the manufacture of pesticides. Risks from pesticides include infertility, miscarriage, small-for-gestational age, preterm delivery, low birthweight, and stillbirth.[121] Epidemiologic evidence associated persistent, flame retardant PBDE chemicals with

damaging male reproductive hormone production.[121] One of the confirmed associations determined for PFOA linked community exposure to pregnancy-induced hypertension,[57] a risk factor for prematurity and low birthweight. Also, the co-occurrence of mercury with PFOA in NHANES population samples was discussed earlier as potentially increasing neurological risks during in utero development.[79] Worker exposure has the potential to be higher than these risks observed among the general population.

The reproductive risks associated with lead are profound, and lead is still a significant occupational exposure. Lead has been associated with miscarriage and premature birth in human studies.[121] Other metals that pose potential human reproductive risks include nickel, cadmium, mercury, and possibly arsenic. Animal studies have also implicated silver nanoparticles with reproductive and developmental toxicities, such as delayed cognitive behavior.[121] Detection of silver nanoparticles in the testes, the placenta, and breast milk following injection has raised concern about their ability to migrate and become bioavailable. Titanium and silver concentrations associated with nanoparticle ingestion have also recently been associated with neural tube defects in offspring.[121] **Figure 6.10** depicts these various categories of occupational reproductive hazards.

6.4 Management of Hazardous Products and Byproducts From Manufacturing

Exposures to the products and byproducts of manufacturing are unevenly distributed, both geographically and socially. This is true of the familiar industrial burdens of resource extraction, manufacturing, and waste disposal. It is true of chemical burdens measured in people and in their microenvironments. And it is true on a global scale, where economic disparities encourage the

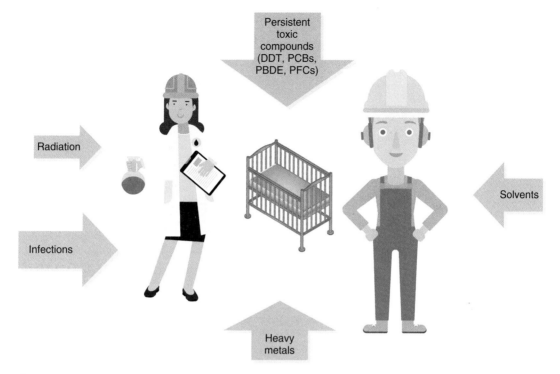

Figure 6.10 Contributors to occupational reproductive risks.
© Visual Generation/Shutterstock; © HappyPictures/Shutterstock

export of hazardous work from more-developed to less-developed countries.

Industrial Pollution and Workplace Exposures in the United States

A large amount of research literature has shown social disparities in exposure to industrial pollution in the United States: both a greater burden on people of color than on Whites and a greater burden on the poor than on the well-to-do. For example, Navajo workers and communities have historically borne the brunt of environmental pollution and occupational hazards associated with U.S. uranium mining, and more than half of U.S. coal is mined in two of the country's poorest states, West Virginia and Kentucky.[123-125] Several studies have documented differential exposure of African Americans to occupational hazards in industry.

An important early study of coke oven workers, for example, indicated that African American men were more likely to hold undesirable jobs at the top of the oven, and this was reflected in their higher exposures to the hazardous chemicals being driven off as fumes.[126]

Outside of the occupational setting, early studies of social disparities in exposure to environmental hazards, undertaken in the 1970s, focused mainly on urban air pollution after the passage of the Clean Air Act in 1970[127-133]; most uncovered both economic and racial disparities. A later nationwide study found that for the 1970 to 1984 period, poor and non-White populations had higher exposures to total suspended particulates, and that the race gap was wider and more consistent than the income gap.[134] Still another analysis focused on interactions between race and poverty, documenting wide disparities in exposure to industrial air pollution between poor non-White populations and nonpoor White populations.[135]

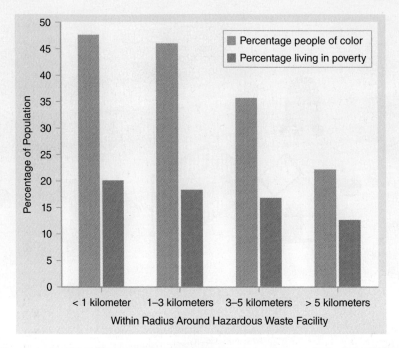

Figure 6.11 Demographic disparities in residential proximity to hazardous waste facilities in the United States, 1990.

Data from Bullard R, Mohai P, Saha R, Wright B. Toxic Wastes and Race at Twenty: 1987–2007. United Church of Christ, Justice & Witness Ministries. 2007; Table 3.1. Available at: www.ejrc.cau.edu/TWART%20Final.pdf. Accessed April 17, 2008.

Through much of the 1980s and 1990s, attention to social disparities in exposure to environmental hazards focused on the disposal of hazardous wastes. In the late 1970s, waste oil contaminated with PCBs was illegally dumped along more than 200 miles of roads in several counties in North Carolina. The State, faced with disposing of a large quantity of PCB-contaminated soil, selected a site— over protest—in a locale with high poverty and a mostly African American population. The planned waste site went through, but a North Carolina congressman called for the U.S. General Accounting Office* (GAO) to examine the question of bias in the siting of hazardous waste landfills. The GAO's 1984 report, a key document in the nascent social movement for environmental justice, documented that three of the four large off-site hazardous waste landfills in the southeastern states were sited in poor,

largely African American communities.[136] The GAO study spurred a nationwide assessment by activists, published in 1987, which reported that zip codes hosting hazardous waste sites had a higher non-White population and, less strikingly, lower income than other zip codes.[137] A 2007 update to the 1987 study, using census data from 1990 and 2000, reported the persistence of this inequity: The proportion of the population made up of people of color, as well as the proportion living in poverty, declined with increasing distance from a hazardous waste facility (see **Figure 6.11**).[138]

The decades following publication of the GAO report have produced many studies, most documenting a differential burden of active and abandoned hazardous waste sites, industrial pollution, or industrial facilities on poor and non-White communities in the United States.[139,140] For example, a 2009 analysis found that industrial facilities and Hispanic populations in Orange County, California, were clustered in the same census tracts.[141] Across Texas cities,

---

*The GAO, renamed the General Accountability Office in 2004, is the investigative arm of Congress.

Hispanic newborns and non-Hispanic Black newborns were found to live in neighborhoods with higher toxic industrial air pollution than non-Hispanic White newborns.[142] Zoning laws can contribute to social disparities in exposure because disenfranchised populations are more likely to live in neighborhoods zoned to allow noxious land uses, resulting in environmental burdens.[143] For example, the burdens associated with waste facilities may include noise, vibration, exhaust, risk of pedestrian injuries from truck traffic, and even illegal dumping of wastes.[144]

The Global Disparity in Protections for Workers

Striking disparities in occupational health risks are apparent on an international scale. Exposures to asbestos and cotton dust, now dramatically decreased in the more developed countries, are on the upswing in less-developed countries. Agate grinders in India work without protections and get silicosis—incurable, progressive, and fatal—after 5 to 10 years of work.[145] And some more developed countries, including the United States, are sending hazardous wastes overseas for processing. This practice of exporting materials for recycling creates jobs in less-developed countries, but most are very hazardous jobs with little or no protection provided for workers.

For example, **shipbreaking**—the dismantling of oceangoing vessels to obtain scrap metal—now occurs mostly on the shores of India and Bangladesh, where there is a market for scrap metal and its price is kept low by the lack of protections for workers. Approximately 25,000 workers at Chittagong in Bangladesh and about 40,000 at Alang in India manually dismantle ships that are run aground on the beach at high tide (see **Figure 6.12**).[146] As of 2009, approximately 500 to 700 large ships each year, and perhaps 3,000 ships per year in total, are being dismantled, and unless worker protections are imposed, the practice is likely to continue as a steady stream of ships reach retirement age.[147] Workers labor without protective gear and use equipment that is not maintained. They suffer falls and physical injuries

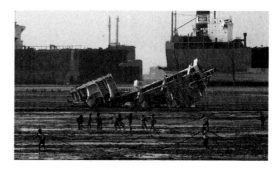

Figure 6.12 Manual laborers break down beached ships on the shore of Bangladesh.
Courtesy of Pierre Claquin.

and are exposed to noise, heat, explosions, fire, and smoke; asbestos; lead and mercury; organic tin compounds formerly used as antifouling agents in marine paints; PCBs; and dioxins from the burning of plastics.[148] It takes about 6 months to take apart a ship by hand, as opposed to about 2 weeks in a mechanized U.S. facility,[146] in which hazardous materials are removed, and useful equipment and valuable materials are salvaged before scrapping begins.[149] In 2012, a tanker ship rechristened *Oriental Nicety*—formerly the *Exxon Valdez*, the source of the 1989 oil spill on the Alaskan coast—was sold for shipbreaking on the Indian coast.[150]

In much the same way, many used computers, after being placed in recycling programs by their owners in more developed countries, are sold in batches and end up being manually dismantled by unprotected workers in less developed countries. (Many others are simply stockpiled or disposed of as trash.) Like the outsourcing of shipbreaking, this practice is driven by the cost of protections for workers in the United States and other more developed countries. In contrast, in China or India, it is often members of an informal labor sector, working without protections, who are exposed to lead, hexavalent chromium, mercury, cadmium, and flame retardants as they break down computers and extract valuable metals from printed circuit boards.[151] It is estimated that the 27 European Union countries produce 8.3 million to 9.1 million metric tons of **electronic waste** or **e-waste**, and the United States produces 2.6 million metric tons, each year; and that 50% to 80% of electronic

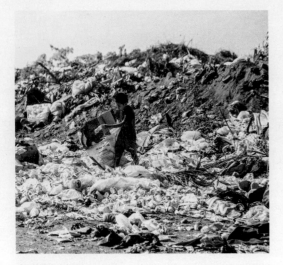

Figure 6.13 E-Waste.

Hermes Rivera/Unsplash.

waste collected for recycling in the United States is exported.[152] The World Health Organization has recently issued an international alert to raise awareness regarding the special vulnerability of children related to e-waste exposure.[153] Much of their risk derives from their developmental susceptibilities to metal toxicities as unsafe recycling activities introduce these toxic agents into their environment's soil, water and food. Unfortunately, many children also receive direct contact with the hazardous components of e-waste as they work alongside their families (refer to **Figure 6.13**)

The Basel Convention on the Control of Transboundary Movements of Hazardous Wastes and Their Disposal is an international agreement that provides a basis for managing the trade in hazardous wastes, including outdated electronics and defunct ships. The United States signed the convention in 1990, but as of 2020 had not approved or ratified it. Some 179 other nations, including the United Kingdom, Germany, and other European nations, have approved or ratified the convention.

Managing Industrial Pollution

The U.S. regulatory framework for the control of industrial pollution, including hazards in the industrial workplace, is an amalgam of laws that have been passed, amended, and reamended over a period of decades. It seems most useful to describe this framework as moving "upstream" in a conceptual sense, beginning with provisions that seek to remediate the effects of past practices and ending with approaches that attempt to head off future hazards.

As described previously, the law known colloquially as **Superfund** was originally passed in 1980 as the Comprehensive Environmental Response, Compensation, and Liability Act (CERCLA; "circla"), and then substantially amended in 1986 as the Superfund Amendments and Reauthorization Act (SARA). This legislation was a response to the widespread problem of hazardous wastes originating from inactive or abandoned industrial sites (see **Figure 6.14**). Superfund created procedures to assess and remediate the pollution at sites, set criteria for identifying parties to be held financially responsible for site cleanup, and established a fund (the "Superfund") to pay for cleanup if no responsible party could be identified.

Hazardous wastes from industry are regulated under the Resource Conservation and Recovery Act (RCRA; "rick-rah"), originally passed in 1976 and substantially amended in 1984. RCRA's provisions apply to any waste meeting one of two criteria. It may be a type of waste listed by the EPA: wastes from a set of common industrial or manufacturing processes; wastes from specific

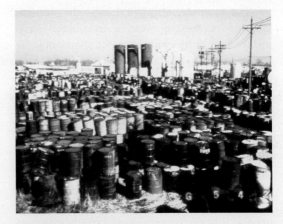

Figure 6.14 Drums of toxic wastes litter a Superfund site in this undated photo.

Courtesy of CDC Public Health Image Library. ID# 1193. Content provider: CDC. Available at: http://phil.cdc .gov/phil/home.asp. Accessed October 15, 2012.

industries, including petroleum refining and the manufacture of pesticides; and certain unused chemical products when they are discarded (e.g., pesticides). Or, it may meet the definition of a **hazardous waste** under RCRA: any waste that is ignitable, corrosive, reactive (chemically unstable), or toxic, as defined by specific criteria.

RCRA incorporates two major types of requirements. First, it requires the use of a "cradle-to-grave" manifest system, discussed in Chapter 3, to track hazardous wastes from the point of generation through transportation and ultimately treatment, storage, or disposal. Second, RCRA sets performance standards and permitting procedures for **hazardous waste landfills** and underground storage tanks. RCRA also includes provisions to promote the recycling of hazardous wastes and to minimize their production. RCRA's provisions not only deal with industrial wastes but also with municipal trash (described later in the context of daily life in communities). In addition, RCRA regulates the underground disposal of liquid wastes, mostly from the oil and gas industries, by injection into deep wells.

Several major laws govern the handling of manufacturing wastes—most of which are liquids or sludges—as they are produced. Industrial discharges of chemicals to outdoor air are regulated under the Clean Air Act. As will be described further in the context of energy production, ambient standards have been established for a small set of Criteria Air Pollutants related mostly to the burning of fossil fuels, and emissions standards have been set for a few hazardous air pollutants, which are less common but more toxic. Emissions from manufacturing facilities are subject to both sets of standards.

Today's Clean Water Act began in 1948 under another name and has been shaped by amendments in 1972 and at several time points since. The provisions of the Clean Water Act not only deal with industrial pollution but also with municipal sewage wastes, also described later in the context of daily life in the community setting. Drinking water quality is regulated under a separate law, also described later. Under the Clean Water Act, the federal government sets standards for ambient water quality and also sets general

requirements for the technology that must be used to achieve the standards. To date, federal water-quality criteria for human health have been set for 126 pollutants, designated *priority pollutants*; this list includes both metals and synthetic organic compounds.[154] The law requires that industrial facilities obtain a permit for any discharge into a body of water and also use "best available technology" to control discharges. The regulatory framework of the Clean Water Act distinguishes between two types of water pollution sources. The first type, called a **point source**, releases waste at a specific location—for example, a pipe releasing industrial wastes, or a sewage outfall. Pollution sources that cover a large area, such as abandoned coal mines, agricultural fields, or paved urban areas, are called **nonpoint sources**.

State governments set permit requirements for individual discharge sources such that the federal ambient standards and technology requirements will be met, and the states also enforce compliance with the permits. This permitting system is known as the National Pollutant Discharge Elimination System. In 1990, the Oil Pollution Act amended the Clean Water Act, setting requirements for oil facilities to develop plans with which to prevent spills as well as plans to respond to spills when they occur.

Readers are referred to Appendix 1 for a table summarizing the major environmental regulatory laws in the United States.

Managing Workers Health

Federal requirements for the protection of workers stem from the Occupational Safety and Health Act, requiring employers to provide a workplace free of "recognized hazards that are causing, or are likely to cause, death or serious physical harm" to employees.[155] The law applies to most employers, but excludes the self-employed as well as family-only farm operations. The law created the Occupational Safety and Health Administration (OSHA), responsible for promulgating and enforcing occupational health standards, as well as NIOSH.

Federal regulations include protections for a wide range of mechanical hazards. Other than mechanical injuries, inhalation exposures are generally of greatest concern in the workplace, and steps to reduce inhalation exposures often reduce the potential for dermal and incidental ingestion exposures. Most occupational health standards take the form of a **permissible exposure limit (PEL)**, which is a concentration of a contaminant in air. OSHA can set up to three distinct types of PELs for a given contaminant: The PEL-TWA (time-weighted average) is a limit on the time-weighted average concentration over an eight-hour work day; the PEL-STEL (short-term exposure limit), intended to protect workers at times when the concentration exceeds the overall daily average, is a limit on the concentration to which workers can be continuously exposed during a 15-minute period (with no more than four such periods per day); and the PEL-C (ceiling) is a concentration that must not be exceeded at any time during the workday.[155,156]

NIOSH produces three types of recommended exposure limits (RELs) that parallel the OSHA standards: the REL-TWA, REL-STEL, and REL-C. Although RELs, published by NIOSH, are intended as the basis for PELs promulgated by OSHA, historically, there has been little connection between the two. Under pressure to set standards quickly after both agencies were established in 1970, OSHA promulgated a set of about 425 interim PELs the next year. Most of these standards were drawn directly from values published in 1968 by ACGIH, an organization founded as the American Conference of Governmental Industrial Hygienists, but whose membership now consists of occupational and environmental safety and health professionals more broadly. In ACGIH terminology, these concentrations were known as **threshold limit values (TLVs)** and, like PELs and RELs, were designated as time-weighted averages, short-term exposure limits, or ceilings.

The process designed to replace these interim standards with permanent ones has essentially failed. In 1989, OSHA, which had promulgated only a few permissible exposure limits since 1971, adopted as PELs more than 400 updated TLVs published by ACGIH, despite the fact that NIOSH had by this time published recommended exposure limits for numerous chemicals. OSHA's 1989 PELs were challenged by the AFL-CIO, the umbrella organization for U.S. labor unions,

and vacated by a federal court in 1992, leaving in force the 1971 PELs.[155,156] Since that time, ACGIH has not only revised many of the TLVs on which OSHA's PELs were based but has also developed TLVs for many additional chemicals: It now publishes TLVs for more than 700 chemicals and physical agents. Currently, the NIOSH REL exposure limits are not legally enforceable but are considered by OSHA when promulgating their legal PEL standards.

OSHA requires that an employer first attempt to meet an exposure limit by modifications of the work environment, such as ventilation. Only if changes to the workspace prove inadequate to meet the PEL can workers be required to wear **personal protective equipment**, such as goggles, ear protectors, or respirators. Workers sometimes find such gear hot, clumsy, and uncomfortable, and do not always comply with a requirement to use it, which is part of the rationale for requiring modifications to the work environment as a first step.

Although mechanical hazards often are obvious to workers, chemical hazards may not be. For this reason, workers are specifically guaranteed access to information about chemical hazards in their workplace. Manufacturers and importers of chemicals must produce a summary of their health effects in the form of a **Material Safety Data Sheet (MSDS)**, and employers are required to provide MSDSs to workers, along with training about the chemicals to which they are exposed.

Regulation of the Manufacture and Use of Chemicals

In principle, the 1976 Toxic Substances Control Act (TSCA; "tosca") empowered the EPA to control toxic chemicals in production and commerce before they become wastes—a precautionary approach. A company desiring to manufacture a new chemical must submit a notice to the EPA 90 days before manufacturing begins, providing information about the chemical and its effects. The EPA can gather additional information about the chemical and can then restrict the manufacture, distribution, or use of a chemical if it poses an "unreasonable" risk to human health or the environment relative to the benefits it offers.

However, progress was slow. As of 2006, about 30 years after the passage of the Toxic Substances Control Act, the EPA had required testing of fewer than 200 of the 20,000 chemicals added to the TSCA inventory since the law went into effect and had issued regulations to limit or ban the production of only five chemicals (or sets of chemicals).[157] There were about 62,000 chemicals in the original TSCA inventory. The painfully slow pace of this work reflected the challenge of showing unreasonable risk while respecting the confidentiality of companies' trade secrets, as well the inadequacy of the EPA's resources for this task. In 2009, the agency announced changes in its approach to managing toxic chemicals under existing laws, with the goal of moving the process forward at a faster pace. Unfortunately, few improvements have occurred during the last decade as political sentiment in the U.S. has discouraged governmental regulatory actions.

As the preceding discussion makes clear, U.S. environmental laws and regulations have had many positive effects on public health, although for the most part without reflecting (or without implementing) a truly precautionary stance. The Pollution Prevention Act of 1990, in contrast, explicitly provided support for **source reduction** (also called **waste prevention**), naming it as the preferred option over treating or disposing of wastes. The act also created the Office of Pollution Prevention in the Environmental Protection Agency, which manages pollution prevention initiatives related to greenhouse gases, hazardous materials, and the use of natural resources, and encourages the development of sustainable policies.

In light of the slow pace of progress in specifically regulating chemicals, in 2009, the EPA initiated fundamental changes in its approach. At the same time that the agency revised its approach to managing toxic chemicals under existing laws, it also announced a set of principles defining how toxic chemicals *should* be managed, with an eye toward reforming U.S. laws.[158] These included a requirement that manufacturers provide the EPA with information demonstrating the safety of chemicals; that actions by both the EPA and chemical manufacturers in reviewing chemicals should be timely; and that regulatory changes should encourage **green chemistry**, require greater transparency on the part of chemical manufacturers, and support public access to information.

Toxics use reduction is a preventive approach to chemical hazards. The basic objectives of this approach are to use chemicals that are less toxic than those currently in use and to reduce the quantities of toxic chemicals that are used. Within this context, **green chemistry** is the scientific work of identifying specific chemicals and processes that achieve these objectives.* Green chemistry takes pollution prevention to the molecular scale: For example, if a process change means that a higher proportion of reactant atoms end up in the product and a lower proportion end up in waste, the change will reduce both the quantity of inputs needed and the quantity of waste produced. **Alternatives assessment** is the broader process of identifying potential substitutes for toxic chemicals in use, weighing their merits, and recommending the best alternative. The practical objectives of alternatives assessment are to eliminate the worst actors altogether; to reduce the overall quantity and toxicity of chemicals produced and used, and wastes generated; and to make products safer.

Much innovation in green chemistry begins in forward-thinking corporations that both anticipate changing markets and help bring them about. Government policies can also encourage green chemistry. In Massachusetts, for example, for more than 20 years, the state-funded Toxics Use Reduction Institute has worked hand in hand with individual businesses that are taking innovative steps to reduce their use of toxic chemicals.

---

*The 12 principles of green chemistry, as first articulated by Paul Anastas and John Warner in *Green Chemistry: Theory and Practice* (Oxford University Press: New York, 1998, p. 30), are provided on the EPA website: www.epa.gov/sciencematters/june2011/principles.htm.

It is sometimes less difficult politically to move forward with precautionary approaches at a more local level. For example, some local and state governments have set regulations to encourage the substitution of water-based cleaning methods for dry-cleaning methods that use solvents. A 2006 California law sets regulations and mechanisms to reduce the state's production of greenhouse gases.[159] Another California measure, passed in 1986, requires the governor to annually publish a list of chemicals known to cause cancer or reproductive toxicity and also requires California businesses to give warnings if their activities cause exposures to these chemicals.[160] Massachusetts passed a law in 1989, the Toxics Use Reduction Act, that sets goals for reducing the production of toxic wastes in the state, and, as a means to achieve this goal, requires firms to document plans to use fewer toxic chemicals in industrial processes.[161] As noted above, the state's Toxic Use Reduction Institute has been effective in promoting the use of alternatives to toxic chemicals through research and training services and technical support.

Toxics use reduction, which benefits the health of both workers and the broader community, is in alignment with the basic preventive stance of public health. In addition, it can generate substantial economic benefits through the creation of new jobs and reduced costs of toxic cleanup.

Study Questions

1. What are the distinctive features of the workplace as a setting where exposure to chemical and physical hazards occurs?
2. What are the specific health effects associated with occupational exposure to synthetic chemicals?
3. Describe some of the health risks associated with occupational exposure to toxic metals.
4. In your view, do people have a right to both a healthy working environment and a healthy ambient environment? Why or why not?
5. In your view, do the more developed countries have any special responsibility in the international trade in hazardous wastes?
6. What factors do you see as barriers to a more precautionary approach in the development and use of new technologies in the United States?

References

1. U.S. Bureau of Labor Statistics. (n.d.). Distribution of workforce population by occupation, 2019. Current Population Survey, Workforce Population Charts. https://wwwn.cdc.gov/NIOSH-WHC/chart/bls-cps/demo?T=ZY&V=C&Y=

2. U.S. Environmental Protection Agency. Toxics release inventory [data]. https://www.epa.gov/toxics-release-inventory-tri-program

3. U.S. Environmental Protection Agency. (n.d.). Dry cleaning emissions standards/basic Information. Retrieved April 7, 2012 from https://www.epa.gov/regulatory-information-sector/dry-cleaning-sector-naics-8123

4. Levin SM, Lilis R. Organic compounds. In Wallace RB, Doebbeling BN, eds., *Maxcy-Rosenau-Last Public Health and Preventive Medicine*. Appleton & Lange; 1998: 509-542.

5. International Agency for Research on Cancer. (2020). Agents classified by the IARC monographs, Volumes 1-128. https://monographs.iarc.fr/agents-classified-by-the-iarc/

6. Russell HH, Matthews JE, Sewell GW. TCE removal from contaminated soil and ground water. *EPA Ground Water Issue*, EPA/540/S-92/002. 1992. https://www.epa.gov/sites/production/files/2015-06/documents/tce.pdf

7. Shea KM. Pediatric exposure and potential toxicity of phthalate plasticizers. *Pediatrics.* 2003;111(6):1467-1474.

8. Toxics Use Reduction Institute. DEHP Facts/Use Nationally and in Massachusetts. (n.d.). Retrieved April 12, 2012 from https://www.turi.org/TURI_Publications /TURI_Chemical_Fact_Sheets/Trichloroethylene _TCE_Fact_Sheet/TCE_Facts/Use_Nationally_and_in _Massachusetts

9. Dodson RE, Nishioka M, Standley LJ, Perovich LJ, Brody JG, Rudel RA. Endocrine disruptors and asthma-associated chemicals in consumer products. *Environ Health Perspect,* 2012;120(7): 935-943.

10. Rudel RA, Camann DE, Spengler JD, Korn LR, Brody JG. Phthalates, alkylphenols, pesticides, polybrominated diphenyl ethers, and other endocrine-disrupting compounds in indoor air and dust. *Environ Sci Technol.* 2003;37(20):4543-4553.

11. Shaz BH, Grima K, Hillyer CD. 2-(Diethylhexyl) phthalate in blood bags: is this a public health issue? *Transfusion.* 2011;51, 2510.

12. Jaeger RJ, Rubin RJ. Contamination of blood stored in plastic packs. *Lancet,* 1970;296(7664):151.

13. Rubin RJ, Ness PM. What price progress? An update on vinyl plastic blood bags. *Transfusion.* 1989;29(4): 358-361.

14. Martino-Andrade AJ, Chahoud I. Reproductive toxicity of phthalate esters. *Molec Nutr Food Res,* 2010;54(1): 148-157.

15. Saillenfait AM, Sabaté JP, Gallissot, F. Effects of *in utero* exposure to di-*n*-hexyl phthalate on the reproductive development of the male rat. *Reprod Toxicol.* 2009;28(4): 468-476.

16. Ormond G, Nieuwenhuijsen MJ, Nelson P, et al. Endocrine disruptors in the workplace, hairspray, folate supplementation, and risk of hypospadias: case-control study. *Environ Health Perspect.* 2009;117(2):303-307.

17. Swan S, Main KM, Liu F., et al. Decrease in anogenital distance among male infants with prenatal phthalate exposure. *Environmental Health Perspectives,* 2005; 113(8):1056-1061.

18. vom Saal F, Hughes C. An extensive new literature concerning low-dose effects of bisphenol A shows the need for a new risk assessment. *Environ Health Perspect.* 2005;113(8):926-933.

19. Grün F, Watanabe H, Zamanian Z, et al. Endocrine-disrupting organotin compounds are potent inducers of adipogenesis in vertebrates. *Molec Endocrinol,* 2006;20(9):2141-2155.

20. Stahlhut RW, van Wijngaarden E, Dye TD, Cook S, Swan SH. Concentrations of urinary phthalate metabolites are associated with increased waist circumferences and insulin resistance in adult U.S. males. *Environ Health Perspect.* 2007;115(6):876-882.

21. Heindel JJ, Blumberg B. Environmental obesogens: mechanisms and controversies. *Ann Rev Pharmacol Toxicol.* 2019;59:89-106.

22. U.S. Food and Drug Administration. (2018). Bisphenol A (BPA): use in food contact application. Retrieved April 12, 2012 from www.fda.gov/newsevents/publichealth focus/ucm064437.htm

23. Moon MK. Concern about the safety of Bisphenol A substitutes. *Diabet Metab J.* 2019;43(1):46-48.

24. U.S. Centers for Disease Control and Prevention. *Fourth National Report on Human Exposure to Environmental Chemicals, Volume 1.* 2019. https://www.cdc.gov/exposure report/index.html

25. Nelson JW, Scammel MK, Hatch EE, Webster TF. Social disparities in exposures to bisphenol A and polyfluoralkyl chemicals: A cross-sectional study within NHANES 2003–2006. *Environmental Health,* 2012;11(10).

26. Rudel RA, Gray JM, Engel CL, et al. Food packaging and bisphenol A and bis(2-ethyhexyl) phthalate exposure: findings from a dietary intervention. *Environ Health Perspect.* 2011;119(7):914-920.

27. Commoner B. *Making Peace with the Planet.* Pantheon Press. 1990.

28. U.S. Agency for Toxic Substances and Disease Registry. *Toxicological Profile for Polychlorinated Biphenyls (PCBs).* U.S. Department of Health and Human Services. 2000.

29. Webster TF, Commoner B. Overview: the dioxin debate. In Schecter A, Gasiewicz T, eds. *Dioxins and Health* [2nd edition,]. John Wiley & Sons, Inc. 2003:1-53.

30. U.S. Environmental Protection Agency. (n.d.). Hudson River PCBs: Background and Site Information. Retrieved November 28, 2012 from https://www.epa.gov/hudson riverpcbs

31. U.S. Environmental Protection Agency. (n.d.). Twelve-Mile Creek/Lake Hartwell, Pickens County, SC. Retrieved July 18, 2020 from: https://www.itrcweb.org /contseds_remedy-selection/Content/Appendix%20 A/A%2077Case%20Study%20Twelvemile%20Creek .htm

32. U.S. Department of Veterans Affairs. (n.d.). Become familiar with Agent Orange and the health of our Vietnam veterans. Retrieved February 8, 2007 from www.va.gov/agentorange

33. U.S. Environmental Protection Agency. (n.d.). NPL Site Narrative for Times Beach Site. Retrieved November 28, 2012 from: www.epa.gov/superfund/sites/npl/nar833.htm

34. Bernard A, Hermans C, Broeckaert F, De Poorter G, De Cock A, Houins G. Food contamination by PCBs and dioxins. *Nature.* 1999;401:231-232.

35. Baccarelli A, Pesatori AC, Consonni D, et al. Health status and plasma dioxin levels in chloracne cases 20 years after the Seveso, Italy accident. *B JD.* 2005;152(3)459-465.

36. Yoshimura T. Yusho in Japan. *Industrial Health,* 2003;41(3) :139-148.

37. BBC News. (2004, December 17). Deadly dioxin used on Yushchenko. http://news.bbc.co.uk/2/hi/europe /4105035.stm

38. U.S. Environmental Protection Agency. (n.d.). Poly-chlorinated biphenyls (PCBs): health effects of PCBs. www.epa.gov/pcb/pubs/effects.html

39. Clapp RW. Polychlorinated biphenyls. In Wallace RB, Kohatsu N, eds. *Maxcy-Rosenau-Last Public Health and Preventive Medicine* (15th ed.). McGraw-Hill. 2008.

40. de Wit CA. An overview of brominated flame retardants in the environment. *Chemosphere*. 2002;46(5):583-624.

41. Fonnum F, Mariussen E. Mechanisms involved in the neurotoxic effects of environmental toxicants such as polychlorinated biphenyls and brominated flame retardants. *J Neurochem*. 2009;111(6):1327-1347.

42. Stapleton HM, Klosterhaus S, Keller A, et al. Identification of flame retardants in polyurethane foam collected from baby products. *Environ Sci Technol*. 2011;45(12): 5323-5331.

43. Hale RC, La Guardia MJ, Harvey E, Mainor TM. Potential role of fire retardant-treated polyurethane foam as a source of brominated diphenyl ethers to the US environment. *Chemosphere*, 2002;46 (5):729-735.

44. Alaee M, Wenning RJ. The significance of brominated flame retardants in the environment: current understanding, issues and challenges. *Chemosphere*, 2002; 46(5) 579-582.

45. McDonald TA. A perspective on the potential health risks of PBDEs. *Chemosphere*. 2002;46(5):745-755.

46. Meironyte D, Noren K, Bergman A. Analysis of polybrominated diphenyl ethers in Swedish human milk. A time-related trend study, 1972-1997. *J Toxicol Environ Health*. 1999;58(6):329-341.

47. Messer A. Mini-review: polybrominated diphenyl ether (PBDE) flame retardants as potential autism risk factors. *Physiol Behav*. 2010;100(3):245-249.

48. U.S. Consumer Product Safety Commission. CPSC Bans TRIS-Treated Children's Garments [press release]. 1977.

49. Shaw SD, Blum A, Weber R, et al. Halogenated flame retardants: do the fire safety benefits justify the risks? *Rev Environ Health*, 2010;25(4):261-305.

50. Calafat AM, Kuklenyik Z, Caudill SP, Reidy JA, Needham LL. Perfluorochemicals in pooled serum samples from United States residents in 2001 and 2002. *Environ Sci Technol*. 2006;40(7):2128-2134.

51. Grandjean P, Clapp R. Changing interpretation of human health risk from perfluorinated compounds. *Pub Health Rep*. 2014;129(6):482-485.

52. Morrison J. Perfluorinated chemicals taint drinking water. *Chem Engineer News*. 2016;94(23):20-22.

53. Giesy JP, Kannan K. Global distribution of perfluorooctane sulfonate in wildlife. *Environ Sci Technol*. 2001;35(7):1339-1342.

54. Kannan K, Koistinen J, Beckmen, K., et al. Accumulation of perfluorooctane sulfonate in marine mammals. *Environ Sci Technol*, 2001;35(8):1593-1598.

55. Organisation for Economic Co-operation and Development. Co-operation on existing chemicals: hazard assessment of perfluorooctane sulfonate (PFOS) and its salts. Joint meeting of the Chemicals Committee and the Working Party on Chemicals, Pesticides and Biotechnology, 2002;88:2.

56. Stahl T, Mattern D, Brunn H. Toxicology of perfluorinated compounds. *Environ Sci Europe*, 2011;23, 38.

57. U.S. Environmental Protection Agency. Technical fact sheet—Perfluorooctane sulfonate (PFOS) and Perfluorooctanoic acid (PFAS). Office of Land and Emergency Management, EPA 505-F-17-001. 2017.

58. World Meterological Organization. Scientific Assessment of Ozone Depletion: 2006, Report No. 50. 2006. www.wmo.int/pages/prog/arep/gaw/ozone_2006/ozone_asst_report.html

59. World Meteorological Organization. Scientific Assessment of Ozone Depletion: 2010. Global Ozone Research and Monitoring Project Report No. 52. 2010. http://ozone.unep.org/Assessment_Panels/SAP/Scientific_Assessment_2010/index.shtml

60. United Nations Environment Programme, Ozone Secretariat. Status of Ratification: Ratification of Vienna Convention by Countries. Retrieved April 20, 2012 from https://ozone.unep.org/treaties/status-ratification

61. Agency for Toxic Substances and Disease Registry. Substance priority list. https://www.atsdr.cdc.gov/spl/index.html#2019spl. 2019.

62. Gidlow DA. Lead toxicity. *Occup Med*. 2004;54(2):76-81.

63. Papanikolaou NC, Hatzidaki EG, Belivanis S, Tzanakakis GN, Tsatsakis AM. Lead toxicity update. A brief review. *Med Sci Monit*. 2005;11(10):RA329-RA336.

64. Gilbert SG, Weiss B. A rationale for lowering the blood lead action level from 10 to 2 µg/dL. *NeuroToxicology*. 2006;27(5):693-701.

65. Bellinger DC. The protean toxicities of lead: new chapters in a familiar story. *Int J Environ Res Public Health*. 2011;8(7):2593-2628.

66. Needleman H, Gunnoe C, Leviton A, et al. Deficits in psychologic and classroom performance of children with elevated dentine lead levels. *N Engl J Med*. 1979;300: 689-695.

67. U.S. Environmental Protection Agency. (n.d.). Lead and compounds (inorganic) (CASRN 7439-92-1). www.epa.gov/iris/subst/0277.htm

68. Wigg NR. Low-level lead exposure and children. *J Paediatr Child Health*. 2001;37(5):423-425.

69. Jones RL, Homa DM, Meyer PA, et al. Trends in blood lead levels and blood lead testing among US children aged 1 to 5 years, 1988–2004. *Pediatrics*. 2009;123(3):e376-e385.

70. Schell LM, Ravenscroft J, Cole M, Jacobs A, Newman J, and Akwesasne Task Force on the Environment. Health disparities and toxicant exposure of Akwesasne Mohawk young adults: A partnership approach to research. *Environ Health Perspect*. 2005;113(12):1826-1832.

71. National Research Council. *Toxicological Effects of Methylmercury*. National Academies Press. 2000.

72. Clarkson TW. The three modern faces of mercury. *Environ Health Perspect*. 2002;110(suppl 1):11-23.

73. Grandjean P, Weihe P, White RF, et al. Cognitive deficit in 7-year-old children with prenatal exposure

to methylmercury. *Neurotoxicology and Teratology*, 1997;19(6), 417-428.

74. Grandjean, P, Budtz-Jørgensen E, White RF, et al. Methylmercury exposure biomarkers as indicators of neurotoxicity in children aged 7 years. *A J Epidemiol*. 1999;150(3):301-305.

75. Debes F, Budtz-Jørgensen E, Weihe P, White RF, Grandjean P. Impact of prenatal methyl mercury exposure on neuroebehavioral function at age 14 years. *Neurotoxicol Teratol*. 2006;28(5):536-547.

76. U.S. Environmental Protection Agency, Great Lakes National Program Office. Great Lakes Binational Toxics Strategy Report on Alkyl-lead: Sources, Regulations and Options. 2000. www.epa.gov/glnpo/bns/lead/Step%20Report/steps.pdf

77. Mahaffey KR, Sunderland EM, Chan HM, et al.Balancing the benefits of n-3 polyunsaturated fatty acids and the risks of methylmercury exposure from fish consumption. *Nutr Rev*. 2011;69(9):493-508.

78. U.S. Agency for Toxic Substances and Disease Registry. Toxicological profile for mercury. 1999. www.atsdr.cdc.gov/toxprofiles/tp.asp?id=115&tid=24

79. Chen L, Luo K, Etzel R, Zhang X, Tian Y. Zhang J. Co-exposure to environmental endocrine disruptors in the US population. *Environ Sci Pollution Res*. 2019;26:7665-7676.

80. Hubbs AF, Mercer RR, Benkovic SA, et al. Nanotoxicology—A pathologist's perspective. *Toxicol Pathol*. 2011;39(2):301-324.

81. Quadros ME, Marr LC. Environmental and human health risks of aerosolized silver nanoparticles. *J Air Waste Manag Assoc*, 2010;60(7):770-781.

82. Witschi HR, Last JA. Toxic responses of the respiratory system. In Klaassen CD, ed. *Casarett & Doull's Toxicology: The Basic Science of Poisons* [5th edition]. McGraw-Hill. 1996: 443-460.

83. Wu, M., Gordon RE, Herbert R, et al. Case report: lung disease in World Trade Center responders exposed to dust and smoke: nanotubes found in the lungs of World Trade Center patients and dust samples. *Environ Health Perspect*, 2010;118, 499.

84. American College of Occupational and Environmental Medicine. The History and future direction of ACOEM and occupational and environmental medicine. 2002 .https://acoem.org/acoem/media/PowerPoints/ACOEMSlides.pdf

85. U.S. Centers for Disease Control and Prevention. (n.d.). NIOSH Worker Health Charts. https://wwwn.cdc.gov/Niosh-whc/

86. Takala J. Editorial: Eliminating occupational cancer. *Indust Health*, 2015;53(4):307-309.

87. National Institute for Occupational Safety and Health. Occupational cancer. https://www.cdc.gov/niosh/topics/cancer/default.html. 2012.

88. Ozonoff, D. Failed warnings: asbestos-related disease and industrial medicine. In Bayer R, ed. *The Health &*

Safety of Workers: Case Studies in the Politics of Professional Responsibility. Oxford University Press. 1988.

89. Case BW. Asbestos, smoking, and lung cancer: interaction and attribution. *Occup Environ Med*. 2006;63(8):507-508.

90. Robinson BS, Musk AW, Lake RA. Malignant mesothelioma. *Lancet*, 2005;366(9483):397-408.

91. Joshi TK, Gupta RK. Asbestos-related morbidity in India. *International J Occup Med Environ Health*. 2003;9(3):249-253.

92. Joshi TK, Gupta RK. Asbestos in developing countries: magnitude of risk and its practical implications. *Int J Occup Med Environ Health*. 2004;17(1):179-185.

93. Burki T. Health experts concerned over India's asbestos industry. *Lancet*. 2010;375(9715):626-627.

94. U.S. Occupational Safety and Health Administration. *Fact Sheet: Cotton Dust*. 1995;2007.

95. U.S. Centers for Disease Control and Prevention. Byssinosis: mortality. Retrieved April 14, 2012 from https://wwwn.cdc.gov/eworld/Data/Byssinosis_Number_of_deaths_crude_and_age-adjusted_death_rates_US_residents_age_15_and_over_19792010/918

96. Wang, X-R, Eisen EA, Zhang H-X, et al. Respiratory symptoms and cotton dust exposure; results of a 15 year follow up observation. *Occup Environ Med*. 2003;60(12):935-941.

97. Saiyed HN, Tiwari RR. Occupational health research in India. *Indust Health*. 2004;42(2):141-148.

98. U.S. Occupational Safety and Health Administration. (n.d.). Safety and Health Topics: Isocyanates. Retrieved November 28, 2012 from: www.osha.gov/SLTC/isocyanates/index.html

99. Burge PS. Recent developments in occupational asthma. *Swiss Med Wkly*. 2010;140(9):128-132.

100. Quirce S, Sastre J. New causes of occupational asthma. *Curr Opin Allergy Clin Immunol*. 2011;11(2):80-85.

101. Eng A, 'T Mannetje AT, Douwes J, et al. The New Zealand Workforce Survey II: occupational risk factors for asthma. *Ann Occup Hygiene*. 2010;54(2):154-164.

102. Vandenplas, O. Occupational asthma: etiologies and risk factors. *Allergy Asthma Immunol Res*. 2011;3(3):157-167.

103. Canadian Centre for Occupational Health and Safety. (n.d.). What are the Health Effects of Hand-Arm Vibration? Retrieved November 28, 2012 from www.ccohs.ca/oshanswers/phys_agents/vibration/vibration_effects.html

104. Canadian Centre for Occupational Health and Safety. (n.d.). Work-Related Musculoskeletal Disorders (WMSDs). Retrieved November 28, 2012 from www.ccohs.ca/oshanswers/diseases/rmirsi.html?print

105. Tak S, Davis RR, Calvert GM. Exposure to hazardous workplace noise and use of hearing protection devices among U.S. workers—NHANES, 1999–2004. *Am J Indust Med*. 2009;52(5):358-371.

106. Carmelo A, Concetto G C, Zirilli A, et al. Effects of cigarette smoking on the evolution of hearing loss caused by industrial noise. *Health*. 2010;2(10):1163-1169.

107. Anonymous. Mick Jagger raises awareness on hearing loss. *Telegraph.* www.telegraph.co.uk/news/celebritynews /2448946/Mick-Jagger-raises-awareness-on-hearing -loss.html. 2008.

108. Estridge B. Loud rock music wrecked my hearing, says Dire Straits star . . . now iPod generation is at risk. *Daily Mail.* www.dailymail.co.uk/health/article-1202105/Loud -rock-music-wrecked-hearing-says-Dire-Straits-star-- Now-iPod-generation-risk.html. 2009.

109. U.S. Centers for Disease Control and Prevention. Worker Health eChartbook [data]. Retrieved April 9, 2012 from https://wwwn.cdc.gov/Niosh-whc/

110. National Institute for Occupational Safety and Health. *Criteria for a Recommended Standard: Occupational Noise Exposure, Revised Criteria 1998,* DHHS (NIOSH) Publication No. 98-126. 1998.

111. Mahboudi H, Zardouz S, Oliaei S, Pan D, Bazargan M, Djalilian HR. Noise-induced hearing threshold shift among U.S. adults and implications for noise-induced hearing loss: National Health and Nutrition Examination Surveys. *European Arch Oto-Rhino-Laryngology.* 2013; 270:461-467.

112. Folmer RL, McMillan GP, Austin DF, Henry JA. Audiometric thresholds and prevalence of tinnitus among male veterans in the United States: data from the National Health and Nutrition Examination Survey, 1999–2006. *J Rehabil Res Develop.* 2011;48(5), 503-516.

113. Smith AP. Effects of noise, job characteristics and stress on mental health and accidents, injuries, and cognitive failures at work [conference presentation]. *10th International Congress on Noise as a Public Health Problem 2011 (ICBEN 2011), London, UK.* 2011:486.

114. Gan WQ, Davies HW, Demers PA. Exposure to occupational noise and cardiovascular disease in the United States: The National Health and Examination Survey 1999–2004. *Occup Environ Med.* 2011;68: 183-190.

115. McMenamin, TM. A time to work: recent trends in shift work and flexible schedules. *Monthly Lab Rev.* 2007;130(12), 3.

116. Straif K, Baan R, Grosse Y, et al. Carcinogenicity of shift-work, painting, and fire-fighting. *Lancet Oncology.* 2007;8:1065-1066.

117. Fonken LK, Nelson RJ. Illuminating the deleterious effects of light at night. *F1000 Medicine Reports.* 2011; 3:18.

118. Spivey A. LIGHT POLLUTION: light at night and breast cancer risk worldwide. *Environ Health Perspect.* 2010;118(2):a525.

119. Fonken LK, Workman JL, Walton JC, et al. Light at night increases body mass by shifting the time of food intake. *PNAS.* 2010;107(43):18664-18669.

120. Gamble KL, Resuehr D, Johnson CH. Shift work and circadian dysregulation of reproduction. *Frontiers in Endocrinology.* 2013. https://doi.org/10.3389/fendo.2013 .00092

121. Rim K-T. Reproductive toxic chemicals at work and efforts to protect workers' health: a literature review. *Safety Health Work.* 2017;8(2):143-150.

122. National Institute for Occupational Safety and Health. Reproductive health and the workplace: solvents. Retrieved July 17, 2020 from https://www.cdc.gov /niosh/topics/repro/solvents.html

123. U.S. Census Bureau. Bituminous coal underground mining. 2004. www.census.gov/prod/ec02/ec0221i 212112.pdf

124. U.S. Census Bureau. Bituminous Coal and Lignite Surface Mining. 2004. www.census.gov/prod/ec02/ec022 1i212111.pdf

125. U.S. Census Bureau. Anthracite Mining. 2004. www .census.gov/prod/ec02/ec0221i212113.pdf

126. Mazumdar S, Redmond C, Sollecito W. Sussman N. An epidemiological study of exposure to coal tar pitch volatiles among coke oven workers. *Journal of the Air Pollution Control Association.* 1975;25(4):382-389.

127. Kruvant WJ. People, energy, and pollution. In Newmand DK, Day D, eds. *The American Energy Consumer* Ballinger Publishing Company. 1975: 125-167.

128. Zupan JM. *The Distribution of Air Quality in the New York Region.* Johns Hopkins University Press for Resources for the Future. 1975.

129. Burch WR. The peregrine falcon and the urban poor: some sociological interrelations. In Richerson P, McEvoy J, eds. *Human Ecology: An Environmental Approach.* Duxbury Press. 1976.

130. Anderson SJ, Gardner BW, Moll BJ, et al. Correlation between air pollution and socioeconomic factors in Los Angeles County. *Atmospher Environ.* 1978;12(6-7), 1531-1535.

131. Freeman AMI. Distribution of environmental quality. In Kneese AV, Bower BT, eds. *Environ Qual Anal.* Johns Hopkins University Press. 1972.

132. Berry BJL. *The Social Burdens of Environmental Pollution: A Comparative Metropolitan Data Source.* Ballinger Publishing Company. 1977.

133. Asch P, Seneca JJ. Some evidence on the distribution of air quality. *Land Economics.* 1978;54(3):278-297.

134. Gelobter, M. Toward a model of environmental discrimination. In Bryant B, Mohai P, eds. *Race and the Incidence of Environmental Hazards: A Time for Discourse.* Westview Press. 1992.

135. Perlin SA, Wong D, Sexton K. Residential proximity to industrial sources of air pollution: interrelationships among race, poverty, and age. *J Air Waste Manag.* 2001;51(3):406-421.

136. U.S. General Accounting Office. *Siting of Hazardous Waste Landfills and Their Correlation With Racial and Economic Status of Surrounding Communities.* Washington, DC: U.S. General Accounting Office. 1983.

137. Chavis BF, Lee C. *Toxic Wastes and Race in the United States.* United Church of Christ, Commission for Racial Justice. 1987.

138. Bullard R, Mohai P, Saha R, Wright B. Toxic Wastes and Race at Twenty: 1987–2007. United Church of Christ, Justice & Witness Ministries. 2007.

139. Mohai P, Bryant B. Environmental injustice: weighing race and class as factors in the distribution of environmental hazards. *University Colorado Law Review.* 1992;63: 921-932.

140. Ringquist EJ. Assessing evidence of environmental inequities: a meta-analysis. *Journal of Policy Analysis and Management.* 2005;24(2):223-247.

141. Romious ALS. *Investigating Environmental Equity in Orange County, California: A GIS-based Spatial Analysis of the Toxics Release Inventory.* [PhD]. University of California, Irvine. 2009.

142. Scharber H. *Three Essays on Racial Disparities in Infant Health and Air Pollution Exposure.* [PhD]. University of Massachusetts, Amherst.

143. Maantay J. Zoning, equity, and public health. *Am J Pub Health.* 2001;91(7):1033-1041.

144. Zota AR, Rudel RA, Morello-Frosch RA, Brody JG. Elevated house dust and serum concentrations of PBDEs in California: unintended consequences of furniture flammability standards? *Environ Sci Technol.* 2008;42(21):8158-8164.

145. Patel J, Robbins M. The agate industry and silicosis in Khambhat, India. *New Solutions.* 2011;21(1):117-139.

146. Bailey, P.J. (2000). Discussion paper: is there a decent way to break up ships? International Labour Organization.

147. International Labour Organization. (n.d.). Ship-breaking: a hazardous work. Retrieved October 15, 2012 from www.ilo.org/safework/areasofwork/hazardous-work /WCMS_110335/lang--en/index.htm

148. U.S. Occupational Safety and Health Administration. (2001). OSHA Fact Sheet: Shipbreaking. www.osha.gov /OshDoc/data_MaritimeFacts/shipbreaking-factsheet .pdf

149. United States Department of Labor. U.S. Occupational Safety and Health Administration. (n.d.). Shipyard Employment/Shipbreaking. Retrieved April 19, 2012 from www.osha.gov/SLTC/etools/shipyard/ship_breaking /index.html

150. NGO Shipbreaking Platform. (n.d.). Media Alert—Toxic Ship Exxon Valdez Sent for Dismantling. Retrieved April 19, 2012 from https://www.shipbreakingplatform.org/ wp-content/uploads/2018/07/TOXIC-SHIP-EXXON-VALDEZ-SENT-FOR-DISMANTLING.pdf

151. Chatterjee S, Kumar K. Effective electronic waste management and recycling process involving formal and non-formal sectors. *Int J Physical Sci.* 2009;4(13): 893-905.

152. Breivik K, Gioia R, Chakraborty P, Zhang G, Jones KC. Are reductions in industrial organic contaminants emissions in rich countries achieved partly by export of toxic wastes? *Environ Sci Technol.* 2011;45(21):9154 -9160.

153. World Health Organization. Raising awareness on e-waste and children's health. Retrieved July 18, 2020 from www.who.int/activities/raising-awareness-on-e-waste-and-children-s-health

154. United States Environmental Protection Agency. CWA Methods/Priority Pollutants. Retrieved April 19, 2012 from http://water.epa.gov/scitech/methods/cwa /pollutants.cfm

155. U.S. Occupational Safety and Health Administration. OSH Act of 1970/Sec. 5 Duties. www.osha.gov/pls /oshaweb/owadisp.show_document?p_table=OSHACT &p_id=3359

156. Lippman M, Cohen BS, Schlesinger RB. *Environmental Health Science: Recognition, Evaluation, and Control of Chemical and Physical Health Hazards.* Oxford University Press. 2003.

157. United States Government Accountability Office. Chemical regulation: actions are needed to improve the effectiveness of EPA's chemical review program (statement of John B. Stephenson). 2006. www.gao.gov /new.items/d061032t.pdf

158. U.S. Environmental Protection Agency. Essential principles for reform of chemicals management legislation. Retrieved April 20, 2012 from https://www .epa.gov/assessing-and-managing-chemicals-under-tsca /essential-principles-reform-chemicals-management-0

159. California Air Resources Board. Greenhouse gas emissions inventory. Retrieved September 13, 2012 from www.arb.ca.gov/cc/ccei.htm

160. California Office of Environmental Health Hazard Assessment. (n.d.). Proposition 65. Retrieved November 28, 2012 from https://oehha.ca.gov/proposition-65

161. Massachusetts Toxics Use Reduction Institute. *An Overview of TURA.* Retrieved September 13, 2012 from http://turadata.turi.org/WhatIsTURA/OverviewOfTURA .html

CHAPTER 7

Producing Energy

LEARNING OBJECTIVES

After studying this chapter, the reader will be able to:

- Define or explain the key terms introduced throughout the chapter
- Describe the fossil fuel cycle, its environmental impacts, and its occupational risks
- Explain why the fossil fuel cycle produces the major air pollutants that it does and describe the major health risks associated with particulates and pollutant gases
- Explain the relationship between particulate size and the fate of inhaled particulates in the body
- Explain in simple terms how pollutant gases increase the temperature of the troposphere and describe the anticipated environmental and human health effects of global climate change
- Describe key approaches to managing the various public health risks associated with reliance on fossil fuels, including the U.S. regulatory framework
- Describe the major stages of the nuclear fuel cycle
- Describe the key sources of exposure to ionizing radiation related to the nuclear fuel cycle
- Describe key approaches to managing the public health risks associated with reliance on nuclear fuels, including the U.S. regulatory framework
- Describe the range of alternatives to traditional fossil and nuclear energy sources, weighing their advantages and disadvantages

7.1 Sources of Energy

The food production practices and manufacturing activities that we rely on in our modern world would not be possible without the consumption of energy and *lots of it*. Ensuring access to fuels to power heavy agricultural equipment and transportation, and to generate the electricity to light and heat our homes and businesses plus run industrial machinery and our electronics, is vital. However, in addition to its benefits, the production of energy exacts a heavy toll on our environmental resources and also poses many direct risks to human health during the stages of acquiring the energy resource, transport and conversion to power, and the disposal of any associated waste. The environmental and human health impacts associated with producing energy from fossil fuels (Section 7.2) and uranium (section 7.3) are presented along with the regulatory frameworks in the United States that have been established to mitigate these hazards. Section 7.4 describes the environmental and health impacts of generating energy from renewable resources, and the chapter

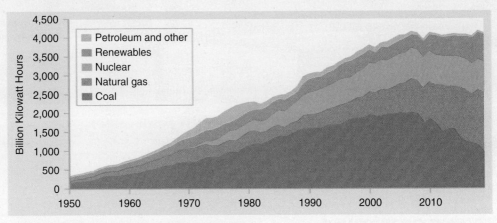

Note: Electricity generation from utility-scale facilities.

Figure 7.1 Electricity generation from 1950 to now by source.

Data from U.S. Energy Information Administration. Monthly Energy Review, Table 7.2a, March 2020 and Electric Power Monthly, February 2020, preliminary data for 2019.

concludes with a discussion of conservation in Section 7.5.

Since the early days of the Industrial Revolution, economic growth and rising standards of living have been driven by carbon-based fuels. Coal deposits near the Earth's surface were mined in Britain in the 12th century, and perhaps even under Roman rule, but it was not until the early 19th century that coal was used on a large scale. By the mid-20th century, petroleum (crude oil) had joined coal as a leading energy source for transportation. Most recently, natural gas has emerged as a dominant source for electricity generation (refer to sidebar on **Electricity Generation** and **Figure 7.1**) as well as heating for half of all homes in the United States. Nuclear power is

Electricity Generation

When an electromagnetic shaft rotates, it creates small currents that are combined into a larger current of electrons or **electricity** that is then transmitted through power lines to consumers. A turbine is used to convert the kinetic energy of a moving liquid or gas into the mechanical energy needed to rotate the electromagnetic generator. Water may be used directly to turn a turbine, as is the case with hydroelectric power generation, or the force of wind as in the case with windmills. Most electricity is generated using heat to boil water and create steam that turns the turbine and rotates the electromagnetic generator. The source of heat comes from the combustion of fossil fuels, such as burning coal or oil, or is released with the fission of uranium in the case of nuclear power or may come from solar radiation.[*] The process of using natural gas to generate electricity is more complicated and involves a hybrid system with a compressor and the generation of *jet air* forces to turn the turbines.

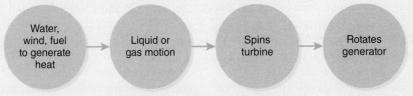

[*] Solar photovoltaic cells directly convert light into electrical current without the use of rotating turbines.

U.S. Energy Information Administration https://www.eia.gov/energyexplained/us-energy-facts/

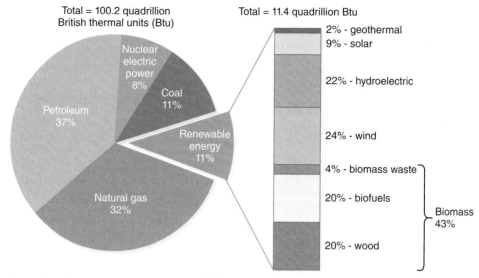

Total = 100.2 quadrillion British thermal units (Btu)

Petroleum 37%

Nuclear electric power 8%

Coal 11%

Renewable energy 11%

Natural gas 32%

Total = 11.4 quadrillion Btu

2% - geothermal
9% - solar
22% - hydroelectric
24% - wind
4% - biomass waste
20% - biofuels
20% - wood

Biomass 43%

Note: Sum of components may not equal 100% because of independent rounding.

Figure 7.2 U.S. 2019 Energy Consumption by Source.

Data from U.S. Energy Information Administration. Monthly Energy Review, Tables 1.3 and 10.1, April 2020, Preliminary Data.

used to generate approximately one-fifth of U.S. electricity. Uranium and the carbon-based fuels mentioned previously are all considered **nonrenewable or finite energy resources**. In contrast, **renewable resources**, such as wind or solar power, also contribute toward the generation of electricity in the United States. **Figure 7.2** provides specific details about the types of renewable energy sources that contributed 11% toward total energy consumption in the United States during 2019.

The total amount of primary energy consumed in the United States in 2019 equaled 100,165,395,000,000,000 British thermal units (BTUs) or about 100.2 quadrillion BTUs. For the first time in over 60 years, U.S. energy production exceeded its consumption.[1] Natural gas production is primarily responsible for shifting the United States from being an importer to an exporter of energy, although annual U.S. crude production was also the highest on record in 2019. Natural gas supplied 35% of all energy produced in 2019, the largest share, followed by petroleum products representing 31% of energy production. The transportation sector consumed

91% of all petroleum products compared with less than 1% of petroleum utilized by the electric power sector. Renewable energy production and consumption also reached record highs in 2019.[1] Nuclear energy production provided 8% of the total in 2019, a level that has been consistent for the past two decades, demonstrating improved production capacity considering there are now fewer nuclear power plants than in 2000. Coal production of energy has declined since its peak usage in the late 1990s to represent only 11% of energy produced in 2019, about half as much energy as coal was responsible for in the past.[1]

7.2 Energy from Fossil Fuels

Fossil fuels—coal, petroleum, and natural gas—are formed from decayed plants and animals that died millions of years ago and were then subjected to heat and pressure underground. The term *fossil fuels* is also used to refer to fuels, such as gasoline, that are derived from coal, oil, or natural gas. Fossil fuels contain **hydrocarbons** and are also known as **hydrocarbon fuels** (see the following sidebar titled, "About Organic Chemicals, Hydrocarbons, and Fuels"). Unlike water and wind power, and even wood fuel, fossil fuels cannot be renewed on the human time scale: They are considered **nonrenewable energy resources**.

As described later in this chapter, the fossil fuel "cycle" is an extension of the natural global carbon cycle. However, on the human time scale, the use of these nonrenewable resources is not a cycle, but rather a one-way process in which fuels are extracted from the earth and then burned. This section addresses the following series of topics:

- How we extract fossil fuels from the earth and how long we can expect to do so
- The environmental impacts of burning fossil fuels, including a well-known suite of air pollutants
- These pollutants' health impacts at both local and regional scales
- The impact of burning fossil fuels on the global climate
- U.S. regulatory approaches to controlling pollution from burning fossil fuels

Extraction of Fossil Fuels

Coal, a solid fuel, is mined from the earth. Petroleum, also called crude oil, is a gooey liquid; it is pumped from underground deposits where it often occurs with natural gas (which is indeed a gas at ordinary temperatures). Workers in coal mines and oil and gas fields face an array of occupational hazards, many of them physical in nature.

Environmental and Health Effects of Coal Mining

Traditionally, coal was mined underground, and many underground mines are still active. In recent decades, however, **surface mining** (also called **strip mining**) has become more common. In surface mining, enormous trucks are used to remove the earth overlying a seam of coal, a process that generates great quantities of dust. In the most extreme form of surface mining, entire mountaintops are removed and neighboring valleys are filled with the earth. In this way, a landscape is

About Organic Chemicals, Hydrocarbons, and Fuels

For the most part, *organic chemicals* are those that contain carbon (there are a few exceptions, including carbon dioxide and carbon monoxide, which are classified as inorganic compounds). Carbon is special: It forms many different compounds because it has the unique ability to bond to itself in long chains, rings, and combinations of these. Some organic compounds, known as *hydrocarbons*, are composed only of hydrogen and carbon. Methane (with one carbon atom), propane (with a chain of carbon atoms), and benzene (with a ring of carbon atoms) are examples of hydrocarbons. Most hydrocarbons are combustible, and our most familiar fuels—coal, oil, natural gas—all contain hydrocarbons. These fuels are referred to both as *hydrocarbon fuels* and as *fossil fuels*, a term that alludes to their prehistoric origins.

altered via leveling, making the long-term stability of the filled valleys uncertain. Underground mines scar the surface landscape: Forests above coal mines have often been cut down for railroad ties and for timbers to shore up the mineshafts.[2] The center of U.S. coal production has shifted in recent decades from Appalachia to the western states, where the coal deposits have lower sulfur content and surface mines can be excavated on a massive scale. The coal is transported by rail in single-cargo, single-destination trains of 100 cars or more.[3] During 2002 through 2008, the peak years for coal usage to power electricity generation, more than 1 billion tons of coal were shipped within the United States, almost two-thirds by rail.[4]

Because any form of coal mining disturbs the Earth's surface and creates waste rock, **acid mine drainage** has become a common problem at both active and abandoned coal mines. Acidic drainage from mines develops because pyrite (iron sulfide) is typically present in the coal and waste rock piled at mine sites (this includes metal mines as well as coal mines). When pyrite in coal or waste rock is exposed to water and air, a chemical reaction produces sulfuric acid, often aided by a species of bacterium that thrives in an acid environment. As a result, rainwater percolating through the waste rock or draining through the mine shafts is made acidic. Because it is acidic, the water mobilizes metals from soils and rock, and it also dissolves minerals, creating suspended solids in the runoff. Thus, acid mine drainage produces a combination of high acidity, high concentrations of metals, and high concentrations of suspended solids (as well as a characteristic orange color resulting from the presence of iron oxide) in the streams or groundwater into which it drains. Acid mine drainage typically originates from a large area, because mines are such sprawling operations, and can continue for decades after a mine is closed or abandoned.

A coal mine is an inherently dangerous working environment. The job of a coal miner carries well-known risks to life and limb, as well as to the lungs. An underground mine in particular, with its blasting and digging, is a dusty environment. Miners are exposed not only to coal dust, but also to silica (quartz) dust because quartz is widespread in the Earth's crust. When particulates lodge in the lungs, tissues react to this physical irritant by forming excessive fibrous tissue (scar tissue). This condition, known as **fibrosis**, makes lung tissues less flexible, and this interferes with breathing. Fibrosis associated with exposure to dust or other particulate matter is known as **pneumoconiosis**; pneumoconiosis associated specifically with coal dust is often called by an older name, **black lung**, and pneumoconiosis associated with exposure to silica is referred to as **silicosis**. Both conditions cause a debilitating loss of lung function. Bands of such scar tissue can form throughout the lungs, but are often concentrated around the small airways (respiratory bronchioles, described later in this chapter).

In the past, miners worked with little or no respiratory protection (see **Figure 7.3**) and were exposed to dust at very high concentrations. In the more developed countries today, there are controls on dust, and miners wear protective gear substantially reducing their exposure to coal and silica dust, although it does not eliminate it. In some less-developed countries, miners still work with little protection. Miners are also at risk of poisoning from carbon monoxide, which can be released from pockets in the coal as it is disturbed by mining.

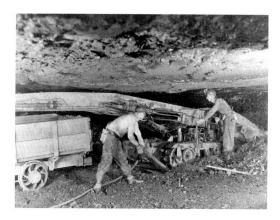

Figure 7.3 U.S. coal miners, circa 1930–1960, wear no respiratory protection as they operate a mechanized coal bin loader.

Courtesy of CDC Public Health Image Library. ID# 9558. Content providers CDC/Barbara Jenkins, NIOSH. Available at: http://phil.cdc.gov/phil/home.asp. Accessed October 14, 2012.

In addition to these inhalation hazards, coal miners are at risk of acute injury and death from accidents involving machinery, cave-ins, and fires or explosions. In the United States, the annual rate of fatal injury among coal miners has been declining since 1984, a year with several mining disasters that killed 206 workers, equal to a rate of 58.4 per 100,000 full-time employees, The average annual rate from 2006 to 2010 (years that also included major mine disasters) was 35.9 per 100,000 workers, to the fatality rate in 2018 of 10.5 per 100,000 workers.[5] The injury rate was roughly doubled in the 2 years in which there was a major accident: at Sago Mine (West Virginia) in 2006 and at Upper Big Branch Mine (West Virginia) in 2010. Of the 24 Upper Big Branch miners on whom autopsies were performed, at least 17 (and possibly 21) had black lung disease; five of the 17 had worked as miners for less than 5 years.[6]

The risk of fire or explosion is ever-present in a coal mine. The elements of the "fire triangle"—the three components that together are sufficient to cause a fire—are fuel, heat, and oxygen. Of these, fuel (the coal itself) and oxygen are already present in a coal mine, so only a source of heat, such as friction or electrical sparks from tools or heavy machinery, is needed to start a fire.[7] The "explosion pentagon" adds two elements to the fire triangle: a confined space and fuel that is finely dispersed and suspended in air. Given that an underground mine is a confined space, if fine coal dust is suspended in the air, only heat is needed for an explosion to occur; and, conversely, if heat is present, all that is lacking is for coal dust to be suspended in the air.[7] The great majority of deaths since 1900 in mining disasters (defined as accidents with five or more fatalities) have been from fire or explosion.[8]

Environmental and Health Effects of Oil and Gas Extraction

Typically, crude oil must be pumped to the surface, although some oil deposits are under pressure so that no pumping is required. Natural gas, which consists mainly of methane, is often extracted along with crude oil from the same geologic formations. Extraction of petroleum produces wastes of oily water and rock fragments, and some liquid wastes are disposed of by injecting them deep underground.

Taking oil and natural gas from the earth requires powerful drilling equipment and releases high-pressure streams of oil and gas. Workers are at risk of accidental injury, overexposure to noise and vibration, and extremes of cold or heat, depending upon location.[9] Hydrogen sulfide (an asphyxiating gas) and radon gas may be mixed in with natural gas.[9] And some components of crude petroleum—still in solution as the oil comes from the earth—will be considered hazardous chemicals after they are separated out at the refinery. Like many other workers, oil and gas workers also use some chemicals on the job—for example, solvents to clean drilling gear.

As more accessible sources of fossil fuels have been drawn down over the decades, resources that are more difficult to extract have become economically viable. For example, some oilfields are now located offshore, so that the oil must be taken from beneath the sea floor, which complicates the extraction process. These operations take place on large offshore platforms for drilling and extracting oil (and natural gas), which is then stored temporarily until it can be taken ashore for refining.

On such a platform in the Gulf of Mexico, on April 20, 2010, the world's largest accidental oil spill occurred. The rig *Deepwater Horizon* had completed the drilling of a new well and was soon to be removed and replaced by a production platform that would extract the oil and gas. But before the drilling rig was removed, the well needed to be secured. During this process, for reasons too complicated to explain briefly, gas and oil and mud exploded up through the wellbore, killing 11 workers on the rig and injuring 17 more.[10] A large fire ensued, and two days after the explosion, the rig sank.

Soon, a growing oil slick on the water's surface indicated an ongoing release of oil. More significant from an ecological perspective was the highly dispersed plume of tiny oil droplets at a depth of roughly 4,000 feet and extending many miles from the rig.[10] The total amount of oil released was estimated at 206 million gallons,[10] a quantity almost 20 times larger than the 1989 *Exxon Valdez* spill described below, yet, by way of context, only about 20% larger than BP's daily worldwide production of 4 million barrels (a barrel contains 42 gallons).[10] The oil released into the gulf, and the dispersant chemicals applied in the attempt to manage the spill, harmed birds and sea animals and their habitats, affected the fishing industry and the livelihoods of those who depend on it, and cost local economies many tourism dollars.

From oil production areas, crude oil is distributed to refineries by ship and also via an extensive pipeline infrastructure. In the United States, the Trans-Alaskan pipeline might be best known because it crosses the pristine Alaskan wilderness and its construction was controversial, but many more miles of pipeline crisscross the continental United States. Pipelines also carry Central Asian oil to ports and Western markets, and pipelines on the floor of the North Sea and the Gulf of Mexico carry oil to shore.

Like the extraction process, deliveries via tanker ship or pipeline come at some cost to the environment. In 1989, after the tanker *Exxon Valdez* ran aground in Prince William Sound, an inlet on Alaska's southern coast, the ship leaked about 11 million gallons of crude oil into the sound over several days. The spill caused extensive environmental contamination and much harm to wildlife, and its lingering effects are still being evaluated. The oilfield at Prudhoe Bay, on

Alaska's north slope near the Alaskan National Wildlife Refuge, has been plagued by spills.

Refined fuel products (such as gasoline and diesel fuel) are distributed from petroleum refineries by rail and truck. Refineries are industrial facilities that not only produce various fuels but also nonfuel products (such as lubricating oils, petroleum jelly, and asphalt) and organic chemicals to be used as inputs to other industries.

Like petroleum, natural gas is often distributed via a pipeline network; in this case, the branching system reaches individual homes and other buildings. When cooled to a very low temperature (about −260°F), natural gas becomes a liquid; such **liquefied natural gas (LNG)** is transported in tanker ships, in which the low temperature can be maintained. When the tanker reaches its destination, the natural gas is warmed to a gaseous state for distribution by pipeline.

A new approach to extracting natural gas has become economically viable, with the extra benefit of also enhancing the recovery of oil reserves that were once too expensive to extract. Natural gas found in some shale formations (sometimes called "shale gas") was once considered unrecoverable, but rising prices for natural gas, along with technological advances in extracting it, have changed this picture. Because the natural gas exists in very small isolated pores in the shale, a preliminary step is needed before a well can start producing. This is **hydraulic fracturing**, or **fracking**, a process that creates many small cracks in the rock and keeps them open so that gas can flow from the well throughout its operational lifetime. The fracturing is achieved by injecting large quantities of a mixture—made up mostly of water and sand, but also containing chemicals[11]—into the well at high pressures. This process may be repeated a number of times at the same well. As a result, the gas that is produced by the well is accompanied by water contaminated by byproducts of the process, and this water must be managed as a waste stream. Formations where natural gas can be obtained in this way, known as shale basins, are widespread across the lower 48 states (see **Figure 7.4**), and fracking is in use in many of these basins.

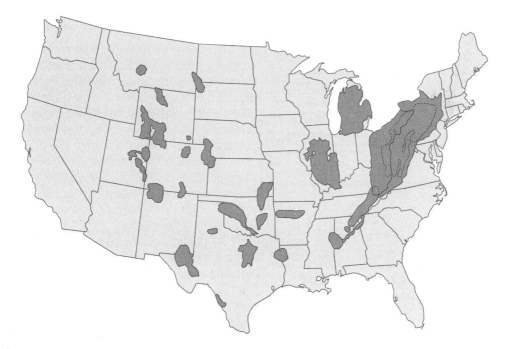

Figure 7.4 Shale basins in the lower 48 U.S. states.

Fracking has become a very controversial process viewed both as a blessing and a curse.[12] The U.S. has been able to become energy independent for both oil and gas primarily due to fracking, reducing reliance on trade with countries that have traditionally not been our allies and which are associated with significant geopolitical tensions. Fracking has also created jobs and generated income in several regions of the country that had become economically depressed with the departure of steel and other industries. As will be discussed subsequently, natural gas is also a cleaner burning fuel to use for electricity generation, reducing emissions of CO_2. However, methane releases associated with fracking contribute to environmental air pollution as well as posing hazards to workers and residents living near fracking sites.[12] Water contamination is another major drawback associated with both the chemicals used during the hydraulic fracturing process as well as allowing for the introduction of naturally occurring radionuclides and metals into drinking water supplies. Perhaps the greatest concern associated with fracking may be related to seismic instability and subsidence in regions with extensive fracking sites.

Although new techniques have allowed for improved supplies of domestic reserves for oil and natural gas, fossil fuels are both nonrenewable and a finite resource. The shift from coal to natural gas to generate electricity should be viewed as an interim solution as research continues to seek more sustainable methods. The economic and political volatility in the oil market since the 1970s also argues for finding an alternative to power our transportation and agricultural sectors. There can be no doubt that the era of unlimited fossil fuel consumption is drawing to a close and that global dependence on these fuels is not a sustainable energy option.

Environmental Impacts of Burning Fossil Fuels

Most combustion products created by burning fossil fuels are released into the atmosphere, becoming air pollution, a term that has traditionally referred to pollution of the troposphere. All combustion is

About Combustion

At its most basic, *combustion* is a chemical reaction that requires a hydrocarbon fuel, the presence of oxygen, and an initial source of heat. Heating causes the hydrocarbon fuel to break down and recombine with the oxygen, forming water (H_2O) and carbon dioxide (CO_2). This oxidation reaction also releases heat energy, causing the combustion to continue as long as fuel remains. Extra heat energy, beyond that needed to maintain the combustion, can be put to use for human purposes. When not enough oxygen is immediately present for a hydrocarbon fuel to burn completely, carbon monoxide (CO) is formed instead of CO_2.

fundamentally the same basic oxidation process (see the following sidebar titled "About Combustion"). However, this simple picture is complicated by both the conditions of burning and the characteristics of the fuel. In particular, combustion under real-world conditions is often incomplete, and fossil fuels are more than just hydrocarbons. Furthermore, some air pollutants from the burning of fossil fuels set in motion complex secondary impacts.

This section describes the sources and environmental fates of key air pollutants from burning fossil fuels, beginning with the most basic products of any combustion; then describing other substances that can be released by burning, depending on the makeup of the fuel; and finally noting the production in the atmosphere of secondary pollutants. Because this picture is already a complicated one, the pollutants' various direct human health effects—many, but not all, respiratory in nature—are presented in a separate section following this one.

The production of electric power, whether derived from fossil or nuclear fuels, also has environmental impacts of a different sort, resulting from the use of water to raise steam to drive a turbine. On the input side, the water is taken from a natural source—for example, a river or a large body of water. After the steam passes through the turbine, it is cooled and condensed back to liquid water, which of course is hot. At some electricity production facilities, this water is released into a nearby body of water, often after some cooling in a pond. In this case, most of the water used in power production is not consumed but is returned to the body of water from which it was originally taken. However, even after cooling, this water is still warmer than the receiving body of water, an effect referred to as *thermal pollution*.

At other facilities, the hot water is pumped to the top of a cooling tower, from where it falls downward through air that is being forced in from the bottom and sides. The air absorbs some of the heat and evaporates a good share of the water; this is the visible steam leaving the top of a cooling tower (four cooling towers appear in Figure 7.15, referenced later). The water that escapes as steam has been removed from the local hydrologic cycle; from the local environmental perspective, this water has been lost. The remaining cooled water is collected at the bottom of the cooling tower and pumped back to be used again to raise steam.

Basic Products of Combustion: Oxides and Particulates

The various combustion processes of an industrial society produce many of the same pollutants, although their profiles vary. As shown in **Table 7.1**, we burn fossil fuels to power vehicles of all types, to generate electricity, and to heat commercial and residential buildings. In addition, some heavy manufacturing facilities, including petroleum refineries, metal smelters, and pulp and paper mills, are powered directly by burning fossil fuels.

Because combustion is oxidation, the combustion of fossil fuels produces several oxides; the most important sources of these pollutants are indicated by check marks in Table 7.1. Carbon dioxide (CO_2), a natural constituent of the atmosphere, is released any time fossil fuels are burned. In contrast, carbon monoxide (CO) is mainly a product of inefficient burning when

Table 7.1 Key Sources of Major Air Pollutants from Burning Fossil Fuels

Pollutant	Sources of Pollutants			
	Vehicles (gasoline, diesel)	Electric Power Plants (coal, oil)	Heating Buildings (oil, natural gas)	Manufacturing (coal, oil, natural gas)
Basic products of the combustion process				
Carbon dioxide (CO_2)	x	X	x	X
Carbon monoxide (CO)	x			
Nitrous oxide (N_2O)	x	X		
Nitrogen dioxide (NO_2), Nitric oxide (NO)	x	X		
Sulfur dioxide (SO_2)		X		(some)
Particulate matter (PM)	x	X	x	X
Other pollutants liberated by combustion				
Mercury (from coal)		X		(some)
Lead (from leaded gasoline)	x			
Volatile organic compounds (from gasoline)	x			

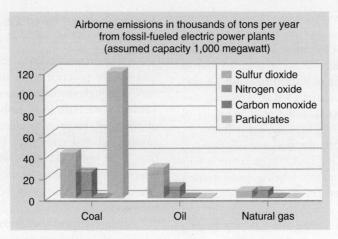

Figure 7.5 Comparison of airborne emissions from coal, oil & natural gas.

Data from Moeller DW. *Environmental Health* (3rd ed.). Harvard University Press. 2005.

vehicles idle; thus, carbon monoxide pollution is primarily attributable to cars.

Nitrogen is plentiful in the atmosphere, and thus oxides of nitrogen—the gases nitrous oxide (N_2O), nitrogen dioxide (NO_2), and, if combustion is incomplete, nitric oxide (NO)—are produced by burning. These reactions occur especially at the high temperatures that are typical of processes that convert one form of energy to another; as a result, cars and power plants are the major sources of these pollutants. Nitrogen dioxide is a brownish gas that is a visible marker of air pollution. In the field of air pollution, NO_2 and NO are together referred to as NO_x, pronounced "nox."

Sulfur is present in most coal and crude oil; however, it is refined out of most fuels derived from crude oil, and the sulfur content of natural gas is very low. As a result, sulfur dioxide (SO_2) gas is produced mainly when coal or sulfur-containing oil fuel is burned, mostly in power plants, but also in aging boilers still being used in manufacturing. Sulfur oxide (SO) may also be formed but does not persist as a stable compound. SO and SO_2 are together known as SO_x ("sox"). Because sulfur is refined out of gasoline and heating fuels, cars and furnaces do not produce SO_x. In the atmosphere, some sulfur dioxide is converted to tiny water-soluble particles known as sulfates.

Finally, burning fossil fuels adds to the burden of particles in the air. In environmental health, and especially in the regulatory context, the term **particulate matter (PM)**, or simply **particulates**, refers to a complex mixture that can include both small solid particles and fine liquid droplets.[*] The actual makeup of airborne particulate matter varies but often not only includes soil particles (dust) but also sulfates, metals, and organic chemicals. A common organic component of particulates is a group of compounds known as **polycyclic aromatic hydrocarbons (PAHs)**; the name describes their structure of multiple carbon rings fused together. PAHs, which are present in petroleum and are also a product of incomplete combustion, are ubiquitous in the environment.

Concentrations of airborne particulate matter are measured as mass per unit volume of air—micrograms or milligrams per cubic meter (ug/m^3 or mg/m^3). Per unit of energy output, the burning of coal produces a much greater mass of particulates than the burning of oil, which in turn produces more than the burning of natural gas (refer to **Figure 7.5** for a comparison of airborne emissions of several pollutants from coal, oil and natural gas).

---

[*]Long, narrow fibers, such as asbestos fibers (not produced by burning fossil fuels), are also considered particulates.

Other Pollutants Liberated by Combustion: Mercury, Lead, VOCs

The burning of fossil fuels not only releases the ordinary products of complete and incomplete combustion but also other substances as well, reflecting the composition of the fuel (Table 7.1). For example, **mercury** is naturally present at low concentrations in most coal as are various other metals. But mercury is easily volatilized at warmer temperatures. This means that, unlike the iron or aluminum found in coal, which remain in the ash when the coal is burned, elemental mercury vaporizes and moves into the atmosphere. The quantity released per ton of coal burned is small, but we burn many tons of coal, and mercury is strongly neurotoxic, as discussed previously.

In contrast to mercury, which occurs naturally in coal, lead was deliberately added to gasoline to improve engine performance. In the early 1920s, General Motors and E. I. DuPont formed a new corporation to produce gasoline to which an organic lead compound, tetraethyl lead, had been added.[13] Tetraethyl lead reduced "engine knock," a premature ignition of fuel in the engine cylinders that makes an annoying sound and causes engine wear and a loss of power. After production began at three plants, a number of workers showed frank lead poisoning—suffering psychosis and hallucinations—and some of them died. There followed a brief hiatus in production and a hearing before the Surgeon General. Foreshadowing future events, scientists like Alice Hamilton expressed concern about dispersing lead so widely in the environment when its health risks short of actual poisoning were not well understood. But political pressure won out: In 1925, a committee appointed by the Surgeon General quickly concluded that leaded gasoline did not pose a health hazard, and production resumed.[13]

This decision ultimately spread lead in the environment wherever people drove cars—for if lead is present in gasoline, it is also present in exhaust. When leaded gasoline is in use, lead is widespread in airborne particulate matter, which is gradually deposited on the ground through settling or with precipitation. Thus, inhalation exposures to airborne lead are important while leaded gasoline is in use but decline fairly quickly after the use of leaded gasoline is discontinued. However, exposures to lead in soil or dust, mostly by incidental ingestion, have continued long after leaded gasoline was banned. The burden of lead in soil is especially heavy in urban areas. (Another important source of lead in soil is deteriorating paint, to which lead was commonly added to increase the paint's durability.) Lead has been phased out as a gasoline additive in most countries of the world—in the United States as of 1996, in the European Union nations as of 2000, and in sub-Saharan Africa and most of Latin America by 2006. As of June of 2011, only six countries worldwide—Afghanistan, Algeria, Iraq, Myanmar (Burma), North Korea, and Yemen—were still using leaded gasoline.[14]

Finally, oil contains some naturally occurring **volatile organic compounds (VOCs)**—organic compounds, such as benzene, that volatilize significantly at ordinary environmental temperatures. Other VOCs are sometimes added to gasoline to improve its performance. Some VOCs are released whenever oil or gas is burned. More are released with any gasoline that escapes unburned through the tailpipe or evaporates from the fuel tank or some other part of a vehicle, contributing to the concentration of these pollutants in ambient air (air in the general outdoor environment).

Secondary Pollutants Formed in the Atmosphere: Ozone, Nitric Acid, Sulfuric Acid

Some of the pollutants listed in Table 7.1 are chemically transformed in the environment, producing **secondary pollutants** that are also important; **Table 7.2** adds these pollutants, with arrows linking precursor pollutants to secondary pollutants. As shown, a chemical soup called **photochemical smog** is created through a complex series of chemical reactions among NO_x, VOCs, and other chemicals in the presence of sunlight. This brand of smog is a particular problem in warm, sunny, and densely urban locales such as Manila, Jakarta, Mexico City, and Southern California. The **ozone (O_3)**

Table 7.2 Key Sources of Major Air Pollutants, Including Secondary Pollutants, from the Burning of Fossil Fuels

Pollutant	Sources of Pollutants			
	Vehicles (gasoline, diesel)	Electric Power Plants (coal, oil)	Heating Buildings (oil, natural gas)	Manufacturing (coal, oil, natural gas)
Basic products of the combustion process				
Carbon dioxide (CO_2)	x	x	x	x
Carbon monoxide (CO)	x			
Nitrous oxide (N_2O)	x	x		
Nitrogen dioxide (NO_2), Nitric oxide (NO)	x	x		
Sulfur dioxide (SO_2)		x		(some)
Particulate matter (PM)	x	x	x	x
Other pollutants liberated by combustion				
Mercury (from coal)		x		(some)
Lead (from leaded gasoline)	x			
Volatile organic compounds (from gasoline)	x			
Secondary pollutants formed in the atmosphere				
Ground-level ozone (O_3) in photochemical smog	x			
Nitric acid (HNO_3)	x	x		
Sulfuric acid (H2SO$_4$)		x		

Note: Arrows link precursor pollutants to secondary pollutants.

that is a key component of photochemical smog is an important secondary pollutant. As noted earlier, the naturally occurring layer of ozone in the stratosphere is valued for the protection it provides against ultraviolet radiation. However, the ozone formed at ground level as a result of pollution is a health hazard. (The term **smog**, originally coined as a combination of *smoke* and *fog*, is sometimes used more generally to refer to any visible air pollution.)

Another indirect environmental effect of burning fossil fuels emerged as a divisive political issue in the 1970s. Through complex chemical reactions in the atmosphere, nitric oxide and nitrogen dioxide are gradually converted to nitrates and nitric acid, and sulfur dioxide is gradually converted to sulfates and sulfuric acid (see Table 7.2). These secondary pollutants are then deposited in precipitation—an outcome originally dubbed **acid rain** and now known more formally as **acid deposition**. In forests, acid deposition acidifies soil and can severely damage the leaves of trees. In some lakes and streams, fish species that cannot tolerate acidic waters have been completely eliminated. Acid deposition also damages buildings and statuary. However, acid deposition does not directly affect human health; in particular, "acid rain" is not so acidic that it causes harm on contact.

Power plants are often built with very tall smokestacks to disperse pollution and avoid local effects, and this can result in acid deposition in distant locations. For instance, coal-burning plants in the Midwestern United States cause acid precipitation in New England and Eastern Canada. Similar problems have arisen in the past between European countries as well as between China and Japan, which bore the brunt of acid deposition from Chinese coal-fired power plants.

Health Impacts of Burning Fossil Fuels

This description of health impacts revisits the set of pollutants listed in Table 7.2, considering the health effects of particulates and key pollutant gases, such as carbon monoxide, nitrogen dioxide, sulfur dioxide, and ozone, of which the last is a secondary pollutant formed in the atmosphere. The fate of these inhaled particulates and pollutant gases in the body, their physiologic effects (mostly in the respiratory system), and their ultimate health impacts are discussed.

Fate of Particulates and Pollutant Gases in the Respiratory System.

In the upper respiratory system, air inhaled through the nose passes from the nostrils through the nasal passages to the throat (see **Figure 7.6**), and of course air can also be inhaled through the mouth. At the larynx, the throat gives way to the cartilaginous **trachea** (windpipe), which is considered a part of the lower respiratory system. Below the trachea, the air passages become more and more finely subdivided. The trachea divides into two **bronchi** (singular bronchus), which are also cartilaginous airways, surrounded by muscles, each serving one lung. The bronchi in turn divide into **bronchioles**—smaller, more flexible airways. Together, all of these elements—nose and throat, trachea, bronchi, bronchioles—form a transport system for moving air in and out of the lungs.

Gas exchange, the real business of breathing, takes place deeper in the lung. Bronchioles divide into **respiratory bronchioles**—very small conducting airways that are a sort of transitional zone—which in turn become **alveolar ducts**. The walls of the alveolar ducts have many outpocketings: clusters of tiny sacs called **alveoli**. A network of capillaries twines around the alveoli, enabling the exchange of gases: diffusion of oxygen from alveoli to bloodstream, and diffusion of carbon dioxide in the reverse direction. The total alveolar surface area in contact with capillaries is approximately 75 square meters, roughly the area of a tennis court.[15]

Particulates and pollutant gases enter the respiratory system with each inhaled breath. In the upper respiratory system, airflow is rapid, and the reversals between inhaling and exhaling are more turbulent than in the lower region. Like a speeding car in a tunnel, an airborne particle in the trachea, bronchi, or bronchioles may careen into a curving wall or strike a wall head-on at a fork in the passageway. With each branching, the total surface area of the respiratory channels increases, trapping more particles. Deep in the lung, where there is less turbulence, particles may simply settle out. Once a particle lodges on an internal surface, it is not readily exhaled, but rather must be removed by some physiological mechanism.

Particles, which come in various shapes and densities, are classified by size using an idealized spherical diameter. The terms **PM$_{10}$** and **PM$_{2.5}$** refer to particulate matter 10 microns or fewer in diameter (about the size of a protozoan cell) and 2.5 microns or fewer in diameter, respectively. As a general rule, particulates 10 microns or fewer in diameter are considered **respirable particulates**. Particulates from 2.5 to 10 microns come mainly from natural or mechanical sources (such as plowing, grinding, or abrasion), whereas **fine particulates** (PM$_{2.5}$) come mostly from

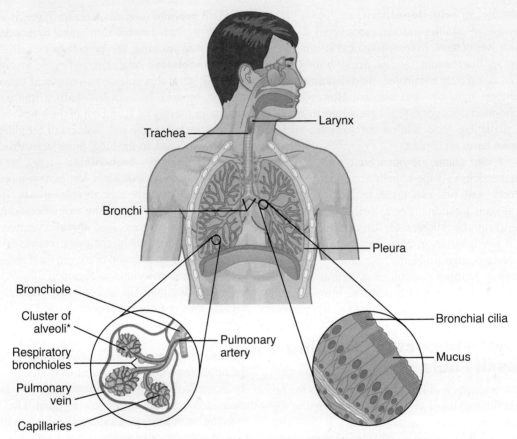

*The alveolar duct itself is hidden by the cluster of alveoli.

Figure 7.6 The human respiratory system.

Data from 2012 American Lung Association. www.lung.org

combustion. **Ultrafine particulates** are those 0.1 microns or fewer in diameter. The most common source of ultrafine particulates is diesel engines, which often idle for extended periods while truckers sleep or while school buses wait for children. Diesel exhaust particulates also have a distinctive chemical makeup. On the whole, the chemical makeup of particulates is variable; for example, it is likely to be different in different locations because the sources are different.

The fate of particulates in the body is mostly determined by their size: Smaller particles stay airborne longer and penetrate deeper before settling out (see **Table 7.3**). In essence, the smaller the particle, the more it behaves like a gas, whether in the airways or in the ambient environment.

Some coarse particles are filtered out by fine hairs lining the nasal passages. These particles may be expelled by sneezing or blowing the nose, or they may be swallowed.

Particulates 2.5 to 10 microns in diameter settle out in the trachea and bronchi, which are lined with **cilia**—tiny, finger-like protrusions of the cells that line the airway. The cilia, which beat in unison, slowly propel a carpet of mucus upward toward the throat, a mechanism known as the **mucociliary escalator**. Particles deposited in this region ride this moving carpet up to the throat, from which the mucus is swallowed or spit out.

Fine particulates can reach the small airways and the alveoli. In the alveoli, macrophages (scavenger cells of the immune system) engulf

Table 7.3 Likely Sources and Fates of Respirable Particulates, by Size Category

Diameter (microns)	Key Sources	Penetration and Fate in Body
2.5 to 10	Natural and mechanical sources	Settle out in trachea and bronchi; are removed via mucociliary escalator
0.1 to < 2.5	Combustion	Reach small airways and alveoli; in alveoli, are removed by macrophages
< 0.1 (ultrafine)	Combustion (especially of diesel fuel)	Can pass through alveolar wall into bloodstream

some particles and remove them via the lymph system. In recent years, it has become clear that ultrafine particulates can pass through the alveolar wall into the bloodstream and circulate throughout the body.[16]

Among the gaseous pollutants, both ozone and its precursor, nitrogen dioxide, penetrate the lower respiratory tract, as does sulfur dioxide if it is adsorbed to particles or aerosols. Carbon monoxide crosses the alveolar boundary into the blood, entering the general circulation.

Physiologic Effects of Particulates and Pollutant Gases

The physiologic mechanisms by which air pollutants cause toxicity are complex and interrelated and are described here only in general terms.

Overall, the organ systems most affected are the respiratory system and the cardiovascular system.

Particulate matter and the major pollutant gases from the burning of fossil fuels have direct irritating effects in the respiratory passages (see **Table 7.4**). Particulate matter and ozone damage the cells lining the respiratory tract.[17,18] Ozone most strongly affects the cells that have cilia; as a result, ozone exposure makes the mucociliary escalator less effective. Particulates and ozone also cause local inflammation.[19,20] As described earlier, chronic inflammation of the bronchi is a feature of asthma, and asthmatics are more susceptible to this effect of air pollutants.

- Sulfur dioxide causes bronchoconstriction (a reduction in the diameter of the bronchi, resulting from muscle contraction),[19,20]

Table 7.4 Key Respiratory Effects of Common Air Pollutants

Pollutant	Effects in Respiratory System			
	Irritating Effects			Impairment of Immune Scavenger Cells in Alveoli
	Damage to Cells Lining the Respiratory Tract	Local Inflammation	Bronchoconstriction	
PM	x	X		x
NO$_2$			(in asthmatics)	x
SO$_2$			x	
O$_3$	x	X	(in asthmatics)	

Data from Bernstein JA. Health effects of air pollution. *J Allergy Clin Immunol.* 2004;114:1116-1123; Chen-Yeung, MN. Air pollution and health. *Hong Kong Med J.* 2000;6:390-398; Costa DL, Amdur MO. Air pollution. In Klaassen CD, ed. *Casarett & Doull's Toxicology: The Basic Science of Poisons* [5th edition]. McGraw-Hill. 1996:857-880; Olivieri D, Scoditti E. Impact of environmental factors on lung defences. *Eur Respir Rev.* 2005;14:51-56.

which hampers airflow and leads to respiratory distress, especially if it occurs along with local inflammation. In people with asthma, the other common pollutant gases, ozone and nitrogen dioxide, can also increase bronchoconstriction,[20] which is a characteristic condition of this chronic disease.

- Finally, fine particulates and nitrogen dioxide can impair the functioning of the immune system's scavenger cells in the alveoli.[17] Evidence of other effects of nitrogen dioxide in healthy individuals is inconsistent,[20] and nitrogen dioxide's greatest impact on respiratory health is as a precursor to ozone.

Airborne particulates and pollutant gases also have important indirect effects on the heart; these effects occur via complex physiological pathways. For example, by increasing systemic inflammation, local lung inflammation can increase the risk of blood clots. Air pollutants can also affect the autonomic nervous system, which controls the heart's rate and rhythm.[21,22] Because ultrafine particulates pass through the alveolar wall into the systemic circulation, they are capable of causing inflammatory responses and health effects elsewhere in the body.[23]

Carbon monoxide, after crossing into the bloodstream in the lungs, binds to hemoglobin in blood. Because carbon monoxide's affinity for hemoglobin is much greater than that of oxygen, it displaces the oxygen that hemoglobin ordinarily carries to the tissues of the body. By denying oxygen to the brain, carbon monoxide causes a loss of alertness and, at high doses, unconsciousness and death.

Health Impacts of Particulates and Pollutant Gases

In the mid-20th century, three episodes of heavy, visible air pollution—in Belgium's Meuse Valley in 1930; in Donora, Pennsylvania, in 1948; and in London in 1952—focused the attention of both scientists and the general public on the hazards of air pollution. In December of 1952, London was blanketed for five days in a smoky, sulfurous fog.[*] A temperature inversion had laid a cap of warmer, less dense air over cooler, heavier air in the London basin, creating stagnant conditions. It had been a cold winter, and perhaps a million coal-burning furnaces were releasing smoke in the area. Londoners were burning high-sulfur coal in these postwar years so that the more desirable low-sulfur coal could be exported to bring cash into the economy. The resulting high concentrations of particulate matter and sulfur dioxide cast a pall over the city—in some locations, the daytime visibility was near zero for two days—and a number of people later reported experiencing the taste of sulfur. Still, in the context of a long history of smoky fog, as well as the recent wartime bombings that had claimed 30,000 lives in London, people for the most part took the smog in stride.

Thus it came as a surprise that about 12,000 deaths over the following 3 months were ultimately attributed to the London Smog. Many sudden deaths occurred at home during the smog, and hospitalizations and emergency-room admissions increased sharply. Autopsies of several adults who died during the smog showed shedding of the bronchial lining, attributed to the extreme acidity of the smog. The majority of deaths were due to pneumonia, exacerbation of emphysema or chronic bronchitis, or cardiovascular causes.

---

*Specifics in this description of the London Smog and its aftermath come from several sources: Bates D. A half century later: recollections of the London Fog. *Environ Health Perspect*. 2002;110(12):A735. Bell M, Davis D, Fletcher T. A retrospective assessment of mortality from the London smog episode of 1952: the role of influenza and pollution. *Environ Health Perspect*. 2004;112(1): 6-8. Black J. Intussusception and the great smog of London, December 1952. *Arch Dis Child*. 2006;88:1040-1042. Davis D, Bell M, Fletcher T. A look back at the London Smog of 1952 and the half century since. *Environ Health Perspect*. 2002;110(12):A734. Dooley E. Fifty years later: clearing the air over the London Smog. *Environ Health Perspect*. 2002;110(12):A748. Whittaker A. Killer smog of London, 50 years on: particle properties and oxidative capacity. *Sc Total Environ*. 2004; 334-335:435-445.

The London Smog was a turning point in public health, not only spurring research on the health effects of air pollution but also the effort to set air pollution standards in the more developed countries. It is estimated that the concentration of total suspended particulates during the London Smog was as high as 7,000 µg/m³. Probably nearly all these particulates were respirable: In samples taken during a 1955 air pollution episode in London, 99% of the total suspended particulates were fewer than 2.5 µg in diameter.[24] By comparison, the current U.S. standards for $PM_{2.5}$ are a 24-hour mean of 35 µg/m³ and an annual mean of 12 µg/m³. That is, $PM_{2.5}$ concentrations during the worst of the London Smog probably approached 200 times the current U.S. daily standard. Even so, the concentration of total suspended particulates during the worst of the London Smog was probably only 10 to 15 times higher than *annual mean* concentrations in some cities in less-developed countries 40 years later (e.g., 400 µg/m³ in Delhi, India, and 800 µg/m³ in Lanzhou, China, in 1995).*,[25]

An extensive epidemiologic literature on the health impacts of air pollution has been generated in locations around the world—from the United States to Europe to Hong Kong. Ambient concentrations of particulates (variously defined), as well as NO_2, SO_2, and O_3, have all been linked to daily (acute) overall mortality and to acute cardiovascular mortality, sometimes lagged by 1 to 5 days after the air pollution measurement.[20,21,26] That is, the mortality rate for a given day may be associated with pollutant concentrations on the same day or on an earlier day. In recent research, satellite imagery has been used to assess particulate air pollution and its links to global patterns of mortality.[27]

In the 1990s, a large study in six U.S. cities linked the ambient concentration of airborne particulate matter to long-term overall mortality, to lung cancer mortality, and to both acute and chronic cardiopulmonary mortality (cardiovascular and nonmalignant respiratory causes grouped together).[28,29] Later follow-up in this study population confirmed these associations and also documented a reduction in mortality associated with a decline over time in fine particulate concentrations.[30] A recent literature review concluded that the body of epidemiologic evidence linking short-term $PM_{2.5}$ exposure to cardiovascular mortality and cardiovascular hospitalizations is strong[31]; and ambient concentrations of particulate matter (PM_{10}) and the major pollutant gases have been linked to acute stroke mortality.[32] More recent work has linked exposure to vehicle exhaust with lung cancer mortality.[33]

Airborne particulates and the same key pollutant gases—NO_2, SO_2, and O_3—have also been linked to acute morbidity in the form of hospital admissions for any respiratory disease and for **chronic obstructive pulmonary disease** (usually chronic bronchitis, emphysema, or both) and also for any cardiovascular disease and specifically for heart failure.[21,22] In urban areas around the world, the same four pollutants have been clearly shown to exacerbate asthma in those who have the disease. Asthma exacerbation has been variously assessed as an increase in symptoms (wheezing and chest tightness), increased hospital admissions or emergency room visits for asthma, increased use of emergency medications by children with asthma, and increased school absences because of asthma.[20,34-38]

All of these findings suggest that air pollution may reduce life expectancy. A 2006 published study of 51 metropolitan areas in the United States estimated an increased life expectancy of 0.61 ± 0.20 years for each 10 mg/m³ reduction in the concentration of fine particulates in air.[39] The estimated effect on the risk of death from lung cancer of elevated $PM_{2.5}$ concentrations at a given point in time has been shown to continue for 2 years, with a gradual decline in the strength of the effect.[40]

---

*Indeed, a young Beijing physician visiting a U.S. laboratory in 2006 commented that she had never before seen lung tissue that was pink, having observed only tissue blackened by particulate pollution (as communicated to the author by toxicologist W. Heiger-Bernays, PhD, in 2006).

Because of air pollution's effects on respiratory and cardiovascular health, susceptible populations are particularly at risk. In newborns, for example, both particulate matter and sulfur dioxide have been linked to low birthweight, and a number of studies have also linked particulate pollution to infant mortality[34] and to respiratory mortality in the postneonatal period.[41]

In recent decades, events have created two natural experiments that have demonstrated the positive health effects of reducing air pollution. In 1990, the Irish government banned the marketing, sale, and distribution of bituminous coal in Dublin. A comparison of mortality before and after the ban revealed a 15.5% drop in respiratory mortality and a 10.3% drop in cardiovascular mortality.[42] A few years later, during the 1996 summer Olympic games, traffic was tightly restricted in the greater Atlanta area. During this period, 30% lower peak daily ozone concentrations were documented, along with a dramatic decline in instances of acute care for asthma.[43]

Finally, it is important to remember that in terms of numbers of deaths, air pollution's greatest impact is through cardiovascular mortality. The original study of six cities reported more than six times as many deaths from cardiovascular disease as from nonmalignant respiratory disease attributed to air pollution.[28] These data are a reminder that cardiovascular disease is the leading cause of death in the U.S. population (nearly 600,000 deaths in 2009),[44] and that any factor that affects the risk of cardiovascular disease has enormous public health implications.

Global Climate Change

The most profound impact of our dependence on fossil fuels is global climate change, and the biggest driver of global climate change is carbon dioxide, a gas that is a natural constituent of the atmosphere and has no direct human health effects. Carbon dioxide has not traditionally been thought of as a pollutant. After all, we exhale it with every breath, and plants depend on it for photosynthesis. Yet, in excess, carbon dioxide has become a pollutant, much as "the dose makes the poison" in toxicology.

Anthropogenic Gases and the Enhanced Greenhouse Effect

As described earlier, carbon dioxide and nitrous oxide, both naturally occurring trace gases in the atmosphere, are known as greenhouse gases because they retain solar energy in the atmosphere, keeping the Earth's climate warm enough for plants and animals to live. But with more of these gases entering the atmosphere from the burning of fossil fuels (see Table 7.2), the resulting *enhanced* greenhouse effect is proving to be too much of a good thing. Ozone from the burning of fossil fuels also makes a significant contribution to global climate change. Methane is not associated with the burning of fossil fuel but is released during the acquisition of oil and natural gas.

Carbon dioxide has the greatest impact because such large quantities are produced through the large-scale burning of fossil fuels by the more developed countries. This impact is truly worldwide because it occurs through effects on the natural **global carbon cycle** (see **Figure 7.7**).

The carbon cycle is the set of processes by which carbon, the fundamental building block of life, moves from the environment through living things and back into the environment. As shown in simplified form in Figure 7.7, green plants take carbon from the atmosphere, incorporating it into glucose through photosynthesis; animals ingest glucose in their food and convert it back to carbon dioxide through cellular respiration. Carbon stored in plant and animal tissue is also returned to the environment through death and decay. (See the following sidebar titled "About Photosynthesis, Respiration, and Decay.")

Where do fossil fuels fit into this continuous cycling of carbon? Fossil fuels are decaying organic matter that, in effect, took a detour into long-term storage (see **Figure 7.8**). For millions

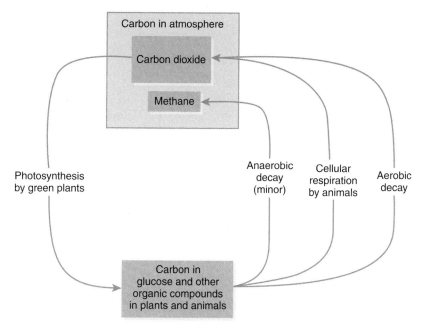

Figure 7.7 The global carbon cycle (excluding fossil fuels).

of years, this stored carbon was not a part of the global circulation of carbon. But now, as fossil fuels are burned, the long-sequestered carbon is being reinjected into circulation in the form of carbon dioxide. In essence, the burning of fossil fuels has converted dead-end storage into a new pathway on one side of the cycle. With no compensating new pathway on the other side, excess carbon is accumulating in the atmosphere in the form of carbon dioxide.

About Photosynthesis, Respiration, and Decay

Photosynthesis, a chemical process that occurs in the cells of green plants, uses energy (from the sun) to convert carbon dioxide (from the atmosphere) and water into glucose and oxygen.

carbon dioxide + water + energy → glucose + oxygen

Plants then convert glucose into the more complex compounds that make up their tissues.

Respiration, a chemical process that occurs in the cells of animals, accomplishes the reverse transformation. Food (actually, glucose from the digestion of food) is the body's fuel. Like combustion, *cellular respiration* converts glucose (which contains hydrogen and carbon) and oxygen into carbon dioxide, water, and energy for the body's use.

glucose + oxygen → carbon dioxide + water + energy

Unlike combustion, cellular respiration is a slow and steady process that occurs at body temperature.

Other organisms in an ecosystem, the decomposers of dead plant and animal matter, accomplish the same chemical transformation through *aerobic decay*. (To a lesser degree, decay also occurs in the absence of oxygen; in this case, methane is produced in lieu of carbon dioxide.)

Together, these processes allow carbon, a fundamental nutrient, to be cycled within ecosystems.

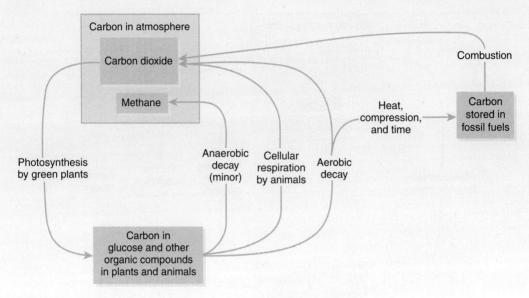

Figure 7.8 The global carbon cycle (including fossil fuels).

The warming effect of anthropogenic greenhouse gases is often quantified as the net gain in radiation energy that results from reducing outgoing terrestrial radiation (heat) relative to incoming solar radiation. The anthropogenic production of carbon dioxide is so great that this gas alone accounted for just over half of the net gain in radiation energy (see **Table 7.5**) as of the late 1990s, despite the fact that the other gases listed are more potent in their warming effects, molecule for molecule.

In 2018, greenhouse gas emissions from the United States were 10% below their 2005 levels, and 81% of carbon dioxide emissions, and most anthropogenic ground-level ozone, were attributable to the burning of fossil fuels.[45] The reduction in U.S. carbon dioxide emissions was associated with the shift to using natural gas for electricity generation, rather than coal. Unfortunately, a life cycle analysis of this shift to using natural gas indicates that it is not as advantageous as hoped due to the amounts of methane released during extraction.[46] The other greenhouse gases listed in Table 7.5, halocarbons and nitrous oxide, come mainly from sources other than the burning of fossil fuels, including industry, agriculture, and community wastes.

Environmental Impacts of Global Climate Change

The notion of global warming was once controversial. Today, however, there is broad scientific consensus that the Earth's climate is warming and also changing in other ways, and the term **global warming** has been supplanted by **global climate change**. Because of the sweeping nature of this environmental issue, in 1988, the World Meteorological Organization and the United Nations Environment Programme jointly established the Intergovernmental Panel on Climate Change (IPCC), an international team of scientists who regularly assess the research data on this matter. The IPCC has published five assessments to date (in 1990, 1995, 2001, 2007, and 2014); the report on the sixth assessment of climate change is expected in 2022.

To date, three basic climate-related environmental changes during the past century have been well documented[47]:

- The global surface temperature rose by approximately 0.74°C—about 1.3°F—from 1906 to 2005, and most of the warmest years have been among the most recent. These figures reflect rising temperatures of both

Table 7.5 Percentage of Net Gain in Energy in the Earth–Atmosphere System from Five Major Greenhouse Gases That Are Attributable to Each Gas

Greenhouse Gas	Percentage of Net Gain
Carbon dioxide	56.5
Methane	16.3
Ozone	10.2*
Halocarbons**	11.6
Nitrous oxide	5.4

*The warming effect of ozone as listed here represents the net effect of an increase in tropospheric ozone (caused mostly by the burning of fossil fuels) and the depletion of stratospheric ozone (caused by certain organic chemicals, described elsewhere).

** Organic compounds containing halogens, such as chlorine or fluorine.

Data from Intergovernmental Panel on Climate Change. Technical summary. In *Climate Change 2007: The Physical Science Basis. Contribution of Working Group I to the Fourth Assessment Report of the Intergovernmental Panel on Climate Change.* Cambridge University Press. 2007.

air near the Earth's surface and near-surface ocean waters.

- There has been a worldwide decline since the mid-1960s in the area covered by snow and glaciers.
- In 2014, global sea level was 2.6 inches above the 1993 average—the highest annual average in the satellite record (1993-present). Sea level continues to rise at a rate of about one-eighth of an inch per year.[48]

These changes are related, as shown in **Figure 7.9**: Warmer surface air contributes to the melting of snow and glaciers, and this meltwater contributes in turn to the rise in sea level. Shrinking icecaps are a marker of rising global temperatures, and the calving of new icebergs (see **Figure 7.10**) speeds melting. Thermal expansion of surface seawater that is warming overall (despite the addition of glacial meltwater) also contributes to the rise in sea level. Finally, the warming of surface air has a circular aspect: Warmer air temperatures result in more evaporation of surface water, increasing the water vapor (a greenhouse gas) in the atmosphere.

Climate data also show an increased frequency of heat waves since the mid-20th century, longer and more intense droughts since the 1970s

(especially in the tropics and subtropics), and more frequent heavy precipitation events in many areas.[47] Climate scientists are currently considering whether episodes of El Niño/Southern Oscillation (ENSO) might be related to global climate change.*[49]

Scientific evidence indicates that most of the warming that has taken place since the mid-20th century is very likely attributable to increased concentrations of greenhouse gases in the atmosphere—that is, it is caused by human activity—and that changes will continue through the 21st century.[47] Using a set of climate models, each based on a set of assumptions about global

---

*El Niño is a change in the surface currents in the Eastern South Pacific: The usual cold, nutrient-rich current is replaced by a warm current that does not support the typically dense populations of fish. Because surface currents are driven largely by friction between air and water, this change occurs when the normal prevailing winds become much weaker or even reverse, which is caused in turn by shifts in atmospheric pressure (the Southern Oscillation). An El Niño event typically occurs every 5 to 10 years and lasts a few months, often around the beginning of the new year.

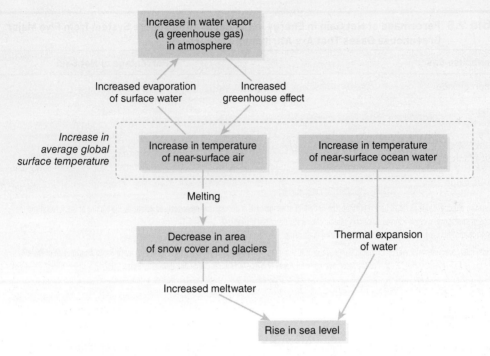

Figure 7.9 Connections among major climate-related environmental changes.

Data from Intergovernmental Panel on Climate Change. Technical summary. In *Climate Change 2007: The Physical Science Basis. Contribution of Working Group I to the Fourth Assessment Report of the Intergovernmental Panel on Climate Change.* Cambridge University Press. 2007.

development, the IPCC has estimated the environmental impacts of a range of emissions scenarios. The most optimistic scenario assumes a world "with reductions in material intensity and the introduction of clean and resource-efficient technologies"[47] and an emphasis on sustainability. The most pessimistic is a sort of business-as-usual scenario that assumes "very rapid economic growth"[47] and a technological emphasis on fossil fuels.

The global average estimates for the end of the 21st century under the optimistic scenario are a temperature increase of 1.8°C and a rise in sea level of 0.18 to 0.38 meters; under the pessimistic scenario, a temperature increase of about 4.0°C and a rise in sea level of 0.26 to 0.59 meters are projected.[50] The environmental impacts of rising sea level include increased coastal erosion, the conversion of coastal marshes to open water, and the intrusion of saltwater into coastal aquifers. Although it is deemed very likely that the deep

ocean thermohaline circulation will slow down, it is deemed very unlikely that there will be a dramatic shift in the global circulation of deep ocean waters before 2100,[50] an effect whose impact on climate would be truly catastrophic. Finally, scientists are increasingly concerned that the ocean's absorption of excess atmospheric carbon dioxide will affect marine ecosystems.

Health Impacts of Global Climate Change

The processes that make up global climate change are complex and interrelated, and there is considerable uncertainty about exactly when, where, and to what degree specific human health impacts will occur. But many of the scenarios that have been modeled converge in predicting certain public health impacts associated with overall rising temperatures, a rising sea level, and more frequent extreme weather events.[51]

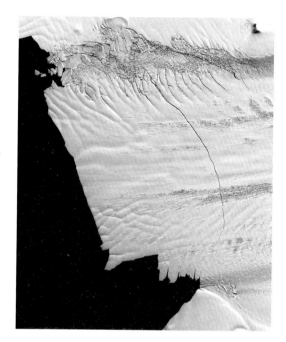

Figure 7.10 Fissure in an Antarctic glacier, 19 miles long, 260 feet wide, and 195 feet deep. It is expected to grow until it causes an iceberg of some 350 square miles to split off.

Courtesy of National Aeronautics and Space Administration. Available at: www.nasa.gov/multimedia /imagegallery/image_feature_2165.html. Accessed March 5, 2012.

Higher overall temperatures will increase the range of major disease vectors[51]—most importantly, mosquitoes—with a corresponding increase in vector-borne diseases, including malaria. Many areas where malaria and other mosquito-borne illnesses are prevalent are in less-developed regions. There may also be an increase in waterborne and foodborne illnesses with increasing temperatures[51]—as is seen now in seasonal fluctuations—because warmer temperatures are more conducive to microbial reproduction. If geographic shifts in temperature occur, corresponding shifts will occur in the regions where specific crops thrive[51]; this will be disruptive and is likely to affect diet and nutrition. Furthermore, in more developed countries, if temperatures rise or intense heat waves occur, livestock being raised in the crowded indoor conditions of modern agriculture may suffer heat stress, resulting in reduced productivity.[52]

A rising sea level will slowly inundate low-lying coastal regions[51]; many of the most heavily populated low-lying areas are in less-developed countries. The change in sea level will affect food supplies, claiming agricultural land and disrupting breeding grounds for fish and shellfish. Saltwater intrusion into freshwater aquifers will affect drinking water supplies. The loss of habitable land will create refugees, potentially in large numbers.

Finally, more frequent extreme weather events will produce familiar impacts on a grander scale.[51] Heat waves will produce crop failures, as well as human deaths from heart attacks and heat stroke. Tornados, hurricanes or typhoons, and floods will cause physical injuries and hunger (perhaps evolving into malnutrition or famine, depending on circumstances). They will also produce conditions conducive to infectious disease, including the emergence of new infectious diseases: flooding that enhances the breeding of mosquitoes, physical disruption that increases contact with rodent vectors, overcrowding that aids the transmission of respiratory illnesses, and damage to the sewage and drinking water systems that ordinarily protect against diarrheal disease. We have only to look at the devastating effects of Hurricane Katrina, a category 5 hurricane in 2005 in the United States—one of the world's wealthiest countries—to appreciate the health impacts and social disruption that can come in the wake of an extreme weather event. And more strong hurricanes have been occurring in the Atlantic with eight category 5 hurricanes from 2000 to 2009, and four from 2016 to 2019.[51]

It is estimated that children will disproportionately experience the health impacts of climate change. Infectious diseases that are important causes of death in children worldwide are also diseases that could become more common with rising temperatures; malnutrition, a key risk factor for infectious disease in children, can also be expected to increase if food supplies are disrupted due to climate change.[53]

International Agreements on Global Climate Change

Through the 1980s, scientists' awareness of the environmental impacts of human activities, and in particular the potential global impacts of carbon dioxide and other greenhouse gases, increased steadily. In 1988, the World Meteorological Association and the U.N. Environment Programme together established a new organization, the Intergovernmental Panel on Climate Change. This group began to assess the science of climate change in order to understand its potential impacts and to consider what might be done to prevent or manage those impacts.

In 1990, a new U.N. committee was created, charged with preparing a "framework convention" on climate change. That is, rather than negotiating specific terms, the committee would establish the core principles by which international action on climate change would move forward. The framework included goals and timetables and acknowledged the distinction in responsibilities of the more developed, and less developed, countries. It also set up the basic procedures for later negotiation of specifics.

The U.N. Framework Convention on Climate Change was opened for signatures at the 1992 U.N. Conference on Environment and Development in Rio de Janeiro—the same conference that produced the first important international articulation of the precautionary principle, as described earlier in the context of preventive regulatory principles. The Framework Convention entered into force in 1994, and as of March 2012, a total of 195 parties, including the United States, had signed and ratified it.[54] However, the terms of the treaty were limited: It encouraged countries to reduce emissions of greenhouse gases to certain targets, but it did not commit them to do so.

The Kyoto Protocol, an agreement linked to the U.N. Framework Convention and adopted in Kyoto, Japan, in December of 1997, committed the countries that ratified it to meet specific targets for the major greenhouse gases. The Kyoto Protocol went into effect in February of 2005 and obligated the countries that ratified it to meet their reduction limits through 2020. The more developed countries that ratified the Protocol agreed to make specific reductions of their emissions of greenhouse gases, for the period from 2008 to 2012, relative to their 1990 emissions.

The United States signed the Protocol, but did not ratify it, and indicated to the United Nations that it did not intend to ratify after all because the U.S. Congress felt that the United States was being treated unfairly.

In order to continue the international agreement process related to curbing climate change, another conference was held in Paris in 2015. The Paris Climate Agreement included a specific target for limiting the increase in global warming to well below 2°C above the pre-industrial levels of 1750.[55] In 2016, China and the United States, representing almost 40% of global emissions, issued a joint statement agreeing to sign the agreement. Altogether, nearly 200 countries made national pledges to reduce their contribution toward climate change, with the more developed countries, including the United States, agreeing to help poorer countries with the costs incurred in meeting their reduction goals. Once again, in 2019, the United States formally notified the United Nations that the U.S. would withdraw from the agreement, after ceasing to implement any federal policies associated with the agreement as soon as the Trump administration took office in 2017, stating that the agreement imposed an unfair economic burden on American workers, businesses, and taxpayers.[56]

Regulation of Air Pollution from the Burning of Fossil Fuels

The first federal air pollution law in the United States was the Air Pollution Control Act of 1955. Coming just a few years after the London Smog, this early legislation mostly supported research. Two laws passed during the 1960s took tentative steps toward controlling air pollution, but it was the Clean Air Act of 1970 that set up a broad framework to do so. The U.S. EPA was created in 1971 to implement the Clean Air Act of 1970. There were two major sets of amendments to the Clean Air Act in 1977 and 1990, and some other laws have addressed specific air-pollution issues.

By its nature, air pollution is challenging to control. The atmosphere is not confined, like a body of water, nor does it respect boundaries drawn on maps. And although power plants and some other important sources of air pollution are stationary, vehicles are highly mobile pollution sources.

In principle, two aspects of air pollution can be assessed: *concentrations* of pollutants in ambient air and *emissions* of pollutants from sources. Ambient concentrations cannot be controlled directly; it is only possible to set a maximum allowed concentration in ambient air and then assess compliance with this standard. The only levers for the control of air pollution are at the source. Here, there are two basic options: either to set a limit on emissions and then measure performance (adherence to the limit) or to require specific technologies that will result in lower emissions. The U.S. regulatory framework for air pollution uses a combination of approaches: ambient standards, performance standards for emission sources, and technology requirements for emission sources.

The EPA sets health-based limits for the concentration in ambient air for a short list of widespread pollutants, known as **criteria air pollutants**. The six criteria air pollutants are carbon monoxide, NO_2, SO_2, particulate matter, lead, and ground-level ozone. All are pollutants from the burning of fossil fuels. For these particulates and gaseous pollutants, the EPA has created a measure of daily air quality called the **Air Quality Index**. Each day, for each of these five pollutants, and for local areas across the country, the EPA publishes a numerical score from 0 to 500 (a lower score indicates cleaner air) and a category rating, ranging from good to hazardous. These ratings indicate the degree of health concern not only for the general population but also for susceptible subgroups of the general population. Many newspapers publish the local Air Quality Index each day, and it can also be accessed online.

For the criteria air pollutants, the EPA sets maximum allowable concentrations. These are the **National Ambient Air Quality Standards (NAAQS, or "nax")**, set at levels intended to protect human health (see **Table 7.6**). Through a State Implementation Plan, each state is required to translate these ambient standards into emissions limits that will enable the state to meet

Table 7.6 Current National Ambient Air Quality Standards

Pollutant	Concentration	Averaging Time
Carbon monoxide	9 ppm 35 ppm	8-hour 1-hour
Nitrogen dioxide	53 ppb 100 ppb	Annual 1-hour
Sulfur dioxide	75 ppb	1-hour
Particulate matter (PM_{10})	150 mg/m³	24-hour
Particulate matter ($PM_{2.5}$)	12 mg/m³ 35 mg/m³	Annual 24-hour
Lead	0.15 mg/m³	Rolling 3-month average
Ozone	0.070 ppm	8-hour

Note: Units of parts per million (ppm) and parts per billion (ppb) are by volume. For additional detail on the form of the standard, see source.

U.S. Environmental Protection Agency. *National Ambient Air Quality Standards (NAAQS)*. Available at: www.epa.gov/air/criteria.html. Accessed July 23, 2020.

the national standards. For purposes of monitoring and enforcement, each state is divided into geographic areas made up of adjacent counties or townships. An area that fails to meet any of the NAAQS is designated as a "nonattainment area" for a given pollutant, and a program of control measures to bring the area into compliance must be agreed upon. Such noncompliance is not uncommon.

In addition to setting ambient standards for a small number of common pollutants, the EPA is charged with setting emissions standards for a long list of less common but more toxic pollutants. This list of 188 hazardous air pollutants (HAPs), also known as "air toxics," includes mercury and its compounds, although most HAPs are volatile organic compounds. For these chemicals, the EPA is charged with setting National Emission Standards for HAPS (NESHAPS) for stationary sources. Some are performance-based standards and others are technology-based standards; neither type is a health-based standard. For example, the standard for mercury emissions is a performance-based standard (emissions from all power plants are capped at a given level), although units of allowed emissions can be traded among regulated facilities as a cost-effective way to reduce mercury emissions from the energy sector as a whole. Citing the shortage of health effects data on many chemicals, the EPA has regulated only seven air toxics to date under NESHAPS (asbestos; the metals mercury, inorganic arsenic, and beryllium; the VOCs benzene and vinyl chloride; and radionuclides). Technology standards under NESHAPS now take the form of a requirement to use either "generally available control technology" or "maximum achievable control technology."

In regulating mobile sources of air pollution (mostly cars and trucks), the EPA has used a range of approaches over the years to address both criteria pollutants and others by regulating tailpipe emissions, engine performance, and fuel. For example, the EPA has set limits on tailpipe emissions of hydrocarbons, carbon monoxide, and nitrogen oxides (specified in grams of pollutant per mile driven). Furthermore, states are required to implement programs to inspect cars to ensure that they meet these emissions limits. The agency also established overall mileage requirements for each auto manufacturer's fleet—the corporate average fuel economy standards, or CAFE (pronounced "café") standards. Finally, in the context of growing scientific appreciation of the health hazards of diesel exhaust, the EPA has set new pollution control technology requirements for heavy-duty trucks and buses, and refineries are producing ultralow-sulfur diesel fuel.

The use of lead as a gasoline additive was gradually reduced between 1973 and 1986 as the EPA phased in new limits. During this period, car manufacturers introduced catalytic converters (devices that reduce the pollutants in exhaust), which were needed to meet emissions limits, and which also sped up the phasing out of lead because lead damaged the converters. Leaded gasoline was eliminated in the United States in 1996. The benefit of removing lead from gasoline is shown clearly in **Figure 7.11**, which tracks the decline of blood lead levels in U.S. children as leaded gasoline was phased out—a public health success story, although a belated one.

A more recent innovation is the development of "reformulated gasoline," which produces less VOC pollution when it is burned, reducing the formation of ozone. Use of reformulated gasoline is now required in urban areas experiencing serious smog problems. Approximately 30% of the gasoline sold in the United States is reformulated.[57] On the whole, the regulation of pollution from cars is a difficult challenge in the United States, where many people live in suburban settings, consider a large car to be a basic necessity, and show little support for higher gas prices, public transit, carpooling, or bicycle lanes.

In the U.S. regulatory framework, acid deposition is controlled through the Clean Air Act's emissions limits on NO_2 and SO_2. The 1990 amendments set a plan for reducing total SO_2 emissions over time, specifically to address the problem of acid deposition, adding a market-based system of trading emission allowances. And, reflecting the transboundary nature of this problem, the United States and Canada have agreed to a joint program to reduce emissions of NO_X and SO_X.

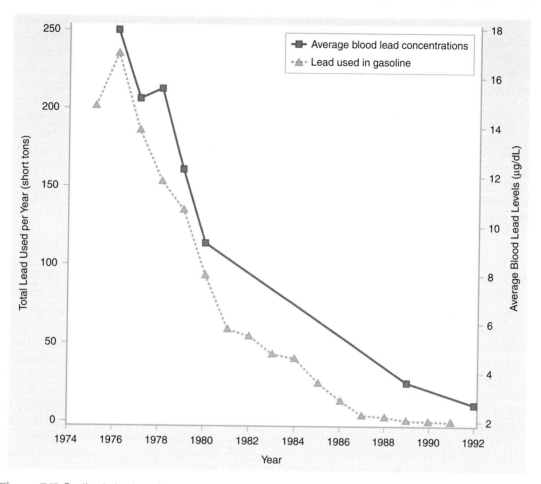

Figure 7.11 Decline in lead used in gasoline, and of average blood levels in U.S. children, 1974–1992.

U.S. Environmental Protection Agency. Great Lakes National Program Office. *Great Lakes Binational Toxics Strategy Report on Alkyl-lead: Sources, Regulations and Options*, 2000. Available at: www.epa.gov/glnpo/bns/lead/Step%20Report /steps.pdf. Accessed April 12, 2008.

Over the years during which global climate change grew into a major environmental policy concern, the EPA declined to regulate carbon dioxide on the grounds that it was not an air pollutant under the Clean Air Act. In 2007; however, the U.S. Supreme Court struck down that interpretation, ruling that carbon dioxide fell within the broad definition of air pollutants under the law, and further, that the EPA must regulate carbon dioxide unless it made a determination that carbon dioxide was *not* a contributor to global climate change.[58] In late 2009, the EPA made a formal determination that carbon dioxide is a greenhouse gas. In March of 2012, the agency presented a draft rule to limit carbon dioxide emissions, by new power plants only, to 1,000 pounds per megawatt-hour of power produced, averaged over a period of 30 years.[59] That is, the rule allows new plants to begin operations at emissions levels greater than 1,000 pounds per megawatt-hour, as long as later reductions make the plant meet the 30-year average requirement. In 2014, the Clean Power Plan was proposed that would slash allowable levels of carbon emissions by more than a third by 2030 in an attempt to encourage utilities to shift away from coal, but this plan was never enacted. As of 2020, the current administration favors loosening the environmental air regulations to help protect the coal industry.

The Clean Air Act also gives the EPA a key role in the implementation of the National Environmental Policy Act (NEPA), signed into law in 1970. As discussed earlier, NEPA requires all federal agencies in the executive branch of government to evaluate and disclose the environmental impacts of their proposed actions (e.g., building an interstate highway or cutting timber) *before* decisions are made or actions are taken. Depending on the complexity of the proposed action, this disclosure may take the form of a full **environmental impact statement (EIS)** or a more streamlined environmental assessment. NEPA adds the explicit consideration of a new factor—environmental impacts—to the traditional criteria of technical and economic feasibility in agencies' decision making, although the law stops short of actually requiring protection of the environment.[60]

In principle, the Environmental Protection Agency must comply with NEPA's requirements as other agencies do. However, many EPA actions (for example, under the Clean Air Act and the Clean Water Act) are exempt from NEPA's requirements in light of the fact that the EPA's own procedures already achieve the same objectives. Furthermore, as alluded to earlier, the EPA has an important role in the implementation of NEPA: The Clean Air Act requires the EPA to review and comment publicly on environmental impact statements by all other federal agencies and evaluate the acceptability of the environmental impacts of the agencies' planned actions.

7.3 Electricity from Nuclear Fuel

In contrast to coal, which people have used as fuel for perhaps a thousand years, **uranium** has only been tapped as a source of energy in the last 60-plus years. Following World War II, during which nuclear weapons were developed and used, serious efforts were made to develop peaceful applications of nuclear technology—in particular, to generate electricity. **Nuclear power** is derived from the controlled splitting of uranium atoms, in contrast to the uncontrolled chain reaction of a nuclear weapon.

Nuclear power was attractive on several grounds. It was "clean," producing none of the combustion products associated with coal- and oil-fired power plants. And, although uranium is a nonrenewable resource, U.S. reserves would serve for many decades. Finally, U.S. plans for civilian nuclear power and military nuclear weapons dovetailed nicely because, at that time, both were managed by the Atomic Energy Commission; for example, radioactive wastes from civilian power plants were to be reprocessed for use in both power plants and weapons.

The early optimism over nuclear power faded as the safety challenges of operating power plants and reprocessing or entombing their radioactive wastes became clear. By the early 1980s, the U.S. nuclear power industry had reached a plateau and was moribund for decades, with no new power plants coming on line, and little progress in resolving the difficult issues around transporting and storing the radioactive wastes that plants produce. Within the growing public acceptance of the reality of global climate change during the early 2000s, nuclear power appeared to fit well into a low-carbon energy strategy, and several new nuclear power plants were proposed. However, since the Fukushima nuclear plant accident in 2011, to be discussed subsequently, enthusiasm for nuclear power has evaporated once again as its risks seem to outweigh its benefits. Nonetheless, in the era of global climate change and dwindling oil reserves, nuclear power clearly remains in the mix of energy technologies for the United States and the world.

The environmental and health impacts of using uranium as a fuel are very different from those associated with fossil fuels. The fundamentals of radiation, including radioactive decay; the electromagnetic spectrum, the important distinction between ionizing and nonionizing radiation; and the specialized units for quantifying exposure to ionizing radiation were presented earlier in the context of naturally occurring radiation. This section treats the following topics:

- The major stages in the nuclear fuel cycle (which, like the fossil fuel cycle, is not really a cycle)

- The health impacts of radiation exposures from the nuclear fuel cycle
- The U.S. regulatory framework for preventing or limiting exposures to ionizing radiation from the nuclear fuel cycle

The Nuclear Fuel Cycle

As it operates in the United States today, the **nuclear fuel cycle** is not actually a cycle but rather a one-way series of events, usually grouped into three stages (see **Figure 7.12**). In the first stage, often called the front end of the process, uranium is mined and ultimately fabricated into a form that can be used as fuel in a power plant. The middle stage is the generation of electricity at nuclear power plants. The last stage, often referred to as the **back end**, is the disposal of the radioactive wastes produced by power plants. If nuclear wastes were to be reprocessed (and some other countries do reprocess these wastes), this partial recycling occurs in the middle of the back end of the cycle and would complete the "cycle" in the term "nuclear fuel cycle."

The Front End of the Nuclear Fuel Cycle

Uranium is widespread in the Earth's crust. For example, it is found at low concentrations in granite and in many coal deposits. However, it is practical to mine only uranium-bearing rock in which concentrations are much higher—that is, uranium ore. Uranium ore has been removed both from underground mines and, especially in the earlier years of the industry, from surface mines. Nearly all uranium deposits in the United States are in the western states, mostly in the Four Corners region where Colorado, Utah, Arizona, and New Mexico come together; and historically, most U.S. uranium mining took place on Navajo tribal lands.

The mining of uranium ore releases radiation into the confined spaces of underground mines and also into the ambient environment. Mining produces waste in the form of crushed rock, known as tailings. Of course, the line between ore that is worth mining and ore that is not worth mining is blurry (and it changes over time with shifts in the market price of uranium), but as a

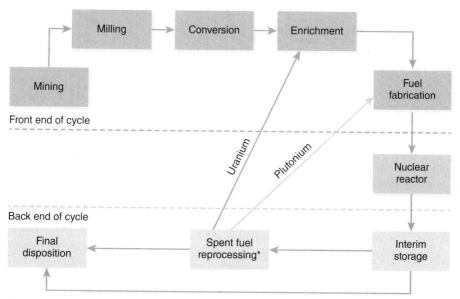

Spent fuel reprocessing is omitted from the cycle in most countries, including the United States.

Figure 7.12 The nuclear fuel cycle.

U.S. Energy Information Administration. Nuclear explained, The nuclear fuel cycle. Available at: https://www.eia.gov/energyexplained/nuclear/the-nuclear-fuel-cycle.php

rule, **uranium mine tailings** contain higher concentrations of uranium than ordinary rock does. Mine tailings are left in large piles on the ground surface near mines. Radon gas is released from tailings to the air, radioactive dust is carried on the wind, and rainwater leaches radioactive constituents into groundwater.

Uranium ore extracted by mining is next processed at a mill. Milling converts the uranium ore to a more concentrated form known as **yellowcake**, which is transported to the Eastern United States for further processing. Milling of uranium also produces large volumes of depleted ore in the form of sandy sludge, known as **uranium mill tailings**.

Such waste is dumped in piles on the ground or placed in walled impoundments. Like mine tailings, mill tailings are a source of radon and radioactive dust. Nevertheless, in the past, mill tailings were sometimes used for construction. For example, in the 1950s, many tons of tailings piled in Grand Junction, Colorado, were given away free to builders, who used them in constructing basements and patios in the area.[61]

During the peak period for nuclear power in the 1980s, there were 26 licensed uranium milling sites in the United States. As of 1996, the 26 licensed sites represented a total of about 200 million metric tons of tailings, and 24 abandoned sites accounted for another 26 million metric tons,[62] mostly in the Western United States (see **Figure 7.13**). Today, there are three remaining uranium mills, and only one is actively operating.[63]

In recent years, it has become common to use an acidic or alkaline solution to dissolve uranium from the ore in which it is embedded, rather than mining; this process is known as **in situ leaching**. When uranium is leached from ore in situ, yellowcake is produced in a single step, along with liquid waste. This waste is placed in a manmade pond and water is allowed to evaporate, leaving behind radioactive sludge. Like mining, in situ leaching takes uranium out of its natural geologic setting, where human exposure to radiation is very limited, into the realm of human activity and exposure.

Most naturally occurring uranium, and, therefore, most of the uranium in yellowcake, is

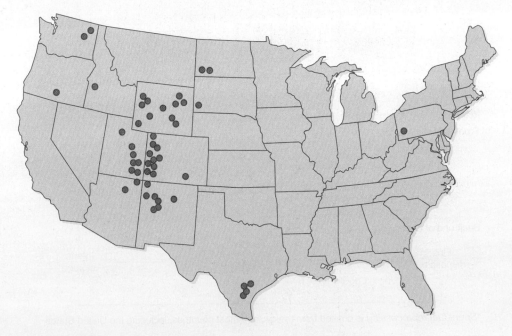

Figure 7.13 Locations of uranium mill tailings piles in the United States.

U.S. Environmental Protection Agency. Uranium mill tailings. Available at: www.epa.gov/rpdweb00/docs/radwaste/402-k-94-001-umt.htm. Accessed: October 14, 2012.

uranium-238. However, it is uranium-235 that can be used as fuel in a power reactor. For this reason, the next step in uranium processing is to increase the ratio of uranium-235 to uranium-238. This step, known as **enrichment**, is actually achieved by *removing* uranium-238 from the yellowcake. This excess uranium-238, called **depleted uranium**, has some uses; in particular, because it is extremely dense, it is used to make military armor and armor-piercing weapons. However, most is treated as waste with a relatively low level of radioactivity.

The final step in preparing uranium for use in power plants is **fuel fabrication**. The enriched uranium is formed into hard pellets, which are placed inside long, thin metal tubes. These loaded tubes are the fuel rods that will be used in a nuclear power plant.

Production of Nuclear Power

At present, there are 96 nuclear power reactors operating at 58 plants in the United States (see **Figure 7.14**),[64] most located far from the environmental disruptions caused by the mining and milling of uranium (see Figure 7.13). Twenty-seven plants have been decommissioned and are no longer operating. The newest reactor is located in Tennessee, which began operation in June of 2016 alongside the next-youngest operating reactor, which entered service in May of 1996.[65]

As already described, in a fossil fuel–driven power plant, coal or oil is burned to generate heat, which is used to produce steam, which drives the turbines that generate electricity. A nuclear power plant operates in the same way, except that the heat used to produce steam is generated by a controlled nuclear chain reaction.

Normal Operations. In the core of a power reactor, tens of thousands of uranium fuel rods stand upright, surrounded by water. The core is bombarded with neutrons. Each neutron striking the nucleus of a uranium atom causes it to split, or fission, into two smaller atoms of different elements, releasing more neutrons along with energy (heat). Any of the neutrons that strikes the nucleus of another uranium atom causes it to split, releasing still more neutrons, and so forth.

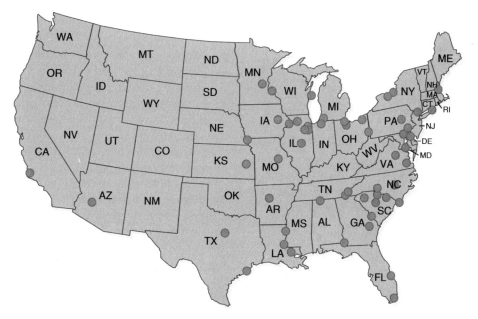

Figure 7.14 Locations of operating nuclear power plants in the United States, 2020.

U.S. Energy Information Administration. Location of U.S. Nuclear Power Plants. Available at: https://www.eia.gov/energyexplained/nuclear/us-nuclear-industry.php

To keep this **nuclear fission** chain reaction from cascading out of control, rods containing a neutron-absorbing material are inserted into slots among the fuel rods. These **control rods** can be moved into, and out of, the core to slow down or speed up the chain reaction. The fission reaction can be shut down rapidly by fully inserting the control rods, although it would then take several months for the heat in the core to be dissipated by the cooling system. The core is shielded to contain the radiation produced by the fission reactions.

In one common design, the water (as liquid or steam) circulates in a loop, passing through the reactor core and the steam turbine. The circulating water has two functions, which are really two sides of the same coin. In the core, it acts as a coolant, removing heat from the nuclear chain reaction; then, having absorbed heat in the core, it is converted to steam, which serves to drive a turbine. After passing through the turbine, the steam is cooled and condensed, returning to the core in liquid form. (This basic design is known as a boiling water reactor; other designs are also used.)

It is critical to keep the core of a nuclear reactor from becoming too hot. Overheating will compromise the structural integrity of the fuel rods, which in turn will prevent the control rods from moving freely into the core. This will result in even greater overheating and damage to the fuel rods. This very dangerous cycle of effects can lead to a partial or full meltdown of the core, with the potential for large releases of radioactivity. The cylindrical, or dome-shaped, containment building that surrounds a nuclear reactor (two are shown in **Figure 7.15**, housing the two reactors) is designed to limit the escape of radioactivity in the event of an accident. The photo also shows the four large cooling towers that reduce the temperature of the water that will be returned to the river; this feature is not unique to nuclear power and was described previously in the context of generating power by burning fossil fuels.

The containment building is only the most visible safety feature of a nuclear reactor. Redundant and flexible safety features are engineered into commercial reactors. A key element is an independent emergency core cooling system that refloods the reactor core in the event that the core

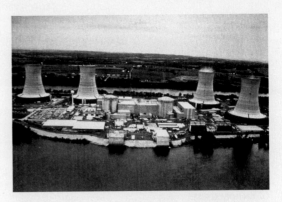

Figure 7.15 The Three Mile Island nuclear power plant in Pennsylvania was the site of the most serious accident at a U.S. commercial nuclear plant.

Courtesy of CDC Public Health Image Library. ID# 1194. Content provider CDC. Available at: http://phil.cdc.gov /phil/home.asp. Accessed October 14, 2012.

loses coolant, although an accident that causes physical damage to the core can render this system ineffective.

During normal operations, a nuclear power plant releases small quantities of numerous radioactive fission products into the air, including iodine-131 and strontium-90, as well as radioactive isotopes of the noble (chemically inert) gases xenon and krypton.

Accidents at Nuclear Power Plants. Nuclear power is an unforgiving technology in two ways: First, if the reactor core is damaged, an accident can spiral out of control, as occurred at the Chernobyl plant in Ukraine (then a part of the Soviet Union) in 1986 and at the Fukushima plant in Japan in 2011; and second, the resulting radiation exposure is long lasting, and its effects are potentially serious. The overall safety significance of nuclear events is classified using a 7-point scale developed by the International Atomic Energy Agency, as follows[66]:

Level 1: Anomaly
Level 2: Incident
Level 3: Serious incident
Level 4: Accident with local consequences
Level 5: Accident with wider consequences
Level 6: Serious accident
Level 7: Major accident

Of course, nuclear power plants are subject to all of the factors that contribute to accidents at other industrial facilities, including aging physical plants, natural disasters, bad design decisions, and human error. The effects of everyday human error can be greatly magnified in a technically complex setting such as a nuclear power reactor. For example, at the Browns Ferry nuclear plant in Alabama in 1975, a maintenance worker who was using a candle flame to identify air leaks accidentally set fire to insulation surrounding some electrical cables.[67] Because this accident happened in a room where cables from all over the plant converged, multiple components were simultaneously disabled, and a serious accident was narrowly averted.[67] However, most mistakes are less significant, and most are discovered and fixed before they pose any risk to the public: for example, tools or protective gear inadvertently left in locations where they could impede the plant's operation; devices turned on or off for routine maintenance, and not turned back off or back on. Such lapses are not new, and they are not unique to nuclear power.

The most serious nuclear event in the United States to date, at the Three Mile Island plant in Pennsylvania in 1979, began when a valve stuck open so that coolant drained out of the core. The operators' instrument panel did not make it clear that the valve was open. It appeared to them that the core had *too much* water, so they shut off the emergency cooling pumps. Although a part of the core melted, the reactor vessel remained intact, and the total radioactive release was relatively low. The incident was classified as a Level 5 nuclear event.[66]

The design of the Soviet reactor at Chernobyl differed from that of Western reactors in important ways, including the lack of a true containment building and the use of graphite to absorb neutrons in the core. At Chernobyl, a complicated series of decisions and actions by the plant's operators resulted in a power surge in the core at a time when the emergency core cooling system had been turned off as part of a test. The fuel rods melted and ruptured, rendering the control rods ineffective, and a steam explosion destroyed the reactor core. The ensuing graphite fire released large quantities of radioactive elements into the air,

creating a plume that spread across Europe. The regions most heavily contaminated by the accident were those now known as Ukraine, Belarus, and the Russian Federation. The 1986 Chernobyl accident is classified as a Level 7 nuclear event.[66]

The events of March 2011 at the Fukushima reactor in Japan began with a natural disaster: a massive earthquake under the Pacific Ocean, the largest ever recorded in Japan, followed about 40 minutes later by a series of seven tsunamis that swept over the Fukushima site.[68] The nuclear installation at Fukushima consisted of six reactors. Reactor units 1, 2, 3, and 4 are located close together, and the three reactors producing power at the time of the accident were all in this cluster. The initial earthquake triggered automatic shutdowns of the nuclear reaction in the three operating units; still, hydrogen explosions occurred in all three of the reactors whose cores were exposed by damage from the earthquake and tsunami, releasing radiation. Because of the extensive destruction in the region, workers at the plant were largely isolated during the aftermath of the accident. Although the tsunami wiped out a substantial part of the site's electrical power, workers managed to inject seawater into the damaged reactors to stop the cores from melting down completely; two workers died in the efforts to control the accident. Like Chernobyl, the Fukushima accident has been classified as a Level 7 nuclear event (a major accident).[69] On the day after the earthquake, people within 20 kilometers of the plant were ordered to evacuate, and those who had survived the tsunami left the area.

The Back End of the Nuclear Fuel Cycle

Over time, the amount of "unburned" uranium-235 in the core of an operating power reactor declines. The reactor is periodically shut down to remove spent fuel and replace it with new fuel rods. The spent fuel is extremely hot, releasing both radiation and heat. It is placed immediately in an underground storage pool at the reactor site; the pool is shielded to prevent the escape of radiation, and circulating water gradually cools the spent fuel. After about a year, spent fuel can be removed from the pool, although it is still highly radioactive.

Embedded in the spent fuel are two types of radioactive materials created by bombarding uranium with neutrons. Fission products—elements lighter than uranium—are created when neutrons *split* uranium nuclei. Alternatively, if an atom *absorbs* a neutron, the atom becomes a different element with a higher atomic number. In this way, plutonium and other elements heavier than uranium are created in the spent fuel. These heavy elements are sometimes called transuranic elements because their atomic numbers are higher than that of uranium.

As noted earlier, the original plan in the United States was to recycle the wastes of nuclear power plants, extracting "unburned" uranium-238 to be fabricated again into fuel pellets. As shown in Figure 7.12, such **reprocessing** of spent fuel would also extract plutonium to be used in making nuclear weapons, and it would create a new waste stream of highly radioactive material, now in liquid form. These liquid wastes of reprocessing would contain uranium and plutonium not captured by reprocessing, as well as the fission products and transuranic elements present in the spent fuel. This waste stream, like the original spent fuel, would require permanent storage in a repository. In the United States, commercial reactor fuel has not been reprocessed for at least 3 decades, for three reasons: (1) It is not clear that reprocessing reduces the waste management challenges of nuclear power; (2) It is also not clear that reprocessed fuel is cheaper than the newly made fuel it is intended to replace; (3) Finally, production of nuclear weapons has declined dramatically, and there is some risk that reactor-grade plutonium, if obtained by terrorists or rogue nations, could be used to make a crude nuclear weapon.*

Nuclear power plants themselves, when they are decommissioned (closed down), become radioactive waste. As of July of 2020, 10 commercial nuclear reactors in the United States have been successfully decommissioned and another 20 plants are in the process.[65] After the plant's works are flushed out to remove radioactive debris, the facility can be dismantled and its components, such as the reactor vessel, can be shipped offsite for permanent disposal as radioactive waste. Federal regulations give plant operators the option of letting the facility stand for some years before being dismantled, to allow radioactivity to decline; decommissioning must be completed within 60 years after the plant closes. To date, most waste from decommissioned U.S. nuclear power plants has been shipped to a commercial radioactive waste facility in Barnwell, South Carolina.

If reprocessing was Plan A for nuclear wastes in the United States, Plan B was to build a single permanent repository for the final disposition of nuclear waste (see Figure 7.12), but this plan, too, has now been abandoned. The Nuclear Waste Policy Act of 1982 mandated that a national repository be established. In 1987, from a starting list of nine sites in six states, Congress directed the Department of Energy (DOE) to consider only Yucca Mountain, in Southern Nevada, as a candidate site; in 2002, the DOE determined that Yucca Mountain was a suitable site. The site is on federally owned land adjacent to the Nevada test site, where decades of nuclear weapons testing took place and so is already highly contaminated with radioactive materials. The population density in the immediate area is low, and the water table is so deep that plans called for the repository to be built 1,000 feet below the surface *and* 1,000 feet above the water table.[70] Eight years after the Nevada site was designated, construction had not yet been authorized; furthermore, it had become clear that the repository's planned capacity would be fully committed by the time it opened.[71]

Finally, local opposition to the Nevada site is strong, and it is rooted in a clear geographic injustice: Like the uranium tailings piles, the site is located in a part of the country not served by nuclear power. Indeed, only eight of the country's 104 operating nuclear plants are in states west of the Rocky Mountains.[72] The site's location also

---

*In contrast to commercial nuclear reactors, the main purpose of military reactors is to produce plutonium to be used in weapons, and wastes from these reactors have always been reprocessed.

raises another thorny issue: Trains would have to crisscross the country to carry spent fuel to Nevada.

In early 2010, by presidential order, the plan to build the Yucca Mountain site was formally cancelled, and a Blue Ribbon Commission on America's Nuclear Future was established under the authority of the DOE. The Commission submitted its final report two years later, with recommendations that do not hinge—one way or the other—on the existence of a repository at Yucca Mountain. Among its recommendations were[73]:

- A new, consent-based approach should be used in siting nuclear waste facilities
- A new organization should have responsibility (and authority and resources) for the management of nuclear wastes
- Work should begin promptly to develop one or more geologic facilities for permanent disposal *and* one or more facilities for interim storage
- Work should begin promptly to prepare for the transport of spent fuel and high-level waste to such facilities

If implemented, these recommendations will redraw the landscape of nuclear waste disposal in the United States and perhaps secure the future of nuclear power in the larger context of declining fossil fuel resources and concern about global climate change. However, it remains to be seen whether it will be less difficult to site smaller facilities in multiple locations than it has been to site a single large facility.

Meanwhile, in the absence of a permanent repository, spent fuel from U.S. nuclear power plants remains in temporary storage at 75 plants in 33 states. Some is still stored in pools at reactor sites. Some spent fuel has been moved to dry storage in steel containers placed in concrete vaults at reactor sites.

Whatever the permanent resting place for spent fuel, the fuel must be sequestered for a very long time—it will take about 300,000 years for its radioactivity to become comparable to the uranium ore originally mined.[74] This very long timeframe greatly amplifies the technical challenges of siting a repository where it will not be compromised. Over so many thousands of years,

hydrologic conditions may change. Earthquakes may occur. Even communicating the hazard to people in the distant future is a challenge.

Low-Level Radioactive Wastes

In addition to leaving highly radioactive spent fuel and reactor components as wastes, nuclear power production also yields wastes with lower levels of radioactivity. These **low-level radioactive wastes** include protective gear worn by workers, used filters and tools, and residues from cleaning the cooling water used in reactors. These wastes emit much less radiation than spent reactor fuel, the wastes of reprocessing spent fuel, and the components of decommissioned reactors. Low-level radioactive wastes are not physically hot and do not require the same shielding as high-level radioactive wastes. And the time required for most low-level wastes to decay to the point at which the radiation they emit is comparable to natural background radiation can be counted in hundreds of years rather than hundreds of thousands of years.

Furthermore, some of the nation's low-level radioactive waste originates outside of the nuclear fuel cycle. For example, some medical and research facilities use radioactive materials for sterilization of equipment, for diagnostic or treatment techniques in patients, or for testing in laboratory animals. Such activities yield radioactively contaminated waste products, such as syringes, glassware, and animal carcasses.

Under a U.S. federal law (the 1982 Low-Level Radioactive Waste Policy Amendments Act, as amended in 1985), each state became responsible for disposing of low-level radioactive wastes generated within the state. The law encourages states to form groups (called compacts), within which one state hosts a waste facility for all of the compact's member states. As of May of 2010, all but 10 states had joined a compact[75]; however, at present, there are only three active facilities to store low-level radioactive wastes. One is in South Carolina (in the Southeast Compact), one is in Hanford, Washington, and one is in Clive, Utah (both in the Northwest Compact). Thus like the management of high-level nuclear wastes, the management of low-level radioactive wastes is facing a predicament.

The Future of Nuclear Power

The story of nuclear power in the United States to date has been one of great expectation followed by great disappointment. As shown in **Figure 7.16**, optimism peaked from 1974 to 1976, with 217 plants in the pipeline, in operation, or retired from service. After 1976, although the number of licensed plants continued to increase for some years, cancellations steadily eroded the number of plants on order, a process hastened by the 1979 accident at Three Mile Island. As public confidence declined, construction and licensing became more drawn out and costly. Since 1996, only one new nuclear reactor has been brought on line and little action has been taken on the proposals for new nuclear power plants. Instead, nuclear plants already under construction have actually been abandoned, as occurred with the V.C. Summer plant in South Carolina in 2017 costing state utilities almost $9 billion.[76]

The United States still operates the largest number of commercial nuclear reactors in the world, followed closely by France, which produces 75% of its electricity from nuclear power.[77] However, the French government hopes to reduce their reliance on nuclear power significantly by 2035. Other countries that also rely on nuclear power significantly today include Russia, China, and Japan, although strong opposition is growing in these countries regarding its continued use. Following the Fukushima accident, Germany opted to completely abandon any further use of nuclear power.

As far as nuclear resources are concerned, two-thirds of the world's known uranium reserves are located in ore deposits in just four countries: Australia (28%), Kazakhstan (15%), Canada (14%), and South Africa (10%); the United States is home to just 3% of this resource base.[78] At the current rate of electricity production, the world's known resources are estimated to be adequate for some 80 years, and similar resources, not yet documented, could add more than 200 years to this time horizon.[78] In principle, though not yet in practice,

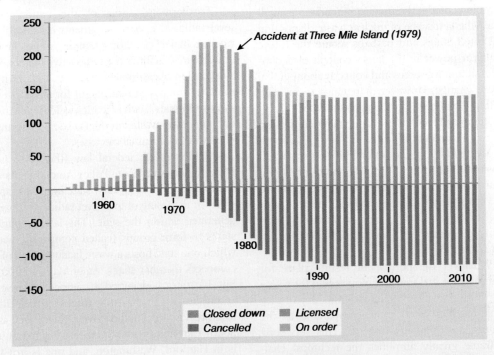

Figure 7.16 Number of nuclear power plants in the United States, 1953–2012.

Data from U.S. Energy Information Administration. U.S. Nuclear Reactors: Reactor status list. Available at: www.eia.doe.gov/cneaf/nuclear/page/nuc_reactors/reactsum.html. Accessed: October 7, 2006; and Wald ML. Federal regulators approve two nuclear reactors in Georgia. New York Times. February 9, 2012; Available at: www.nytimes.com/2012/02/10/business/energy-environment/2-new-reactors-approved-in-georgia.html. Accessed November 19, 2012.

uranium could also be extracted from tailings at gold and phosphate mines and even from seawater, an enormous potential resource.[78] Specialized reactors have been developed to convert naturally occurring thorium into a fissile isotope of uranium (U-233, not a naturally occurring isotope),[78] and of course it would be possible to reprocess nuclear wastes already generated. It is impossible to know at present which of these potential resources will be realized as technology, costs, and health concerns are weighed in coming decades.

Health Impacts of the Nuclear Fuel Cycle

People have exposures to ionizing radiation throughout the nuclear fuel cycle. At the front end, miners and mill workers are exposed to the natural decay products of uranium; as described earlier in the context of naturally occurring ionizing radiation, radon is a known human carcinogen (IARC Group I). Nuclear power plants release products of nuclear fission—at low levels as routine emissions and at much higher levels in the event of an accident. At the back end of the nuclear fuel cycle, failures and accidents (during transportation or storage of wastes) could result in exposures to radiation from the decay of wastes containing unfissioned uranium, fission products, and transuranic elements.

Health Impacts at the Front End

Uranium miners' and mill workers' exposures to radon and radon progeny carry some risk of cancer; in particular, excess lung cancer has been well documented among uranium miners. Studies in uranium miners and other populations also indicate a synergistic effect between radon exposure and cigarette smoking in increasing lung cancer risk.[79]

In the early decades of the industry, radon exposure was unregulated, and exposures were much higher than is allowed today. In a bleak chapter in the history of occupational health in the United States, early uranium miners in the Southwest during the 1940s and 1950s, many of whom were either Navajo or Hispanic, worked without ventilation or protective gear. At the time, uranium mining was known to carry a high risk of lung cancer, although the specifics of radon and radon progeny had not yet been elucidated. Later research, focusing on miners active between 1956 and the early 1990s, found that the lung cancer risk of miners with the highest radon exposure was 29 times that of miners in the least exposed group.[80] Furthermore, in a somewhat later cohort of Navajo miners (who smoked little), nearly three-quarters of lung cancer cases were attributable to their occupational exposure to radon.[81] These extraordinary risks reflect the miners' very high radon exposures compared with those of the general population. Uranium miners, like coal miners, are also exposed to silica dust and risk of physical injury.

The uranium mining on Navaho lands also left behind its legacy of mill tailings and radioactive waste, causing members of the community to be exposed. Environmental runoff from the tailings contaminated drinking water supplies with elevated levels of uranium, arsenic, and other heavy metals. Children were also exposed while playing in these tailing piles.[82] Additionally, initial efforts to promote the use of these leftover materials for housing construction created domestic exposures to uranium and its associated decay products. Ongoing epidemiologic studies have implicated these exposures not only to elevated lung cancer rates but also to other chronic diseases, including kidney disorders associated with uranium's toxicity as a heavy metal.[83,84] Mice studies demonstrating that uranium exhibits estrogenic endocrine disruption have also raised concern that the doses received by these mice may be similar to the environmental exposures possible for communities in the American Southwest living near these legacy uranium mining and milling wastes.[85]

Health Impacts of Accidents at Power Plants

In nuclear power plant accidents, the profile of radionuclides released varies somewhat but typically features the fission products iodine-131 (half-life of about 8 days) and strontium-90 and cesium-137 (both with half-lives of about 30 years). All three elements emit beta radiation and thus pose both an internal and external radiation hazard. Emissions from a nuclear power plant accident can also include plutonium-238 (an alpha emitter) and other transuranic elements that are byproducts of nuclear fission.

When iodine-131, strontium-90, and cesium-137 are released into the environment, people are exposed mostly through ingestion of water and food. Radioactive iodine and strontium, for example, can accumulate on leafy vegetables that people eat; when cows eat contaminated grass, iodine-131 appears in their milk. In addition, iodine-131 in gaseous form can be inhaled. Precipitation brings contaminated airborne dust to earth, creating additional exposures through water and food.

In the body, iodine-131 is taken up by the thyroid gland, causing thyroid cancer. In fact, iodine-131 is concentrated by the thyroid gland, such that the radiation dose to the thyroid may be more than 1,000 times the average dose to the whole body.[86] Preexisting iodine deficiency increases the uptake of radioactive iodine; iodine pills taken promptly when an accident occurs can reduce uptake. Strontium-90 displaces calcium and is deposited in bone, irradiating the marrow and causing leukemia. Exposure to other radioactive isotopes produced by a nuclear accident carries an increased risk of solid tumors other than thyroid cancer.

In terms of known public health impacts, the most serious accident at a nuclear power plant to date was the Chernobyl event in Ukraine in 1986. The challenges of doing epidemiologic research on cancer related to the Chernobyl accident are substantial. They include patchy data on exposure in the first months and years after the accident and, more broadly, social disorganization in the wake of this devastating event. Populations were dislocated and medical care was disrupted, as were food supplies and many basic social services. These factors make it harder to conduct any epidemiologic study. Changes in medical care reflect increased concern about radiation-related health effects since the accident. These changes are likely to result in more complete reporting of cases than before the accident, a source of bias in surveillance studies. At the same time, because most solid tumors have long latencies, it was difficult to document associations in individual-level studies during the first years after the accident. Given that mechanistic data leave little doubt that ionizing radiation, however low the dose, poses a risk of cancer, the real question in such a situation is what can be discerned through epidemiology.

Now, 25 years after the 1986 Chernobyl accident, a dose-related increase in thyroid cancer has been clearly documented in children and adolescents. Three epidemiologic studies of children in Ukraine, Belarus, and/or Russia (the areas most affected by the accident) have shown an approximately fivefold increased risk of thyroid cancer per Gray of exposure.[87] This is not a surprising outcome. Children are more sensitive to the effects of ionizing radiation on the thyroid than adults,[86] and they also tend to be more highly exposed to iodine-131 because they drink more milk. There is also evidence of an increased incidence of leukemia among Chernobyl's cleanup workers, who were exposed as adults.[87] Psychological impacts, specifically depression and posttraumatic stress disorder, have also been documented among cleanup workers and among mothers whose children were young at the time of the accident.[88]

Similar psychological impacts have been reported for the tsunami survivors who lived within 20 kilometers of the Fukushima nuclear power plant and were ordered to evacuate on the day following the accident. Additionally, many people suffered physical distress associated with the combined hazards of experiencing an earthquake, tsunami, and nuclear accident evacuation.[89] Longer-term effects of exposures to radiation will not be known for years and will be difficult to assess given the broad social disruption that followed the accident as well as discerning a radiation-caused cancer from background cancer rates, particularly among adults. Nonetheless, the United Nations Scientific Committee on the

Effects of Atomic Radiation (UNSCEAR) has been tasked with conducting risk assessments for both the displaced community members as well as the nuclear reactor workers.[89]

No acute radiation health effects were documented, and the majority of the workers as well as the evacuated population are thought to have received exposures at doses far below concerns for latent, deterministic risks.[89] Thirteen workers did receive absorbed doses that increases their deterministic risk for hypothyroidism as well as their latent risk for thyroid cancer. Overall, only 173 workers (0.7% of the workforce) received effective doses of 100 mSv or more, and among this group, a small increased risk of cancer would be expected.[89] Among the general public, radiation exposures were low and any increase in cancer incidence would not be expected to be discernable over baseline levels. However, UNSCEAR specifically highlighted concern with infants and children and their risks for the subsequent development of thyroid cancer or leukemia, although indicating that special follow-up would be required to discern these cancers from background rates.[89]

Health Impacts at the Back End

The safe storage of nuclear waste must isolate it, by use of engineered and perhaps also natural barriers, over many, many years. In the absence of a permanent storage site (or sites) for spent reactor fuel in the United States, it is currently stored at reactor sites around the country. Both cooling pools and dry casks are constructed to prevent the escape of ionizing radiation, but they are not designed to last for the radioactive lifetime of the wastes. The design of many commercial nuclear reactors also involved creating large lakes for cooling, and there is now concern about the integrity of their dams, especially associated with disrupting stored spent fuel canisters. Furthermore, the power plant sites are not in isolated locations, and in fact many are located in heavily populated areas.

If a permanent repository (or repositories) is built to hold spent fuel from nuclear reactors, releases to air or contamination of groundwater are unlikely in the short term, but could occur over the very long life of such a facility, especially in the event of a geologic disturbance such as an earthquake. Another challenge is devising effective and long-lasting warnings to alert and inform future generations about the stored radioactive hazards. Protecting these radioactive wastes from those who would wish to use it to cause alarm and public panic is also a matter of national security.

Waste from Coal-fired Electricity Production

The recent attention addressing the integrity of dams associated with power plants actually occurred because of dam failures at two plants generating electricity with coal. In 2008, a dam failure at the Kingston Fossil Plant in Tennessee released more than 5 million cubic yards of coal ash into the Emory River, eventually pouring over 300 acres of land and damaging 40 homes.[1] The spill in Tennessee, now considered one of the largest environmental disasters ever in the United States, was followed by another accident six years later in North Carolina when about 39,000 tons of coal ash spilled into the Dan River after two large drainpipes underneath a coal ash impoundment collapsed.[2] The cost associated with this spill that blanketed seven miles of the river is estimated to be almost $300 million when ecological damage, recreational impacts, effects on human health with consumption of water or fish from the river, and aesthetic value losses are combined.[2]

Where could so much waste material come from? The answer is that generating electricity using coal for over a century has required billions of tons of coal to be burned, producing extensive amounts

(continues)

Waste from Coal-fired Electricity Production *(continued)*

of coal combustion residual byproducts, including waste ash. The EPA estimated that 130 million tons of coal combustion residuals were generated in 2014 alone, with 60% of it being coal ash.[3] Although a significant portion of coal ash may be reused for construction and road materials, electric utilities have had to find a way to store massive quantities of coal ash year after year. The EPA estimates in 2014 determined that coal ash was stored in over 310 active landfills and 735 active surface impoundments across 47 states.[3] These impoundments were typically located near the coal-fired power generator to allow for coal ash slurry to be directly disposed of via a pipeline. Electricity generation also requires a nearby source of water for cooling purposes, meaning that large impoundments of coal ash waste grew up behind dams near large lakes and rivers. The 2014 EPA report determined that 75% of the coal ash storage sites were 25 years old and 10% were more than 50 years old.[3]

So far, the major hazards associated with coal ash spills involve the ecological damage associated with *smothering* a body of water with massive amounts of debris, resulting in fish kills and coating river banks and bottoms with several feet of ash deposits that permanently alter riparian habitats.[2] However, coal ash can contain various levels of several toxic metals, such as arsenic, selenium, and chromium to name just a few, depending on where the coal originated. Furthermore, as air pollution mitigation technologies have improved associated with coal power electricity generation, more of these metals that once might have left as airborne emissions are now entrained in the solid waste residuals, essentially trading one form of pollution for another.[1] Human exposure to these toxic metals in coal ash could occur when drinking water is contaminated from these large surface water spills or if water from coal ash storage sites leaches into groundwater drinking supplies. According to EPA estimates, a person living within one mile of an unlined coal ash disposal site has a 1 in 50 lifetime risk of cancer associated with arsenic contamination.[1,4]

These newly emerged concerns about the waste associated with using coal to generate electricity only add to the pressure to shift away from using coal that already exists related to air pollution and climate change. However, the United States still generates a quarter of its electricity using coal, meaning that thousands of railroad cars of coal are still consumed daily with its residual wastes. Then there is the immense volume of legacy coal ash waste left over from the past century. The regulatory response to growing environmental health concerns regarding coal ash has primarily supported improvements in coal ash disposal management. In 2014, the EPA established minimum national standards addressing disposal placement locations, liner design criteria, groundwater monitoring and corrective action requirements, and improved recordkeeping and disclosure notifications.[4] Much to the dismay of environmentalists, the EPA also designated coal ash as nonhazardous waste under Subtitle D of the Resource Conservation and Recovery Act instead of using the Subtitle C hazardous waste designation.[4] Since many feel that the federal rules have established too low of a level for risk protection, state environmental agencies and environmental advocacy groups continue to legally demand more stringent standards. Of course, the cost to generate electricity using coal will increase as its disposal costs more accurately account for environmental and human health impacts—a cost that will surely be passed along to consumers.

1. Sierra Club. Coal Ash: A Danger to Our Nation's Health. 2014. https://coal.sierraclub.org/sites/nat-coal/files/report-dangerous-water-coal-ash-crisis.pdf
2. Lemly AD. Damage cost of the Dan River coal ash spill. *Environmental Pollution*. 2015;197:55-61. http://dx.doi.org/10.1016/j.envpol.2014.11.027
3. Sears CG, Zierold KM. Health of children living near coal ash. *Global Pediatric Health*. 2017;4:1-8.
4. Connors E. Coal-ash management by U.S. electric utilities: Overview and recent developments. *Utilities Policy*. 2015;34:30-33. http://dx.doi.org/10.1016/j.jup.2015.03.004

Regulation of Activities in the Nuclear Fuel Cycle

As described earlier, the Atomic Energy Commission (AEC) had mixed military and civilian roles in the years following World War II: It was responsible for developing both nuclear weapons and nuclear power. Even within the realm of civilian nuclear power, the AEC had two faces, in that it was responsible for both *promoting* and *regulating* the nascent nuclear power industry. This conflict of interest was resolved by the Energy Reorganization Act of 1974, which dissolved the AEC and created a new agency, the Nuclear Regulatory Commission (NRC), responsible only for the safety of nuclear power plants. When the DOE was established in 1977, it assumed responsibilities for overseeing nuclear weapon production and managing the associated environmental legacy from weapons production.

The NRC licenses nuclear power reactors, controlling both site permits and operating licenses, and sets emissions limits for radionuclides under normal plant operations. It oversees routine operations, and plant operators are required to monitor and report on radioactive emissions. The NRC also responds to incidents or accidents at nuclear power plants and regulates the storage of spent fuel at reactor sites around the country. Finally, the NRC is responsible for preventing the theft or diversion of nuclear materials.

As detailed earlier, the Nuclear Waste Policy Act of 1982 mandated that a national repository be established, but the process stalled with a single designated candidate site, Yucca Mountain in Nevada, and that plan has now been abandoned. If work on a repository (or repositories) does move forward, at least three federal agencies are likely to be involved: the DOE to design, construct, and operate the facility or facilities; the EPA to develop environmental standards; and the NRC to license the repository or repositories and develop regulations to implement the EPA's standards.[90]

The NRC is also responsible for implementing the Low-Level Radioactive Waste Policy Amendments Act of 1982, as amended in 1985. As described earlier, this law calls for states to form compacts for the management of these wastes. And, under a 1978 set of amendments to the Atomic Energy Act named the Uranium Mill Tailings Radiation Control Act, the EPA sets standards for the management of abandoned mill tailings sites by the Department of Energy. Active tailings sites are licensed by the NRC.

7.4 Energy from Renewable Resources

Our current degree of dependence on fossil fuels is not sustainable—that is, it cannot be maintained over the long future that we would like to imagine for the human race. Instead, we will use up reserves of coal, oil, and natural gas within a few generations, and the ecological impacts, including the effects of global climate change, will far outlive these resources. A reliance on nuclear fuels would be sustainable for a longer period since so much less is required to produce the same amount of electricity. For example, less than one-tenth of a pound of uranium can generate enough electricity to power a lightbulb for one year compared with the 143 pounds of natural gas needed or the 714 pounds of coal—both more than a factor of five times greater than using nuclear fuel.[91] But generating electricity using nuclear power poses significant concerns about doing so safely and uranium is still a finite resource.

Some energy sources are sustainable, and also *renewable*: Such a **renewable energy source** is either continually renewed in nature (e.g., wind or water) or can readily be renewed through human effort (e.g., by planting trees to replace those burned as fuel). The major renewable energy sources are wind power, water power (*hydropower*), solar energy, tidal energy, underground heat sources (*geothermal energy*), and fuels derived from trees or other plants (collectively called *biomass fuels*).

Many renewable energy technologies, although they can be incorporated into centralized systems, lend themselves to a decentralized energy sector.

This is in striking contrast to the current infrastructure for producing and distributing energy. Reserves of the major fossil fuels—coal, oil, and gas—are concentrated geographically, and large quantities must be moved to locations where power is to be generated. The transport of coal takes advantage of ordinary railroad lines, but oil and gas must be moved via dedicated pipelines, terminals, and tankers. Nuclear materials must also be transported and processed, and although the quantities involved are much smaller, the safety and security issues are pressing. Electric plants are tied into an extensive power grid of interconnected generating plants and transmission lines.

Such large-scale energy systems are inherently vulnerable. All of their major elements—pipelines, oil and gas terminals, tankers, electric power plants, and transmission lines—are susceptible to disruption. Indeed, the centralized power system has long been criticized as inherently "brittle."[92] That is, the system is designed to reliably handle predictable problems rather than to be resilient in the face of the unexpected. Even an ordinary event—a lightning strike, an everyday mistake, or a software failure—can ripple through a complex and brittle system in unexpected ways. In 2003, for example, some trees that had grown up in a right-of-way came into contact with electrical power lines in Ohio, becoming a contributing cause of a cascading blackout that left 50 million people in the Eastern United States and Canada without power for up to 3 days.[93]

In contrast to fossil fuels and nuclear power, renewable energy technologies use resources that are local and widely available, although not available evenly across all locations. Both power production and environmental impacts are more dispersed, and this makes it somewhat easier to achieve an equitable sharing of benefits and burdens. With coordination and some redundancy at the local and regional scales, such technologies can form flexible and resilient power networks.

This discussion of alternatives to fossil and nuclear fuels begins with addressing biomass fuels since almost half the world relies on biomass energy to heat their homes and cook their meals. The options that harness the energy of the Sun

or Earth without the use of any type of fuel are discussed next, and this section concludes with a brief description of U.S. regulatory supports for alternatives to fossil and nuclear fuels.

Biomass and Biomass Fuels

Biomass energy is simply energy stored in plant material or animal dung (**biomass**). It originates as the energy in sunlight; through photosynthesis, this energy is stored in plants. If plant material (such as wood or crop residues) or animal dung is burned, this energy is released. Such **biomass fuels** produce a small quantity of energy for the quantity burned, compared with, for example, natural gas. On a larger scale, plant materials can be burned to produce steam, which in turn is used to generate electricity via a turbine. In the United States, this occurs mostly at pulp and paper mills because they both produce large quantities of wood waste and need power for industrial processes.[94]

Using complex technologies, vehicle fuels can be derived from biomass (or from mixes including organic wastes from municipal waste streams). Such fuels, also referred to as *biomass fuels*, can be gaseous (e.g., *biogas*, which is about 60% methane) or liquid. Biogas can be burned directly in some industrial processes, but if it is to be used as natural gas, it must be purified, and if the natural gas is to be used as a fuel for vehicles, it must be compressed to make a liquid fuel. *Ethanol* (an alcohol fuel) is a liquid, as is *biodiesel fuel*. Biodiesel fuel, made from animal fats and vegetable oils (including used cooking oil from restaurants), burns cleaner than diesel fuel does. Mixed with standard diesel fuel, it can be used in most diesel engines. The key advantage of such biomass-derived fuels over fossil fuels is that they are *carbon-neutral*. That is, the carbon released as carbon dioxide from the combustion of biomass fuels was captured from the atmosphere by plants through photosynthesis only a short time before, much as in the carbon cycle shown in Figure 7.7.

All biomass fuels face a fundamental limitation as an energy option. If these fuels are to be produced on a large scale, then fuel crops, such as sugar cane or corn, will need to be grown on a large scale as raw material. Any plan for such "energy plantations" would require vast tracts of land, as well as enormous quantities of water. Indeed, on a global scale, such a strategy would require that very large areas of land now used for food crops be converted to energy crops.[94] The U.S. Department of Agriculture reports that the production of ethanol is claiming an increasing share of the U.S. corn crop—from 7.5% in 2001 to 22.6% in 2007 to an anticipated 35% in 2016.[95]

Some nontraditional fossil fuels are blends of fossil fuel and a biomass fuel—for example, mixed diesel and ethanol, or mixed gasoline and ethanol. Other nontraditional fuels for vehicles are derived from fossil fuels: compressed natural gas and liquefied natural gas (both methane), liquefied petroleum gas (propane), and the alcohol fuel methanol, derived from coal or natural gas. These alternatives to gasoline and diesel produce less pollution (but also less energy) per gallon consumed. Although some alternative fuels, from fossil or biomass sources, have found a niche in the energy market, it has proved challenging to integrate them into a marketplace dominated by familiar fuels and products designed to use them.

Although biomass fuels are considered alternative fuels from the perspective of the world's dependence on fossil fuels, this does not mean that all biomass fuels are benign. Perhaps half of the world's population, mostly in rural areas of less-developed countries, burns biomass fuels for heating and cooking. The fuels used in this way include wood, charcoal, peat, straw, brush, and the dung of cattle or other herbivores—all fuels that are much less expensive than oil or gas (or electricity) used in more developed countries.[96] These biomass fuels are typically burned in simple stoves or open fires indoors, resulting in high concentrations of particulates and irritant gases in indoor air. For example, researchers have reported 24-hour average particulate concentrations (PM_{10}) of 200 to 5,000 mg/m^3 indoors, and as high as 50,000 mg/m^3 near stoves.[97] Research has also documented higher exposures for girls and women because they spend more time near the fire as they cook.[98] These hazardous air pollutants

ranked second only to high blood pressure in terms of healthy years of life lost among women worldwide.[46] In research studies, exposure to indoor air pollution from the burning of biomass fuels has been clearly linked to respiratory tract infections, especially acute respiratory infections in children, to chronic obstructive pulmonary disease, and to tuberculosis; other possible health effects include asthma, lung cancer, cardiac events, cataracts, and low birthweight.[99-102] Overall, a comparative risk assessment published in 2010 estimated that approximately 3.5 million premature deaths were caused by household cooking with biomass fuels.[46]

The majority of households that must rely on biomass fuels are poor and experience what has been termed "energy poverty," in contrast to households that have "energy security" meaning ample access to safer sources of energy to cook and condition the air within their homes.[46] The health risks associated with energy production for those who are energy secure are felt at the community level in terms of regional air pollution hazards, rather than directly facing health risks within their homes. This shift in energy source from biomass to fossil fuels is dependent on the level of economic development and exemplifies the environmental health risk transition from household to community level health risks discussed earlier. The environmental hazards associated with climate change represent the health threats related to increased wealth and energy consumption that now threaten all humans on the planet. Another type of alternative fuel is discussed in the case study, **The Hydrogen Fuel Cell**.

Freedom from Fuels

Wind power, hydropower (including tidal energy), solar energy, and geothermal energy are renewable sources of energy that are freely available in nature. For the most part, these technologies capture some available energy as it passes by, in contrast to technologies that extract energy from fuel. Of course, building and maintaining renewable energy facilities requires inputs of materials and energy. Otherwise, these technologies do not rely on a supply of fuel.

The Hydrogen Fuel Cell

The **hydrogen fuel cell** (see depiction below) relies on a simple chemical reaction in which hydrogen (provided as fuel) and oxygen (from the atmosphere) are combined to produce electricity (a flow of electrons) and, as a byproduct, water. The fuel cell technology itself is environmentally benign. The key questions are: Where does the hydrogen fuel come from? And how much energy does it take to produce the hydrogen fuel?

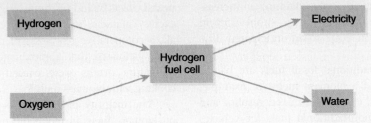

Although the concept of the hydrogen fuel cell is simple, obtaining hydrogen fuel is not. In particular, although we are surrounded by hydrogen, it is not present as hydrogen gas but rather in chemical compounds, many of which are fossil fuels (hydrocarbon fuels). Today, hydrogen for fuel cells is derived mostly by stripping hydrogen atoms from natural gas, whose production, like that of all fossil fuels, creates pollution. In the future, it may become practical to obtain hydrogen from water, which would produce no pollution. But of course water itself is a valuable resource, and in any event, the timeline for developing such technology is unclear. At a more mundane level, the use of hydrogen fuel cells raises difficult engineering challenges: The hydrogen gas must either be greatly compressed or else deep-chilled to a liquid form; and an entire infrastructure of storage facilities, distribution tankers, and fueling stations is needed.

Finally, whatever the source of the hydrogen, the energy required to produce the hydrogen fuel is greater than the energy that is obtained when the fuel cell is put to use. Thus, the hydrogen fuel cell makes sense only if the energy used to produce the hydrogen comes from a source that we can use freely—that is, a source, such as water power, which is continually renewed in nature. For some time now, Iceland has been using geothermal energy to produce hydrogen for fuel cells that power three buses in Reykjavik, a program planned as the first step toward large-scale use of this technology.[1] However, in the difficult economic climate of recent years, the initiative has not expanded as planned.

1. Natural Resources Defense Council. *Building the Hydrogen Boom*. 2005.

Wind power captures the energy of moving air. When wind strikes the blades of a wind turbine (the modern version of a windmill), it causes the shaft of the turbine to turn, converting the wind's kinetic energy into mechanical energy. The shaft is connected to a generator, which converts the mechanical energy into electrical energy.

Traditionally, the mechanical energy was not converted to electricity but was put to use directly. For example, before rural areas in the great plains of the United States had electric power, many farms and ranches had windmills that pumped groundwater up to the ground surface (see Figure 7.17). Wind power can still be used on a microscale to provide either mechanical energy or electricity.

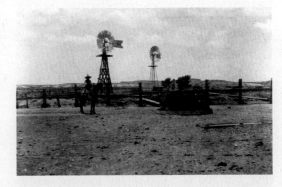

Figure 7.17 Windmills like the one in this undated photo from Presidio County, Texas, are typical of traditional 19th- and 20th-century construction.

Courtesy of U.S. Geological Survey; ID #2247. Undated photo by G.K. Gilbert. Available at: http://libraryphoto .cr.usgs.gov/. Accessed September 13, 2007.

However, wind turbines are now often installed in rows or rectangular grids; such groupings are called **wind farms** and contribute electricity to a power grid. Modern wind turbines can be hundreds of feet tall and are streamlined in shape and usually white in color (see **Figure 7.18**). Wind turbines cause zero environmental pollution, in the usual sense of the term, but they do make noise. At a distance of 1,000 feet, the sound of a wind farm is sometimes compared with that of a home refrigerator or of a car on a highway some distance away. Given that wind farms are sited in windy locations, the "whooshing" sound of the whirling blades is sometimes masked by the sound of wind in trees and around buildings. The research literature on the health aspects of noise from wind turbines is limited but suggests that both annoyance and sleep disturbance are associated with the noise exposure from living near these turbines.[103]

A wind farm occupies a sizeable area, either on land or offshore. Wind turbines are prominent features of a local landscape; in fact, if they are located on land, they are often sited on ridges to capture wind energy most efficiently. Again, reactions are mixed: Some people feel that wind turbines cause "visual pollution," while others find their simple functionality elegant and visually pleasing.

Unlike people, birds in flight appear to have difficulty seeing wind turbines. This is because, although modern turbines rotate slowly, the blades are long and; therefore, the tips move at up to 150 miles per hour, making them difficult to see.[104] As a result, birds sometimes fly directly into the blades and are killed. Designers are working to minimize this hazard (e.g., testing the visibility of patterned blades),[104] but it seems likely that wind turbines will always pose some risk to birds.

On the other hand, the general perception of this risk is exaggerated; early reports of the problem came from a site with unusual turbines and large populations of birds of prey, such as hawks and eagles. The National Wind Coordinating Committee (a collaborative that includes representatives from electric utilities, wind developers, environmental organizations, and others) has estimated that 10,000 to 40,000 birds are killed in the United States each year by wind turbines, compared with 50 to 80 million killed by vehicles, and some 100 million (if not many more) that fly into buildings or windows.[105] Most of the birds killed by wind turbines are the more common species, including house sparrows, European starlings, and pigeons.[105] In 2006, the Massachusetts Audubon Society supported a wind farm proposed for Nantucket Sound off the state's shoreline, noting that the potential harm to birds was outweighed by the ecological benefits of using a renewable energy source.[106] Furthermore, wind power is not the only kind of energy production that poses a risk to birds: Oil pollution kills some birds every year, but public attention focuses on the problem only when there is a major spill such as the 1989 grounding of the oil tanker *Exxon Valdez* in Alaska or the 2010 *Deepwater Horizon* spill in the Gulf of Mexico.

Like wind power, **hydropower** can be used on a microscale; for example, a water wheel can power a small mill that grinds grain into flour or a turbine that generates electricity. Small hydroelectric plants are usually "run-of-river" operations; that is, they operate either with no dam at all or

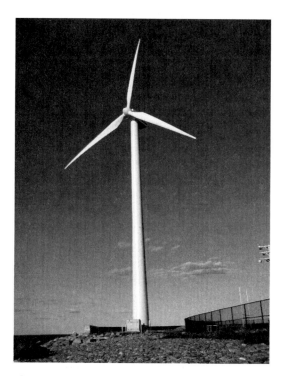

Figure 7.18 This modern wind turbine is one of two now generating electricity for the coastal town of Hull, Massachusetts.

with a small diversion that holds perhaps a day's backup supply of water.*

Unlike a small hydroelectric plant, a large hydroelectric plant relies on a strong, predictable, and adjustable flow of water. This is achieved by storing a large volume of water behind a dam (see **Figure 7.19**), and then releasing it at a rate that supports the generation of power as it is needed. Thus, large-scale hydropower, although it meets the definition of a renewable, alternative energy option, does more than simply capture some of the freely available energy of a watercourse as it passes by, and a large hydroelectric plant, like a coal-fired power plant, is tied into a centralized power grid.

A large hydroelectric dam can also take a heavy environmental and social toll. For example, China's massive Three Gorges Dam on the Yangtze River, completed in 2006 and now filled to capacity, provides electrical power for millions, mostly in urban areas; it will also help to control flooding and manage irrigation, and locks allow ships to reach locations that were previously inaccessible. But the winding 410-mile-long reservoir, which flooded many towns and villages (along with several archaeological sites), has also caused problems and raised concerns.[107,108] The project displaced some 1.4 million people, many of them farmers who were moved to urban areas and whose resettlement has not gone smoothly. Downstream farmers are concerned that lands below the dam will no longer receive the rich silt once left by natural flooding, while engineers are concerned about the accumulation of silt behind the dam. Garbage and algae have accumulated on the reservoir's surface. Finally, there is some concern that the sheer weight of the water behind the dam may increase the probability of an earthquake, raising the specter of a catastrophic failure and a public health disaster.

In the United States, 93 dams have a capacity (the volume of water stored behind the dam) of greater than 500 million cubic meters.[109]

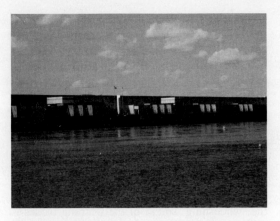

Figure 7.19 The water stored behind this dam will be used to generate electric power.

Construction of the great majority of these large dams was completed more than 40 years ago; only 13 dams (representing 8% of capacity) have been completed since 1970, and none since 1983. The lifespan of any dam, although it may be long, is finite, partly because of long-term deterioration of the materials used to build it, but also because sedimentation behind the dam gradually reduces the volume of water that can be stored behind it.[110] In coming decades, engineers will certainly face the challenge of safely removing aging dams.

Ultimately, both water power and wind power derive from the Sun; solar energy causes snowmelt and also evaporation of water, feeding the rainfall that fills rivers and streams; and differences in the solar heating of air masses cause the movements that we call wind. The Sun's energy can also be harnessed directly, although oddly enough, this direct **solar power** approach is more challenging. For one thing, sunlight is intermittent and variable: It is available only during the day, the number of daylight hours varies with location and season, and the Sun is sometimes obscured by clouds. In addition, unlike a rushing river or a stiff wind, sunlight is a diffuse, low-intensity energy source.

For this reason, a relatively large area is needed to collect enough solar energy to be useful. For small-scale heating of domestic water or indoor space, flat solar collection panels (usually installed on the roof) can be used to absorb the

---

*It is also possible, in certain locations, to capture energy from tidal movements near coastlines or in estuaries.

Sun's radiation and heat a fluid, which then circulates through a heating system. On a large scale, an array of solar collectors can be used to gather and concentrate the Sun's energy and then generate electricity by heating water (or another fluid), creating steam that drives a turbine. However, such an approach is feasible only in a large empty area in a high-sunlight location—most often a desert. The concentrated commercial solar power plant depicted on the cover of this textbook demonstrates the size of the *"footprint"* needed with its 640-foot tower and nearly two-mile wide field of mirrors.*[111]

A solar collection panel is composed of many individual **photovoltaic cells** (also called **solar cells**); this is the device that converts sunlight directly into electrical energy. Photovoltaic cells capture less than one-third of the solar energy that falls on them, but they can be combined in modular fashion to form arrays of any size. To date, the practical challenges of solar energy, along with the economics of the energy market, have not favored large-scale adoption of solar technologies in most locations, but this may change.

Although solar energy is a renewable resource, the technology for capturing this energy has environmental costs. The most widely used semiconductor material in photovoltaic cells at present is silicon. Mining of silica requires large expenditures of energy (resulting in carbon dioxide emissions) and also generates silica dust, a respiratory hazard to miners. Furthermore, the manufacture of silicon wafers uses substantial quantities of several relatively scarce metals.[112] Production of silicon also requires the use of sulfur hexafluoride, the most potent greenhouse gas evaluated to date by the Intergovernmental Panel on Climate Change.[113] The gas is used in a closed system, but because it is some 20,000 times more potent than carbon dioxide as a greenhouse gas and there are no known natural sinks,[113] even leaks are of

concern. The production process also generates some carbon dioxide emissions, although much less than those from burning fossil fuels.[112] Newer semiconductor technologies for photovoltaic cells use cadmium, a highly toxic metal that will be present in wastes from manufacturing solar panels and also in the panels themselves when they become waste at the end of their useful lives. Finally, very large arrays of solar panels, placed in uninhabited areas, have a negative effect on wildlife habitat.[112]

Geothermal energy is the Earth's internal heat energy, emerging in the form of hot water and steam at geysers or steam vents. Hot water and steam can be carried in pipes and circulated through buildings to heat interior spaces. This heat source can be used only where local geology makes it possible (e.g., in parts of Iceland, Japan, and New Zealand), and the steam or water is usually transported over short distances. Less commonly, steam from a geothermal source is used to drive a turbine generating electricity.

Regulatory Support for Alternatives to Fossil and Nuclear Fuels

The Energy Policy Act of 2005, enacted as a comprehensive update of the U.S. energy strategy, includes some supports for alternative energy sources. For example, it provided for tax credits against the corporate income tax of energy producers that generate electricity from wind, biomass, solar power, geothermal energy, and tidal energy. It also required that by 2013 the federal government obtain 7.5% of its power from renewable sources, not an ambitious goal, and there was no parallel requirement for electric utilities to increase their use of alternative energy sources. The law also provided substantial support for traditional energy sectors, with the twin goals of expanding nuclear power and increasing domestic production of fossil fuels.

The Energy Policy Act provides grants to state and local governments to buy hybrid vehicles and to help school districts reduce the diesel emissions of their school buses. It supports

---

*The Crescent Dunes facility in Nevada, similar to the solar power plant on the cover, also addresses the problem of generating power when the sun is not shining by storing the sun's heat in molten salt that may generate steam to run a turbine 24 hours a day.

research on the use of hydrogen as a fuel. At the individual level, the act offers tax credits against the personal income tax of those who buy hybrid vehicles or cars that use alternative fuels. Tax credits are also available for certain home improvements that reduce energy consumption, such as insulation, replacement windows, and some solar heating systems.

7.5 Energy Conservation

The preceding sections have highlighted the environmental and human health costs associated with producing energy from different sources. However, humanity has also benefitted economically from its ever-increasing consumption of energy. But now there is evidence that after a point, there is little to be gained in terms of better health from using more energy.[46] Also, the energy consumptive practices in most of the developed countries are simply not possible to further the economic development elsewhere. And there is nothing to be gained from wasting energy. Conservation of energy is often referred to as the "*Fifth fuel,*" and represents an inexpensive, silent, and nonimpactful way to address energy concerns.

Many aspects of the middle-class American lifestyle are extravagant in terms of energy consumption, even if they fit within individual budgets. **Energy conservation**—simply reducing the amount of energy we consume—and **energy efficiency**—getting more out of the energy we do consume—are twin strategies for reducing vulnerability to potential shortages and to the cost increases that will certainly occur in the future. In homes and offices, for example, we can conserve energy by setting our thermostats lower in the winter and higher in the summer, and turning off lights and computers when they are not being used.

To increase energy efficiency, buildings should be well insulated, and windows in older buildings should be replaced with modern windows dramatically reducing energy losses. Mechanical systems—heat, air conditioning, hot water—should be efficient and well maintained. Energy-efficient devices, from appliances to electronics to light bulbs, are now available and can replace inefficient devices as they wear out. All these things require an initial outlay of money, of course, and older buildings will be upgraded only over a period of years. On its website, the EPA provides extensive information about energy conservation, and the agency gives an "Energy Star" rating of the energy efficiency of many appliances, windows, and light bulbs.

Once an energy-efficient compact fluorescent light bulb lights up, it uses about one-quarter the energy of a traditional light bulb, and its life is about six times that of a traditional bulb.[114] Thus these bulbs offer savings at the household level while also reducing society's overall energy consumption. Unfortunately, each bulb contains about four milligrams of elemental mercury[115]; if the bulb is broken, mercury is released in a powdery residue. For the consumer, this means that these energy-efficient bulbs pose a hazard (and a cleanup challenge) if broken accidentally; moreover, they should not be discarded as ordinary trash. On its website, the EPA offers guidance on how to clean up a broken mercury-containing bulb.[116] The most energy-efficient lighting available today are the light emitting diode (LED) bulbs.

The potential gains from both energy conservation and increased energy efficiency are particularly apparent in the transportation sector. For example, the sprawling pattern of suburban and exurban development that is common in the United States, along with limited (or lack of) mass transit in many urbanized areas, contributes to our dependence on cars. In 2009, Americans logged 2.5 trillion vehicle-miles, and 4.2 trillion passenger-miles, in their personal vehicles; this averages out to almost 14,000 miles for every man, woman, and child.[117]

The fundamental inefficiency of our reliance on cars is exacerbated by the low fuel economy of the U.S. fleet of light vehicles. In 2009, the average fuel economy of all U.S. passenger cars was 23.8 miles per gallon; the average fuel economy of 2009 model-year passenger cars was higher at 32.9 miles per gallon.[118] As shown in **Figure 7.20**, from 1980 through 2005, a time during which the United States' decreasing energy security was widely publicized, the share of the U.S. light vehicle market held by SUVs increased steadily, and even within this class there was a shift to larger vehicles. Wagons, pickups, and vans also gained market share. Meanwhile, the market share held by cars steadily declined, and within this class, too, there was a shift to larger models. In 2010, for the first time, a change appears: as a group, wagons, pickups, and vans lost ground, and small and midsize cars made modest gains. The data do not reveal whether this change in buying habits reflects a fundamental change in values or is simply a reaction to the general economic downturn.

However, the U.S. buying public is beginning to embrace hybrid technologies. The **hybrid car** makes use of both a gasoline-powered combustion engine and electric power. The hybrid is an attempt to find a marketable balance between the electric car's high energy efficiency and zero emissions (but short range because of the limitations of relying on a battery) and the combustion engine's greater range and power. Cars powered

entirely using electricity have increased in popularity but require improvements to accessing electricity or recharging stations, if these vehicles are to be practical for longer distance travels. Life cycle analyses of both hybrid and all electric vehicles also raise concerns with the toxicity of the chemicals in the batteries required to run the cars, and with the fate of their disposal.

The modern lifestyle thrives on the consumption of energy. However, the environmental and human health costs associated with producing energy have not been well accounted for in the price that society pays for its power. In addition to considering the costs of these *externalities*, a more comprehensive accounting should incorporate the benefits associated with mitigating pollution from energy production, such as healthcare savings from reduced asthma attacks in children. And we should all feel a sense of urgency to find a more sustainable energy plan for the sake of not only ourselves but also our planet.

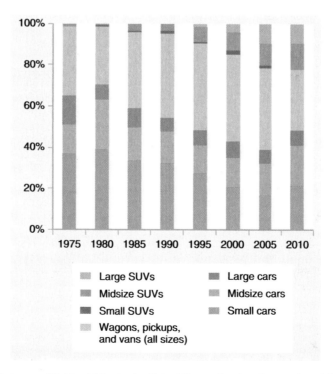

Figure 7.20 Market shares of light vehicles in the United States, by size class and model year, 1975–2010.

Data from U.S. Department of Energy, Transportation Energy Data Book. Available at: http://cta.ornl.gov/data/download31.shtml. Accessed October 14, 2012.

Study Questions

1. Create a table comparing the various sources for energy production in terms of their environmental and human health impacts across the life cycle from acquisition, power generation, and waste disposal.

2. One important lever in the effort to control global climate change is an overall reduction in emissions from the burning of fossil fuels. Consider why the United States has reversed itself twice now in terms of international climate change agreements—what do you think are fair and realistic expectations of the world's more developed and less developed countries in this effort?

3. Describe social disparities, past and present, in the burden of health risks from the nuclear fuel cycle in the United States.

4. Make an argument in favor of either a centralized disposal facility for high-level radioactive wastes or a decentralized approach to managing these wastes in the United States.

5. Consider how much energy you consume and the source of the electricity you use. What specific actions could you take to use less energy?

References

1. U.S. Energy Information Administration. *Energy explained: your guide to understanding energy*. Retrieved July 25, 2020, from https://www.eia.gov/energyexplained/

2. Buckley GL. The environmental transformation of an Appalachian valley, 1850–1906. *Geographical Review*, 1998;88(2):175-198.

3. U.S. Energy Information Administration. *Coal production in the United States: an historical overview*. Retrieved January 25, 2007 from www.eia.doe.gov/cneaf/coal/page/coal_production_review.pdf

4. U.S. Energy Information Administration. (n.d.). *Coal explained: coal imports and exports*. Retrieved July 25, 2020 from https://www.eia.gov/energyexplained/

5. U.S. Centers for Disease Control and Prevention. *Number and rate of occupational mining fatalities by year, 1983–2018*. Worker Health Charts. 2020. Retrieved July 20, 2020 from: https://wwwn.cdc.gov/NIOSH-WHC/chart/bls-fw/injury?T=ZS&V=C&D=RANGE&Y1=2018&Y2=2018

6. Governor's Independent Investigation Panel. Upper Big Branch: Report to the Governor. 2011. Retrieved June 20, 2012 from https://media.npr.org/documents/2011/may/giip-massey-report.pdf

7. Stephan C. *Coal Dust Explosion Hazards*. U.S. Mine Safety and Health Administration. 1998.

8. U.S. Centers for Disease Control and Prevention, National Institute for Occupational Safety and Health. *All Mining Disasters: 1839 to Present*. Retrieved March 28, 2012 from https://www.cdc.gov/niosh/mining/statistics/content/allminingdisasters.html

9. Haight J. Occupational health risks in crude oil and natural gas extraction. In Cleveland C, ed. *Encyclopedia of Energy*. Elsevier. 2004;4:477-487

10. National Commission on the BP Deepwater Horizon Oil Spill and Offshore Drilling. *Deep Water: The Gulf Oil Disaster and the Future of Offshore Drilling. Report to the President*. 2011. Retrieved June 20, 2012 from https://www.govinfo.gov/content/pkg/GPO-OIL COMMISSION/pdf/GPO-OILCOMMISSION.pdf

11. ExxonMobil. *About Natural Gas: Hydraulic Fracturing and Horizontal Drilling*. Retrieved July 9, 2012 from https://corporate.exxonmobil.com/Energy-and-environment/Tools-and-processes/Hydraulic-fracturing

12. Meng Q. The impacts of fracking on the environment: a total environmental study paradigm. *Sci Total Environ.* 2017;580:953-957.

13. Needleman HL. Clamped in a straitjacket: the insertion of lead into gasoline. *Environ Res.* 1997;74(2):95-103.

14. The Lead Group. (2011, June 17). *Countries where leaded petrol is possibly still sold for road use*. Retrieved March 23, 2012 from www.lead.org.au/fs/fst27.html

15. Vander A, Sherman J, Luciano D. *Human Physiology* [6th edition]. McGraw-Hill. 1994.

16. Nemmar A, Hoet PH, Vanquickenbourne B, et al. Passage of inhaled particles into the blood circulation in humans. *Circulation.* 2002;105:411-414.

17. Olivieri D, Scoditti E. Impact of environmental factors on lung defences. *Eur Respir Rev.* 2005;14:51-56.

18. Costa DL, Amdur MO. Air pollution. In Klaassen CD, ed. *Casarett & Doull's Toxicology: The Basic Science of Poisons* [5th edition]. McGraw-Hill. 1996:857-880.

19. Bernstein JA. Health effects of air pollution. *J Allergy Clin Immunol.* 2004;114:1116-1123.

20. Chen-Yeung, MN. Air pollution and health. *Hong Kong Med J.* 2000;6:390-398.

21. Routledge HC, Ayres JG, Townend JN. Why cardiologists should be interested in air pollution. *Heart.* 2003;89(12):1383-1388.

22. Vermylen J, Nemmar A, Nemery B, Hoylaerts MF. Ambient air pollution and acute myocardial infarction. *J Thromb Haemost.* 2005;3(9):1955-1961.

23. Delfino RJ, Sioutas C, Malik S. Potential role of ultrafine particles in associations between airborne particle mass and cardiovascular health. *Environmental Health Perspectives*, 2005;113(8):934-946.

24. Whittaker A, BéruBé K, Jones T, Maynard R, Richards R. Killer smog of London, 50 years on: particle properties and oxidative capacity. *Sci Total Environ*. 2004;334–335: 435-445.

25. Davis D, Bell ML, Fletcher T. A look back at the London Smog of 1952 and the half century since. *Environ Health Perspect*. 2002;110(12):A734-A735.

26. Brook RD, Franklin B, Cascio W, et al. Air pollution and cardiovascular disease: a statement for healthcare professionals from the Expert Panel on Population and Prevention Science of the American Heart Association. *Circulation*. 2004;109(21):2655-2671.

27. Evans J, van Donkelaar A, Martin RV, et al. Estimates of global mortality attributable to particulate air pollution using satellite imagery. *Environ Res*. 2012;120:33-42.

28. Dockery DW, Pope CA, Xu X, et al. An association between air pollution and mortality in six U.S. cities. *N Engl J Med*. 1993;329:1753-1759.

29. Pope CA, Thun MJ, Namboodiri MM, et al. Particulate air pollution as a predictor of mortality in a prospective study of U.S. adults. *Am J Respir Crit Care Med*. 1995;151 (3, pt 1):669-674.

30. Laden F, Schwartz J, Speizer FE, Dockery DW. Reduction in fine particulate air pollution and mortality. *Am J Respir Crit Care Med*. 2006;173(6):667-672.

31. Brook RD, Rajagopalan S, Pope III CA, et al. Particulate matter air pollution and cardiovascular disease: an update to the scientific statement from the American Heart Association. *Circulation*. 121(21):2331-2378.

32. Hong, Y-C, Lee J-T, Kim H, Ha E-H., Schwartz J, Christiani DC. Effects of air pollutants on acute stroke mortality. *Environ Health Perspect*. 2020;110(2): 187-191.

33. Garshick E, Laden F, Hart JE, et al. Lung cancer and vehicle exhaust in trucking industry workers. *Environ Health Perspect*, 2008;116(10):1327-1332.

34. Trasande L, Thurston GD. The role of air pollution in asthma and other pediatric morbidities. *The Journal of Allergy and Clinical Immunology*. 2005;115(4): 689-699.

35. Peden DB. Influences on the development of allergy and asthma. *Toxicology*. 2002;181-182:323-328.

36. Sunyer J, Spix C, Quénel P, et al. Urban air pollution and emergency admissions for asthma in four European cities: the APHEA Project. *Thorax*. 1997;52(9):760-765.

37. Chew FT, Goh DY, Ooi B, Saharom R, Hui J, Lee B. Association of ambient air-pollution levels with acute asthma exacerbation among children in Singapore. *Allergy*. 1999;54(4):320-329.

38. Thompson AJ, Shields MD, Patterson CC. Acute asthma exacerbations and air pollutants in children living in Belfast, Northern Ireland. *Arch Environ Health*. 2001;56(3):234-241.

39. Pope CA III, Ezzati M, Dockery DW. Fine-particulate air pollution and life expectancy in the United States. *N Engl J Med*, 2009;360:376-386.

40. Schwartz J, Coull B, Laden F, Ryan L. The effect of dose and timing of dose on the association between airborne particles and survival. *Environ Health Perspect*. 2008;116(1):64-69.

41. Šrám RJ, Binková B, Dejmek J, Bobak M. Ambient air pollution and pregnancy outcomes: a review of the literature. *Environ Health Perspect*. 2005;113(4):375-382.

42. Clancy L, Goodman P, Sinclair H, Dockery DW. Effect of air-pollution control on death rates in Dublin, Ireland: an intervention study. *Lancet*. 2002;360(9341):1210-1214.

43. Friedman M, Powell KE, Hutwagner L, Graham LM, Teague WG. Impact of changes in transportation and commuting behaviors during the 1996 Summer Olympic Games in Atlanta on air quality and childhood asthma. *J AMA*. 2001;285(7):897-905.

44. U.S. Centers for Disease Control and Prevention. Leading causes of death. Retrieved July 9, 2012 from www.cdc .gov/nchs/fastats/lcod.htm/

45. U.S. Environmental Protection Agency. Inventory of U.S. Greenhouse Gas Emissions and Sinks: 1990–2018. Retrieved July 21, 2020 from https://www.epa.gov /ghgemissions/inventory-us-greenhouse-gas-emissions -and-sinks-1990-2018

46. Smith KR, Frumkin H, Balakrishnan K, et al. Energy and health. *Ann Rev Public Health*. 2013;34:159-188.

47. Intergovernmental Panel on Climate Change. Summary for policymakers. In *Climate Change 2007: The Physical Science Basis. Contribution of Working Group 1 to the Fourth Assessment Report of the Intergovernmental Panel on Climate Change*. Cambridge University Press. 2007.

48. National Ocean Service. *Is sea level rising? Yes, sea level is rising at an increasing rate*. National Oceanic and Atmospheric Administration. 2019. Retrieved July 25, 2020 from https://oceanservice.noaa.gov/facts/sealevel .html

49. Intergovernmental Panel on Climate Change. Historical overview of climate change science. In *Climate Change 2007: The Physical Science Basis. Contribution of Working Group 1 to the Fourth Assessment Report of the Intergovernmental Panel on Climate Change*. 2007. Cambridge University Press.

50. Intergovernmental Panel on Climate Change. Technical summary. In *Climate Change 2007: The Physical Science Basis. Contribution of Working Group 1 to the Fourth Assessment Report of the Intergovernmental Panel on Climate Change*. Cambridge University Press. 2007.

51. Intergovernmental Panel on Climate Change. Summary for policymakers. In *Climate Change 2007: Impacts, Adaptation and Vulnerability. Contribution of Working Group II to the Fourth Assessment Report of the Intergovernmental Panel on Climate Change*. Cambridge University Press. 2007.

52. Kuczynski T, Blanes-Vidal V, Li B, et al. Impact of global climate change on the health, welfare and productivity

of intensively housed livestock. *Int J Agri Biol Engineering*. 2011;4(2):1.

53. Sheffield PE, Landrigan PJ. Global climate change and children's health: threats and strategies for prevention. *Environ Health Perspect*. 2011;119:291-298.

54. United Nations Framework Convention on Climate Change. Status of ratification of the convention. Retrieved March 31, 2012 from http://unfccc.int/essential _background/convention/status_of_ratification /items/2631.php

55. My Climate. *What are the Kyoto Protocol and the Paris Agreement?* Retrieved July 25, 2020 from https://www .myclimate.org/information/faq/faq-detail/what-are -the-kyoto-protocol-and-the-paris-agreement/

56. Pompeo MR. *On the U.S. Withdrawal from the Paris Agreement*. U.S. Department of State Press Release. 2019. Retrieved from: https://www.state.gov/on-the-u-s -withdrawal-from-the-paris-agreement/

57. United States Environmental Protection Agency. Reformulated Gasoline (RFG). Retrieved March 31, 2012 from www.epa.gov/otaq/fuels/gasolinefuels/rfg/index .htm

58. Greenhouse L. Justices say E.P.A. has power to act on harmful gases. 2007. *New York Times*. https://www .nytimes.com/2007/04/03/washington/03scotus .html?hp=&p

59. Barringer F. For new generation of power plants, a new emission rule from the E.P.A. 2012. *New York Times*. https://www.nytimes.com/2012/03/28/science/earth /epasets-greenhouse-emission-limits-on-new-power -plants.html?_r=1&hpw=&pagewant%20%20/%203

60. Black, H. Imperfect protection: NEPA at 35 years. *Environ Health Perspect*. 2004;112(5):A292-A295.

61. Ripley, A. Radioactive building sand stirs dispute. 1971. *New York Times*.

62. U.S. Environmental Protection Agency. Uranium mill tailings. Retrieved March 23, 2012 from https://www .epa.gov/radiation/health-and-environmental-protection -standards-uranium-and-thorium-mill-tailings-40-cfr

63. Uranium Producers of America. Conventional mining and milling of uranium ore. 2014. Retrieved July 25, 2020 from http://www.theupa.org/uranium_technology /conventional_mining/

64. U.S. Energy Information Administration. *Nuclear Explained: U.S. Nuclear Industry*. Retrieved July 25, 2020 from https://www.eia.gov/energyexplained/

65. U.S. Energy Information Administration. *Decommissioning nuclear reactors is a long-term and costly process*. 2017. Retrieved July 25, 2020 from https://www.eia.gov /energyexplained/

66. International Atomic Energy Agency. INES: The International Nuclear and Radiological Event Scale. Retrieved June 20, 2012 from https://www.iaea. org/resources/databases/international-nuclear-and -radiological-event-scale

67. U.S. Nuclear Regulatory Commission. Bulletin No. 75-04A: Cable fire at Browns Ferry nuclear power station. Retrieved April 1, 2012 from www.nrc.gov/reading -rm/doc-collections/gen-comm/bulletins/1975 /bl75004a.html

68. Institute of Nuclear Power Operations. (n.d.). Special Report on the Nuclear Accident at the Fukushima Daiichi Nuclear Power Station. 2011;INPO 11-005. Retrieved October 15, 2012 from: www.nei.org /resourcesandstats/documentlibrary/safetyandsecurity /reports/special-report-on-the-nuclear-accident-at-the -fukushima-daiichi-nuclear-power-station

69. Nuclear Energy Institute. (n.d.). Resources & Stats: Fukushima, Chernobyl and the Nuclear Event Scale. Retrieved October 15, 2012 from https://www.nei .org/resources/fact-sheets/comparing-fukushima-and -chernobyl

70. U.S. Department of Energy, Office of Civilian Radioactive Waste Management. (2006). Overview: Yucca Mountain Project. https://www.energy.gov/listings/list-yucca -mountain-archival-documents

71. Sproat E.(Statement of Edward F. Sproat, III, Director for the Office of Civilian Radioactive Waste Management, U.S. Department of Energy, before the Subcommittee on Energy and Air Quality, Committee on Energy and Commerce, U.S. House of Representatives. 2006. Retrieved October 13, 2020 from https://www.nrc.gov /docs/ML0620/ML062010544.pdf

72. U.S. Energy Information Administration. U.S. Commercial Nuclear Reactors: Reactor Status List. 2019. Retrieved April 6, 2012 from: www.nrc.gov/reading-rm /doc-collections/nuregs/staff/sr1350/

73. Blue Ribbon Commission on America's Nuclear Future. (2012, January). Disposal subcommittee report to the full commission (updated report). Retrieved October 13, 2020 from https://www.energy.gov/sites/prod/files /2013/04/f0/brc_finalreport_jan2012.pdf

74. Ryskamp JM. (2003). Nuclear Fuel Cycle Closure. U.S. Department of Energy, Idaho National Engineering and Environmental Laboratory.

75. U.S. Nuclear Regulatory Commission. Low-level waste disposal oversight. (2017). Retrieved December 8, 2020 from: www.nrc.gov/waste/llw-disposal/oversight.html

76. Plumer B. U.S. nuclear comeback stalls as two reactors are abandoned. 2017. *The New York Times*.

77. World Nuclear Association. (2020, July). *Nuclear power in France*. Retrieved July 25, 2020 from: https:// www.world-nuclear.org/information-library/country -profiles/countries-a-f/france.aspx#:~:text=France%20 derives%20about%2075%25%20of,billion%20per%20 year%20from%20this

78. Herring J. Uranium and thorium resource assessment. In Cleveland C, ed. *Encyclopedia of Energy*. Elsevier. 2004.

79. Frumkin H, Samet J. Radon. *CA: A Cancer Journal for Clinicians*. 2001;(6):337-344.

80. Gilliland FD, Hunt WC, Archer V, Saccomanno G. Radon progeny exposure and lung cancer risk among non-smoking uranium miners. *Health Physics*, 2000;79(4):365-372.

81. Gilliland FD, Hunt WC, Pardilla M, Key CR. (2000). Uranium mining and lung cancer among Navajo men in New Mexico and Arizona, 1969 to 1993. *J OccupEnviron Med*. 42(3):278-283.

82. Arnold C. Once upon a mine: the legacy of uranium on the Navaho Nation. *Environ Health Perspect*. 2014;122(2):A44-A49.

83. Yazzie SA, Davis S, Seixas N, Yost MG. Assessing the impact of housing features and environmental factors on home indoor radon concentration levels on the Navaho Nation. *Int J Environ Res Public Health*. 2020;17(8), 2813-2830. https://doi.org/10.3390/ijerph17082813

84. Hund L, Bedrick EJ, Miller C, et al. A Bayesian framework for estimating risk due to exposure to uranium mine and mill waste on the Navajo Nation. *J R Statist Soc. A*. 2015;178(part 4):1069-1091.

85. Raymond-Whish S, Mayer LP, O'Neal T, et al. Drinking water with uranium below the U.S. EPA water standard causes estrogen receptor-dependent responses in female mice. *Environ Health Perspect*. 2007;115(12):1711-1716.

86. Williams D. Cancer after nuclear fallout: lessons from the Chernobyl accident. *Nat Rev Cancer*. 2002;2:543-549.

87. Cardis E, Hatch M. The Chernobyl accident—an epidemiological perspective. *Clin Oncol*. 2011;23(4):251-260.

88. Bromet EJ, Havenaar JM, Guey LT. A 25 year retrospective review of the psychological consequences of the Chernobyl accident. *Clin Oncol*. 2011;23(4):297-305.

89. United Nations Scientific Committee on the Effects of Atomic Radiation. Sources, effects and risks of ionizing radiation: report to the General Assembly with scientific annexes. Volume I: Scientific Annex A. United Nations. 2014.

90. U.S. Nuclear Regulatory Commission. High-Level Waste Disposal/What We Regulate. 2011. Retrieved September 12, 2012 from www.nrc.gov/waste/hlw-disposal.html

91. Stenger E. Infographic: a light bulb shows how solar and wind beat coal. Retrieved July 27, 2020 http://www.edouardstenger.com/2014/12/01/infographic-coal-solar-light-bulb/

92. Lovins AB, Lovins LH. *Brittle Power: Energy Strategy for National Security*. Brick House Publishing. 1982.

93. U.S. Canada Power System Outage Task Force. Final Report on the August 14th, 2003 Blackout in the United States and Canada: Causes and Recommendations. 2004. Retrieved September 12, 2012 from https://www3.epa.gov/region1/npdes/merrimackstation/pdfs/ar/AR-1165.pdf

94. Kammen DM. Renewable energy: Taxonomic overview. In Cleveland C, ed. *Encyclopedia of Energy* Elsevier. 2004; 5: 385-412.

95. U.S. Department of Agriculture. Amber waves/growing crops for biofuels has spillover effects. Retrieved April 6, 2012 from https://www3.epa.gov/region1/npdes/merrimackstation/pdfs/ar/AR-1165.pdf

96. Maxwell NI. Environmental injustices of energy facilities. In Cleveland C, ed. *Encyclopedia of Energy* Elsevier. 5.

97. Ezzati M, Kammen DM. The health impacts of exposure to indoor air pollution from solid fuels in developing countries: knowledge, gaps, and data needs. *Environ Health Perspect*. 2002;110(11):1057-1068.

98. Ezzati M, Saleh H, Kammen DM. The contributions of emissions and spatial microenvironments to exposure to indoor air pollution from biomass combustion in Kenya. *Environ Health Perspect*. 2000;108:833-839.

99. Balakrishnan K, Ramaswamy P, Sambandam S, et al. Air pollution from household solid fuel combustion in India: an overview of exposure and health related information to inform health research priorities. *Glob Health Act*. 2011;4(1):10.

100. Fullerton DG, Bruce N, Gordon SB. Indoor air pollution from biomass fuel smoke is a major health concern in the developing world. *The Royal Soc Trop Med Hygiene*. 2008;102(9):843-851.

101. Po JY, Fitzgerald JM, Carlsten C. Respiratory disease associated with solid biomass fuel exposure in rural women and children: systematic review and meta-analysis. *Thorax*, 2011;66(3):232.

102. Kim K, Jahan SA, Kabir E. A review of diseases associated with household air pollution due to the use of biomass fuels. *Journal of Hazardous Materials*, 2011;192(2):425-431.

103. Pedersen E. Health aspects associated with wind turbine noise—results from three field studies. *Noise Control Engineering*. 2011;59(1):47-53.

104. Morrison ML, Sinclair K. Environmental impacts of wind energy technology. In Cleveland C, ed. *Encyclopedia of Energy*. Elsevier. 2004;6.

105. Erickson WP, Johnson GD, Strickland DM, Young Jr, DP, Sernka KJ, Good RE. *Avian collisions with wind turbines: a summary of existing studies and comparisons to other sources of avian collision mortality in the United States*. National Wind Coordinating Committee. 2001. Retrieved February 7, 2008 from www.osti.gov/energycitations/servlets/purl/822418-vE68OX/native/822418.pdf

106. Daley B. Audubon review supports wind farm. *Boston Globe*. 2006.

107. Wines M. China admits problems with three gorges dam. *New York Times*. 2011.

108. Wong E. Three Gorges dam is said to hurt areas downstream. *New York Times*. 2011.

109. National Aeronautics and Space Administration, Goddard Space Flight Center. Dams, Lakes and Reservoirs Database for the World Water Development Report II [data]. Retrieved May 12, 2012 from http://gcmd.nasa.gov/KeywordSearch/Metadata.do?Portal=GCMD&KeywordPath=%5BKeyword%3D%27reservoirs%27%5D&EntryId=UNH_WWRDII_DAMS&MetadataView=Data&MetadataType=0&lbnode=mdlb5

110. Poff NL, Hart DD. How dams vary and why it matters for the emerging science of dam removal: an ecological classification of dams is needed to characterize how the tremendous variation in the size, operational mode,

age, and number of dams in a river basin influences the potential for restoring regulated rivers via dam removal. *BioScience,* 2002;52(8):659-668.

111. Dieterich R. 24-hour solar energy: molten salt makes it possible, and prices are falling fast. 2018. *Inside Climate News.* https://insideclimatenews.org/news/16012018 /csp-concentrated-solar-molten-salt-storage-24 -hourrenewable-energy-crescent-dunes-nevada

112. Hogan MC. (2011). Solar Power. In National Council for Science and the Environment, (Eds.), *Encyclopedia of Earth.*

113. U.S. Environmental Protection Agency. (n.d.). Science /High GWP Gases and Climate Change.

114. Energy Star Program. Light Bulbs/Did You Know? Retrieved April 3, 2012 from www.energystar.gov /index.cfm?fuseaction=find_a_product.show ProductGroup&pgw_code=LB

115. U.S. Environmental Protection Agency. Compact fluorescent light bulbs (CFLs). Retrieved April 6, 2012 from www.epa.gov/cfl/cfl-hg.html

116. U.S. Environmental Protection Agency. (n.d.). Cleaning Up a Broken CFL.

117. Davis SC, Diegel SW, Boundy RG. *Transportation Energy Data Book: Edition 30,* ORNL-6986. 2011. Available at: http://info.ornl.gov/sites/publications/files/Pub31202 .pdf

118. Bureau of Transportation Statistics. (n.d.). National Transportation Statistics/Table 4-23: Average Fuel Efficiency of U.S. Light Duty Vehicles. Retrieved April 5, 2012 from https://www.bts.gov/archive/publications /national_transportation_statistics/table_04_23

CHAPTER 8

Living in the World We've Made

LEARNING OBJECTIVES

After studying this chapter, the reader will be able to:

- Define or explain the key terms introduced throughout the chapter
- Describe how various types of municipal waste are consolidated into waste streams that are treated
- Describe the problem that combined sewer overflows are intended to address and how they do so
- Describe the typical steps in municipal wastewater treatment, along with the objectives of each step
- Explain the key principle behind a sustainable approach to sanitation, whether in more-developed or less-developed countries
- Describe the potential hazards of land application of treated sewage sludge
- Explain how the objectives of drinking water treatment are met through the treatment processes
- Describe the U.S. regulatory framework for managing the public health risks associated with municipal wastewater and drinking water
- Identify the four major approaches to handling municipal solid waste and describe the challenges of managing this mundane waste stream
- Describe the environmental health hazards of megacities in less-developed countries
- Describe the environmental health hazards of urban or suburban settings in more-developed countries and some of the specific hazards of the modern home
- Explain the concept of the ecologic footprint and its implications for the sustainability of current development patterns

Although human beings are just one of many animal species, we are unique in the extent of our deliberate modification of the natural world. Especially in the more developed countries, we have built complex systems to produce food, manufacture goods, and generate power. These systems consume raw materials and produce wastes in vast quantities.

This chapter is about living in the world that we have created and in understanding our impact. Section 8.1 begins by describing the major flows into and out of communities, followed by three sections describing the challenges and health concerns of handling sewage (Section 8.2), providing safe drinking water (Section 8.3), and managing trash and other types of solid waste (Section 8.4). Section 8.5 briefly takes up these same concerns in the setting of the world's less-developed countries. Returning to the more developed countries, Section 8.6 discusses the environmental health issues associated with the construction of our modern-day environment and our consequential household lifestyles. Section 8.7 concludes with a discussion of the nonsustainable character of modern development and suggests strategies to mitigate future global risks.

8.1 The "Metabolism" of Communities

If we think of a city or town as an organism, then its water supply, sewage, and trash are the inputs and outputs of a kind of "urban metabolism."[1] The metabolism of today's cities, although incorporating some thoroughly modern features, still reflects some 19th-century decisions regarding infrastructure.

Urban Metabolism in the 19th Century

The development of systems to handle water and waste followed a similar pattern in the majority of cities in the United States and Europe. Through the early years of the 19th century, urine and feces were collected either in pits located below privies or in larger underground vaults known as cesspools. These had to be emptied periodically and the contents carried away. In some cities, there were also sewer pipes to carry away rainwater that collected in the gutters.

By the mid-19th century, it had become possible to supply urban homes with running water from a tap. This led to the development of the water closet, in which water was used to flush human waste through pipes into a privy pit or cesspool. This addition of water to the waste stream meant that a much larger volume of waste was now going to storage vaults, which suddenly seemed too small. The need to more frequently empty these storage vaults was both inconvenient and expensive.

Faced with this crisis, in the latter half of the 19th century, many cities opted for the same technological solution—the use of water to carry away sewage.[1] And as engineers designed sewer systems, they faced a key decision: whether to channel sewage waste and street runoff into one sewer system or to build separate systems for the two waste streams. Separate systems would have been more costly, so most U.S. communities opted for combined sewer systems, which emptied wastewater into a nearby body of water.[1]

Over the next decades, science demonstrated that contamination of a downstream city's drinking water intake by an upstream city's sewage could cause disease in the downstream city. During the same period, filtration technologies were developed that could dramatically reduce microbial contamination of water. Now cities faced another decision[1]: Was it enough for a city to treat its drinking water, or should it also treat its wastewater? Again, most cities took the less expensive option, treating only drinking water. It was not until the 20th century that it became common for cities to treat their wastewater in even a limited fashion.

As will be described later, the processes used to treat sewage and drinking water have costs and side effects, and we might like to imagine different technological decisions, past or future. Nevertheless, these methods have been strikingly successful overall in holding the incidence of waterborne illness to a low level in the more developed countries.

In contrast to sewage, trash as we know it today is largely a phenomenon of the 20th century. Before that time, material goods were scarce and were scavenged and reused as a matter of course.[2] It is only in the era of the *consumer economy* that ordinary people are encouraged to buy many new items simply because they want them, and they continually throw out the old to make way for the new.

Community Metabolism Today

The modern metabolism of U.S. communities is shaped by three factors so fundamental that we rarely think about them. First, on the intake side, we have a unified water supply, not separate supplies of **potable water** (water deemed suitable for drinking) and nonpotable water. There is a strong public health rationale for this approach: It avoids cross-contamination of the potable supply and various mistakes that would lead to waterborne illness. Nevertheless, the result is that we water our lawns and wash our cars with water that has been treated to drinking water standards. And indeed, the second fundamental fact of community metabolism is that, on the outgoing side, we use potable water to carry away sewage.

The third fundamental fact of modern community metabolism is the sheer scale of its inputs and outputs. The most recent national data available indicate that in the United States in 2016, a typical family of four used approximately 300 gallons of water each day with roughly 70% being used indoors.[3] Flushing wastes down the toilet is the single largest indoor use of water (see **Figure 8.1**); other major uses are washing clothes, taking showers, and using water from the faucet for various purposes. To a varying degree, leaks add to the total volume of water consumed. Encouragingly, residential consumption of water has decreased by 22% since 1999 when various

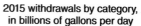
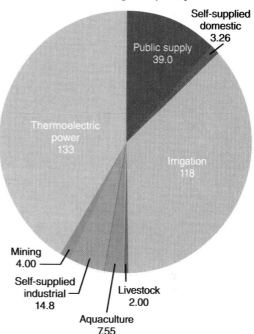

Figure 8.2 Use of water in the United States by sector, 2015.

U.S. Geological Survey. 2015 Withdrawls by Category, in Gallons per day. Available at: https://www.usgs.gov/mission-areas/water-resources/science/total-water-use?qt-science_center_objects=0#qt-science_center_objects

low-flow devices came onto the market.[4] However, water supplied for public use represents a much smaller use of water withdrawals in the United States than the water consumed by thermoelectric power generation or irrigation. **Figure 8.2** provides the percentage of water consumed by each of the sectors in the United States in 2015.[5]

Trash, too, is a high-volume waste stream: In the United States today, each person generates approximately 4.5 pounds of trash each day, on average.[5] And per capita trash generation is increasing each year, in contrast to the moderate declines in water usage. Thus, domestic wastewater, although it is still the most basic human waste stream, is now accompanied by large quantities of trash, and in fact there is some overlap in the contents of these two waste streams. Furthermore, once domestic wastewater enters the municipal system, it may be mixed with two other waste streams: storm runoff from paved surfaces

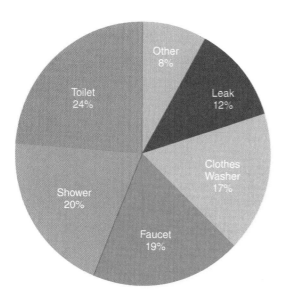

Figure 8.1 Estimated indoor use of water in the United States, 2016.

Reproduced from Water Research Foundation, Residential End Uses of Water, Version 2, 2016.

and liquid wastes from industry. The various connections among waste streams are described here.

Municipal Wastewater and Municipal Solid Waste

The typical household produces three basic types of wastes: urine and feces; food waste; and a mixture of other wastes that includes chemical products and items made of glass, metal, plastic, paper, and other materials. As shown in **Figure 8.3**, these wastes are consolidated into two waste streams, commonly known as **sewage** and **trash**. At the community level, these two waste streams are often referred to as **municipal wastewater** and **municipal solid waste**.

Although these are separate municipal waste streams, there is some overlap in their contents so because each is simply a different mix of the same basic types of waste. Wastewater consists of anything that goes down a drain, not only from toilets but also from sinks, bathtubs, washing machines, and dishwashers. As a result, in addition to urine and feces, wastewater contains paper and cotton products; soap, shampoo, and other personal care products applied to the body; laundry detergents and fabric softeners; and dishwashing products. Other items also go down the toilet: outdated medications, used condoms, dead goldfish, children's toys, jewelry, and so on. More of these same items are discarded as trash, along with a great variety of other household items, large and small. At the same time, a small proportion of fecal waste goes out as trash—mainly in disposable diapers, which in 2010 made up 1.5% by weight of the U.S. municipal solid waste stream.[6] The fate of food waste varies: Some goes down the drain and some into the trash. If a household has a garbage disposal in the kitchen, a much greater share of its food waste enters the municipal wastewater stream. Alternatively, food waste can be composted, a form of recycling.

Municipal Wastewater and Storm Runoff

As noted earlier, many older cities channel storm runoff from gutter drains into the sanitary sewers. This urban runoff, mainly shed from streets and other impervious surfaces, is different from municipal wastewater in two important ways. First, its makeup is different. It may carry small quantities of animal waste, so its overall burden of fecal waste and pathogens is very low. However, it may also contain a heavy load of sediment, as well as oil and grease, road salt, heavy metals, and yard chemicals—including some chemicals deliberately dumped. Second, storm runoff is episodic, surging during and after storms, whereas the municipal waste-water stream is relatively constant, day in and day out. This creates a problem: Treatment plants are designed to handle a steady flow of municipal wastewater and will often be overwhelmed when a storm surge is added to the normal flow.

For this reason, overflow valves, called **combined sewer overflows (CSOs)**, are built into a combined sewer system "upstream" of the treatment plant. When the combined flow of municipal wastewater and storm runoff exceeds the treatment plant's capacity, these overflow valves open, releasing untreated wastewater directly into a random body of water (see **Figure 8.4**, which

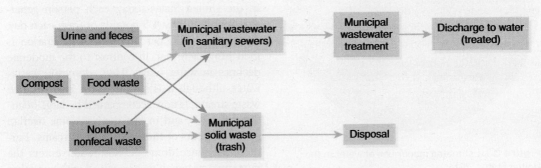

Figure 8.3 Contributors to municipal wastewater and municipal solid waste streams.

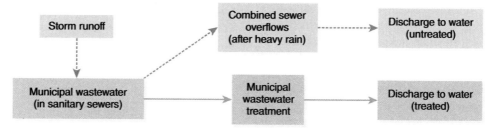

Figure 8.4 Use of combined sewer overflows to handle storm runoff.

zooms in on the municipal wastewater stream in Figure 8.3 and adds new elements). The treatment plant continues to operate at full capacity, but some wastewater never passes through it.

In 2018, about 40 million people in the United States lived in more than 860 communities having combined sewer overflows.[7] These overflows are found mostly in older cities, in areas of relatively dense population and high rainfall; almost no CSOs are found, for example, in the Great Plains or Rocky Mountain states or in the arid Southwest. Modifications to such an infrastructure are difficult and expensive. In Greater Boston, for example, where the sewage system handled 350 million gallons of sewage per day in 2010,[8] and served 2.55 million people in 61 cities and towns, some 70 combined sewer overflows once released untreated sewage into Boston Harbor and the three rivers flowing into it. Although it is not feasible to completely restructure the system, the

regional water authority has taken an incremental approach, and work on controlling the system's CSOs is ongoing. Municipal wastewater and storm water have been separated in some local areas, and in some other locations, CSOs have been consolidated so that the combined waste stream can at least be screened and chlorinated before being released. And during a rainstorm, some wastewater can be held in storage so that it can later go to the treatment plant.[9]

Municipal Wastewater and Industrial Wastes

Although industrial wastes are sometimes treated and discharged separately from municipal wastewater (called a **direct discharge** of industrial wastes to the receiving body of water), they are sometimes discharged via the municipal wastewater stream (an **indirect discharge**); Figure 8.5

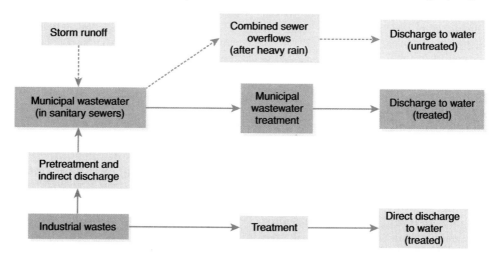

Figure 8.5 Direct and indirect discharge of industrial wastes.

adding this waste stream to the municipal sewage and storm runoff waste streams of Figure 8.4. In the latter case of an indirect discharge, industrial wastes pass through a system that is not designed to treat them, and; therefore, the wastes should undergo **pretreatment** before entering the municipal wastewater stream. Without pretreatment, acidic industrial wastes can damage sewers or the wastewater works, and pesticides, or other toxic chemicals in industrial wastes, may kill the bacteria that are used in wastewater treatment (described later). In addition, metals or synthetic chemicals in industrial wastes can end up in the residual material (called sludge) that remains after sewage treatment.

8.2 Management of Sewage Wastes

The biological processes involved in returning human waste safely to the environment are similar in all settings. However, the systems needed to serve a large city are very different from those that serve people in more sparsely populated areas. This section addresses these major topics:

- The treatment processes used at municipal wastewater treatment plants, which receive wastewater from homes, businesses, and other institutions
- Smaller-scale systems to handle the wastes of individual homes, or clusters of homes, in less densely populated areas
- The U.S. framework for the regulation of municipal wastewater treatment

Municipal Wastewater Treatment

In most cities and towns, sewage treatment comprises a very similar set of processes, most of which are long-established. After outlining the objectives of sewage treatment, this section describes those basic processes, concluding with the common, but still controversial, step of spreading the residuals of sewage treatment on land.

Objectives of Sewage Treatment

As already noted, more than just sewage goes into a city's sanitary sewers, and the term *municipal wastewater* captures this reality. However, municipal wastewater's most prominent component— the component that demands prompt treatment in order to prevent infectious disease, and for which treatment is designed—is sewage. Sewage treatment has three major objectives. The first is to remove most pathogens, thereby preventing waterborne illness in those whose drinking water source is downstream from a sewage outfall.

The second objective is to remove organic matter, thereby decreasing the ecological impact of sewage waste: a decline in dissolved oxygen in the receiving water. This is precisely the same effect seen when large quantities of animal manure are released from concentrated animal feeding operations (CAFOs). As described earlier in more detail, dissolved oxygen in the receiving water declines as oxygen is consumed by bacterial digestion of both fecal waste and the detritus of algal overgrowth. Similarly, if a large quantity of sewage is released into a body of water, bacterial decomposition can deplete oxygen in the water, causing fish and other aquatic organisms to die. This impact of sewage is measured as its **biochemical oxygen demand (BOD)**: the demand for oxygen created by the biochemical process of decomposing organic matter.[*]

The third objective of sewage treatment is to remove suspended solids. Sewage-laden water, even if it is free of floating solids, carries a heavy load of suspended solids, making the water cloudy. Suspended solids are assessed as **turbidity** (cloudiness), which is a measure of how much the transmission of light through water is impaired. Suspended solids not only make water cloudy

---

[*]BOD is measured (in mg/L) as the amount of dissolved oxygen consumed as microorganisms break down the waste in a given volume of water in a given time period, usually either five or 10 days (referred to as BOD5 and BOD10). An alternate test, which takes less time to complete, uses chemical reactions as a surrogate measure of biological decomposition, assessing chemical oxygen demand (COD) in lieu of BOD.

but they also harbor pathogens and interfere with disinfection; moreover, because suspended solids consist partly of organic matter, they contribute to BOD. Thus removing suspended solids also serves the first two objectives of sewage treatment: removing both pathogens and organic matter.

Basic Processes of Sewage Treatment

Basic sewage treatment consists of primary and secondary treatment, although other treatments are frequently added (see **Figure 8.6**; this diagram is an expansion of the municipal wastewater treatment step that appears in the preceding three diagrams). **Primary sewage treatment** is a mechanical process during which ever-finer materials are removed from the waste stream by employing a sequence of steps. Primary treatment begins with a **bar screen**—wastewater flows through a set of parallel bars that screen out relatively large objects, such as children's toys and dead rats. In most modern sewage treatment works, materials captured by the bar screen are removed mechanically; in the past, these materials were raked away by workers. Next, the waste stream passes through a grinder (sometimes called a **comminutor**), ensuring that nothing in the waste stream is large enough to clog up the works.

In the two remaining steps of primary treatment, materials are simply allowed to settle out of the waste stream. First, in the **grit chamber**, heavier particles such as sand settle out; this grit will be landfilled. Then, in the **primary clarifier**, a large uncovered vat, suspended solids containing organic matter are allowed to settle out. These solids are **sewage sludge**, which itself must be treated and disposed of. Materials that float (scum) are skimmed off for further treatment along with the sludge.

The next major step, **secondary sewage treatment**, is the heart of sewage treatment. This is a biological process—an accelerated version of natural decomposition in which bacteria digest organic wastes in an aerobic environment. One of two methods is employed to accomplish this. In the more traditional approach, wastewater is sprayed over a **trickling filter**—a bed of rocks coated with bacteria-containing slime; as the water trickles downward, the bacteria decompose organic matter. Using newer technology, sewage is primed with bacteria and then agitated in large, well-aerated tanks. Either process is followed by a resting stage in which fine matter settles out, becoming sludge, and floating scum is removed to be treated along with the sludge.

Some wastewater treatment systems, particularly in large urban areas, include **tertiary sewage treatment** tailored to specific needs. For example, very fine suspended solids might be removed (generating more sludge); or a carbon filter might be utilized to remove synthetic organic chemicals. Another optional step may follow tertiary or secondary treatment: **disinfection** of the waste stream, usually by chlorination.

How do these processes accomplish the basic objectives of sewage treatment? As exhibited in **Table 8.1**, most pathogens survive primary treatment, unless they are simply unable to survive for long outside of the human body. Although secondary treatment does not specifically target pathogens, many bacteria may die simply because they run out of food; viruses are more likely than bacteria to survive secondary treatment. If disinfection is used at the end of sewage treatment, it is used with the intention of killing pathogens that remain in the waste stream. Although disinfection was used routinely in the past, it is used less commonly today because of concerns about the impact of chlorine in the aquatic environment. Also, given that pathogens enter water from other sources, including farmland, the disinfection of municipal wastewater does not completely eliminate bacterial contamination of waterways.

The objective of removing organic matter from the waste stream is accomplished by removing finer and finer solids, in primary and secondary (and sometimes tertiary) treatments (see Table 8.1). In contrast, primary and secondary treatments do not remove chemicals from the waste stream; this is accomplished, if at all, through optional tertiary treatment designed for this purpose. Primary and secondary treatments are the core processes of treating sewage; it is only

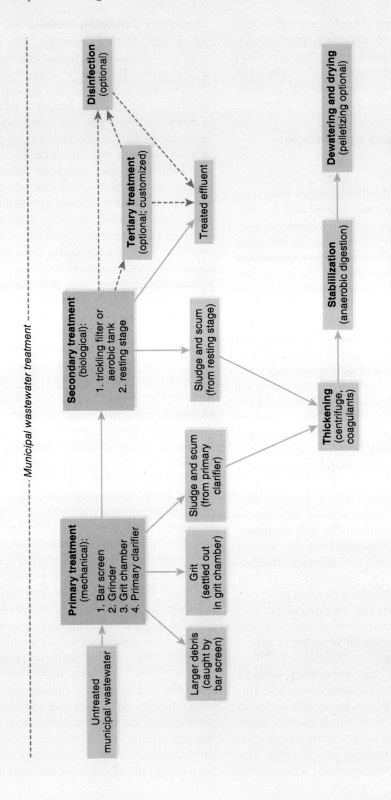

Figure 8.6 Steps in the treatment of municipal wastewater and sewage sludge.

Table 8.1 Objectives and Effects of Municipal Wastewater Treatment

Objectives	Effects of Steps in Municipal Wastewater Treatment			
	Basic Treatment Steps		Additional Optional Steps	
	Primary (mechanical)	Secondary (biological)	Tertiary Treatment	Disinfection
Remove pathogens	Most survive	Many die off	—	Is effective
Remove organic waste (BOD)	Some is removed	Most is removed	Depends on treatment	—
Remove suspended solids	Some are removed	Most are removed	Depends on treatment	—
Remove chemicals	—	—	Depends on treatment	—

in tertiary treatment that other components of the waste stream may be addressed.

As described earlier, some steps in the treatment of wastewater produce sludge as a byproduct. Therefore, the final step in sewage treatment is to treat this sludge (see Figure 8.6). Although "sludge" sounds solid, the sludge that results from sewage treatment is actually mostly water, and the first step in treatment is **thickening**, usually achieved either by centrifuging or by adding coagulants. The next step, **stabilization**, is the heart of sludge treatment. In this process, the sludge is digested by anaerobic organisms in a warm, well-circulated environment; such **sludge digesters** appear in **Figure 8.7**. This process reduces both the volume of sludge and its odor. Stabilization also kills many pathogens as a result of the anaerobic environment and the intense competition for food, but it is not designed to specifically rid sludge of all pathogens. Finally, the sludge is dewatered and dried; treated sludge is a soil-like material and it is sometimes formed into pellets (see **Figure 8.8**). The odor of treated sludge is variable, but often reflects the presence of compounds that contain sulfur or ammonia.

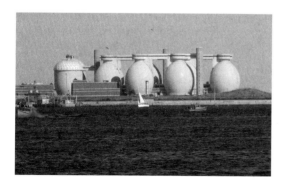

Figure 8.7 Pleasure boats and seabirds pass by the large egg-shaped sludge digesters of Greater Boston's Deer Island Sewage Treatment Plant.

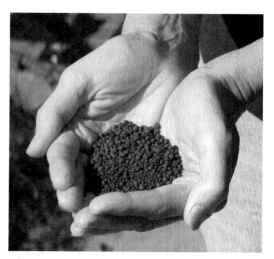

Figure 8.8 Treated sewage sludge, shown here in pellet form, is often used as a fertilizer.
Courtesy of Keith J. Maxwell

Land Application of Treated Sewage Sludge

In the United States, some treated sludge is handled as a waste product—landfilled or incinerated—and some is applied to agricultural land as a soil additive or fertilizer. It would be feasible to landfill all sewage sludge in the United States as it would amount to about 5% of the dry weight of the solid waste that is already being landfilled.[10] The idea of spreading treated sewage sludge on agricultural land may sound alarming, but many view this approach as beneficial. After all, it is an organic waste, rich in nutrients, and spreading it on land solves a big disposal problem. Unfortunately, treated sludge may be contaminated with pathogens and also with metals, including lead, as well as organic chemicals present in the original wastewater stream and concentrated in the residue of treatment.*

Although a potential exposure pathway clearly links sewage to treated sludge to crops or grazing animals consumed by people, it is difficult to quantify the human health risk of pathogens or chemicals in treated sewage sludge—and indeed, the risk is likely to be highly variable. Computer modeling has suggested that the risk of human infection from several common fecal pathogens is low.[11] On the other hand, field studies have drawn direct links between fecal pathogens (e.g., *Salmonella*) isolated from people and from treated sludge.[12] Antibiotic-resistant pathogens in treated sludge are spread in the environment (much as they are in CAFO wastes),

creating the opportunity to spread resistance through bacterial gene swapping.[12] An analysis in the United Kingdom of the bovine spongiform encephalopathy (BSE) risk to cattle grazing on land to which sewage sludge had been applied (evaluated because sewage could contain prions from slaughterhouse wastes) indicated that the risk of infection was too low to sustain BSE in the U.K. cattle herd;[12] even so, it serves as a reminder of the multiple connections among pathogens, wastes, and food.

Chemical analyses of sludge have documented the presence of dioxins,[13] flame retardants,[14] estrogenic breakdown products of alkyphenol ethoxylates found in detergents,[14] and pharmaceuticals.[15] The perfluorinated chemicals PFOS and PFOA, which are in wide use despite the limited understanding of their human toxicity, have also been identified in treated sewage sludge.[16] Unlike most persistent toxic pollutants, these chemicals are somewhat water-soluble, and if present in treated sludge, might be taken up by grass and then bioaccumulated in grazing animals.[16]

The Environmental Protection Agency (EPA) has estimated that as of 2019, almost 5 million dry metric tons of sewage sludge were being produced annually in the United States,[17] and 51% of treated sludge was being applied to land, not only in agriculture and horticulture but also in forests and on reclamation land. **Figure 8.9** provides the use and disposal pathways for biosolids in the United States in 2019.

Smaller-Scale Systems for Sewage Treatment

Although approximately two-thirds of the U.S. population is connected to a municipal wastewater treatment system, this arrangement is not necessary or cost-effective in areas of low population density. Instead, septic systems are widely used in rural areas. In addition, the composting toilet (described in detail in the context of infectious disease as an approach to sanitation in less-developed countries) has found a niche in some U.S. settings.

---

*In the early 1990s, the sewage industry coined a new term for treated sewage sludge, **biosolids**, to be used in marketing this product (Rampton S. Let them eat nutri-cake. *Harper's Magazine*, November 1998;48–49), and the term is now widely used. This term connotes a natural organic material while avoiding reference to either its sewage heritage or its nonsewage chemical constituents. Similarly, the land application of biosolids is sometimes referred to as a "beneficial reuse" of a waste product, although the benefits are accompanied by risks. This text uses the neutral descriptive terms *treated sewage sludge* (or *treated sludge*) and *land application*, asking the reader to bear in mind that municipal wastewater contains more than just sewage.

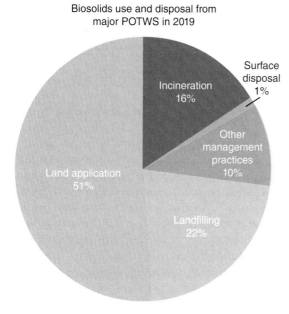

Biosolids use and disposal from
major POTWS in 2019

Surface
disposal
1%

Incineration
16%

Other
management
practices
10%

Land application
51%

Landfilling
22%

Figure 8.9 Biosolid disposal.

U.S. Environmental Protection Agency. Biosolids Use & Disposal from Major POTWS in 2019. Available at:
https://www.epa.gov/biosolids/basic-information-about-biosolids

Septic Systems and Constructed Wetlands

A **septic system** consists of a septic tank and a leach field. The **septic tank** is a buried steel or concrete vault that receives wastewater from a house (see **Figure 8.10**). This holding tank allows some material to float on the surface as scum, while other material sinks and accumulates as sludge on the floor, leaving a liquid layer in the middle. Fecal bacteria are present in all of these layers. The sludge that accumulates in the tank must be pumped out periodically and disposed of. Liquid from the middle layer flows out from the septic tank as it is displaced by water entering the tank. The system is passive, driven by gravity.

The effluent leaving the septic tank is distributed over a rather large area, called a **leach field** or **drainage field**, through a buried system of branching perforated pipes, also driven by gravity. Water trickles out through the perforations and then downward through the soil to the water table. In the process, pathogens carried along with the water are adsorbed onto soil particles or become mired in bacterial slime; they gradually die off due to temperature changes and lack of food.[18] These processes do not work well if the soil is wet. Therefore, the leach field must be located well above the local water table so that wastewater can drain properly. In an extreme situation, if the local water table rises high enough to intrude into the leach field, ponds of untreated wastewater can form on the surface. This poses an immediate health hazard as well as impeding the biological processes of the septic system.

In a variation on the typical septic system, an artificial wetland can be constructed between the septic tank and the leach field so that the effluent is much cleaner when it reaches the leach field. Such a **constructed wetland** is a man-made marsh designed to act as a wastewater treatment system. A constructed wetland consists of a lined

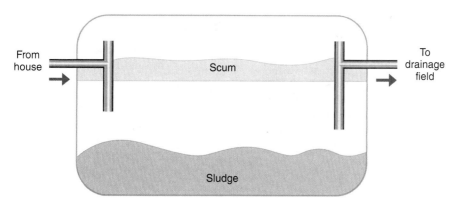

From
house

Scum

To
drainage
field

Sludge

Figure 8.10 Schematic drawing of a septic tank (not to scale).

basin and a layer of soil, sand, or gravel in which plants are rooted. In some constructed wetlands, the water level is above the soil surface, and water flow occurs mostly above ground; in others, the water level is below the soil surface, and water flow occurs mostly below ground.[19] In either case, the vegetation slows down the flow of water, allowing settling and filtering to occur. The plants also provide an environment in which microorganisms can thrive, and it is this microbial community that digests organic wastes. (This process is not unlike a traditional secondary sewage treatment, with its bed of slime-coated rocks.) The combined septic-system-plus-constructed-wetland approach can be employed not only for single homes but also for clusters of homes or apartment units.

Finally, in a variation on the constructed wetlands approach, an enclosed artificial ecosystem can be created for the purpose of decomposing toilet wastes. For example, Vermont has installed such a system at a rest stop on the Vermont Turnpike, where poor drainage had made it difficult to construct an effective septic system.[20] A specially designed greenhouse holds a dramatic array of plants (see **Figure 8.11**). Within this carefully constructed ecosystem, microorganisms digest organic wastes; the cleaned water is recycled to be used in the rest area's toilets.

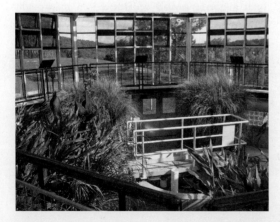

Figure 8.11 This artificial ecosystem, known as a Living Machine, treats toilet wastes at a rest stop on the Vermont Turnpike.

Courtesy of Keith J. Maxwell

The Composting Toilet

In recent decades, the most fundamental sewage management decision of the 19th century in the more developed countries—the decision to use potable water to carry sewage—has been challenged. This challenge rests on two points.[21] First, clean water is a valuable resource that should not be used to carry away urine and feces, especially in an era of increasing water scarcity. Second, human waste is itself a valuable resource, one that should not be mixed in the same waste stream with commercial and industrial discharges carrying metals and organic chemicals. Once these wastes have been mixed together in the municipal wastewater stream, the makeup of the end products—sewage sludge and treated wastewater—cannot be controlled or even predicted. Effective technologies for any *sustainable* approach to sanitation must rest on the understanding that both clean water and human excreta are valuable resources and should be kept separately.

In this spirit, composting toilets can also be useful in some settings in more developed countries, even if our overall dependence on the use of water to carry sewage is unlikely to change. In the United States, for example, continuous composting toilets such as the Clivus Multrum, although not common, are to be found in some "green" homes and even office buildings but more commonly in parks, camps, and other recreation areas.

Regulation of Municipal Wastewater Treatment in the United States

Under the Clean Water Act, the federal government sets standards for the quality of ambient water as well as the technological requirement to use secondary sewage treatment—that is, primary sewage treatment alone is considered inadequate. Municipalities discharging their wastes must meet permitting requirements (under the National Pollutant Discharge Elimination System), which include both effluent limitations and requirements to use specific control technologies, much as for industrial wastes. Standards for a facility are designed to maintain the quality of the receiving waters. The key effluent standards for treated sewage waste are for bacteriological quality (limiting the number of fecal coliform bacteria per volume of effluent) and biochemical oxygen demand, or BOD (limiting the burden of organic matter in the effluent). *Coliform bacteria* are a group of bacteria, widespread in the environment, living in water, soil, or the intestines of warm-blooded animals; the subgroup known as *fecal coliform bacteria* are those which enter the environment in the feces of warm-blooded animals. Although the federal government has ultimate enforcement authority, most of the regulatory activities to ensure that waterways are both *swimmable* and *fishable* are undertaken by the states. One specific strategy is the requirement for the states to identify and prioritize the permitted allocations to discharge for point and non-point contributions to waterways exceeding total daily maximum loads (TDML) thereby trying to reduce not only the total amount of pollution in a body of water but also its composition.

Under federal regulations, treated sludge that is to be applied to land must meet certain standards for pathogens and metals.[22] These regulations recognize the realities that some pathogens survive sludge treatment and that metals do not break down in the environment. There are also restrictions on the land application of treated sludge related to the timing of crop harvesting or animal grazing, for example, as well as requirements for recordkeeping and reporting. There are no restrictions regarding the various organic compounds present in sludge; in particular, the EPA announced in 2003 its decision to not regulate dioxin concentrations in sewage sludge applied to land and this is still true at present.[23]

8.3 Drinking Water: Public Systems and Private Wells

The EPA estimates that almost 55,000 community water systems serve some 264 million people in the United States[24]—about 90% of the U.S.

population. Most of the people relying on private water supplies live in rural areas and have their own wells, from which water is piped into their homes. However, U.S. Census data indicated that an estimated 0.5% to 1% of U.S. residences in 2007 did not have piped water.[25] For example, a lack of piped water is not uncommon in some Native American communities in Alaska and the southwestern states, or in the informal settlements along the border with Mexico, which are known as *colonias* and are made up mostly of illegal immigrants.[25]

Public Water Supplies

Community drinking water is of critical importance in public health due to the fact that it is a mechanism for delivering healthful water to a large number of people or, at times, for spreading a health hazard to the same group of people. Pathogens (protozoa, bacteria, and viruses) and chemical contaminants are of particular concern in this regard. Like wastewater treatments, technologies for the purification of drinking water have traditionally focused on the control of pathogens. The need to remove synthetic organic chemicals is a more recent development, and many communities are developing new and specialized treatments to manage chemical contaminants.

Many large cities rely on water from surface sources because cities require a large daily supply, as well as a surplus to get through dry periods without any interruption in supply. Both Boston and New York City, for example, rely on large reservoirs located in less-populated areas of their respective states. Chicago gets its water from Lake Michigan. Los Angeles draws water from rivers farther north in the state and also from the Colorado River, which forms the border between California and Arizona. The city also draws groundwater from beneath the Los Angeles basin.[26]

Smaller communities and rural areas often rely on groundwater sources. There is considerable variation in the treatment necessary to ensure that this source water is safe to drink. In particular, some groundwater sources may require little treatment (if land uses do not compromise water quality) because groundwater undergoes natural filtering as it moves through an aquifer. As noted elsewhere in the context of agriculture, the production of both crops and animals can increase nitrate concentrations in groundwater in rural areas; specialized treatments are required to remove nitrates from water.

This description of public drinking water supplies focuses mainly on treatments to prevent waterborne illness and reduce tooth decay, but it begins with the story of an early decision that continues to have widespread detrimental impacts on health.

Lead Pipe in Drinking Water Distribution Systems

Lead damages cognitive functioning, has broad neurological impacts, and is linked to both elevated blood pressure and mortality. Indeed, lead has been known for centuries to be neurotoxic and to cause poisoning at high exposures. Nevertheless, by the late 1800s, lead was used in public water service systems in most large U.S. cities, including, in 1900, New York, Chicago, Philadelphia, and Boston.[27] Some pipes were made completely of lead; others were made of iron lined with lead. Although lead was expensive, it was malleable and not prone to corrosion (and, therefore, had a long lifetime), and people's concerns about drinking water at the time were mainly focused on infectious disease.

Gradually, and over a long period, many lead water pipes have been replaced with copper or plastic pipe, but a 2018 assessment estimated that between 6.3 to 9.3 million homes are still served by lead service lines.[28] Under U.S. regulation, the 1991 Lead and Copper Rule set requirements for lead testing by community water systems and defined an action level of 0.015 mg/liter for lead, based on the 90th percentile of tap water samples. A concentration above the action level triggers requirements that may include monitoring, public education, actions to control corrosion, and replacement of pipe.[29] In 2018, following the concern with lead in Flint, Michigan's drinking water, a revision to the Lead Rule has been proposed, although it does not alter the specific action lead level. Rather, the proposed Lead Action Plan calls for a renewed EPA regulatory commitment to replacing lead service lines and provides funding opportunities to improve drinking water infrastructure specifically for small, disadvantaged communities. The new ruling also calls for voluntary testing of drinking water in schools and childcare centers.[28]

Basic Treatment of Drinking Water

Most of the common technologies to treat community drinking water are not new and share similarities to the processes described for treating municipal wastewater. A typical sequence of steps begins with allowing large particles to settle out by gravity. After this initial settling step, tiny particles of silt or clay remain suspended in the water. Such turbidity is of concern because the suspended particles can harbor pathogens and interfere with disinfection. Owing that the fineness of the particles and that they are negatively charged, they tend to repel one another and remain suspended in the water. The second treatment step, called **coagulation and flocculation**, is designed to overcome this problem. In this step, alum (aluminum sulfate) is added to the water, which is then mixed in; the alum neutralizes the particles' charge, allowing them to stick together when they collide, forming clumps known as **flocs**. A **sedimentation** step then allows the flocs to settle out by gravity. Both the initial settling step and the later sedimentation step create sludge, which must be disposed of. Often this sludge, which is mostly water, is simply discharged into a municipal sewer system. Alternatively, it can be dried and disposed of in a landfill.

After sedimentation has cleared the water of many fine suspended particles, the water is filtered. The usual technology is a **sand filter**: The water trickles gently through a bed of sand, driven only by gravity. At regular intervals, the sand filter is cleaned by backwashing from below, using clean water under pressure. Carbon filters may also be used. These steps are very effective in reducing the turbidity of the water and thereby removing many, though not all, pathogens.

Disinfection of Drinking Water

The final step in drinking water treatment is disinfection—that is, treatment with the specific objective of killing pathogens. In the United States, chlorination is the most common method used for drinking water disinfection. Chlorination is highly effective against bacteria but somewhat less effective against viruses and protozoa. In particular, the protozoan parasites *Giardia lamblia* and *Cryptosporidium parvum* are resistant to chlorine. These organisms can be removed by filtration or by disinfection using ozone.

When chlorination is used as the method of disinfection, residual chlorine is deliberately left in the water as it leaves the treatment plant. This is essential to maintain disinfection throughout the distribution system. Particularly in the aging infrastructures of older cities, water mains often have cracks that allow soil and groundwater to enter or rough patches where microbes can collect (see **Figure 8.12**).

Unfortunately, the residual chlorine is also available to combine with organic matter present in water that comes from surface sources—for example, from the decomposition of leaves that have fallen into an open reservoir. These reactions create organic compounds known as **disinfection byproducts (DBPs)**. The most common disinfection byproducts belong to a group of chemicals called **trihalomethanes (THMs)**. (The "*halo*" in *trihalomethane* indicates that these compounds contain a halogen, such as chlorine.) Chloroform (trichloromethane) is by far the most common of the trihalomethanes found in drinking water, as described in an earlier Case Study. Exposure to trihalomethanes in drinking water does not pose an acute health risk, but epidemiologic research has documented an association between chronic exposure and increased risk of bladder cancer.[30, 31] Studies of a possible association between maternal exposure to disinfection byproducts and low birthweight or preterm delivery have not shown a clear link.[32–36]

Some municipal water systems use chloramine (created by mixing chlorine and ammonia) rather than chlorine for residual disinfection. Chloramine is more stable in the distribution system than chlorine is, providing longer-lasting protection and creating fewer disinfection byproducts.[37] As noted earlier, treatment with ozone is another alternative to chlorination as a method of disinfection. Ozone is effective against protozoa and viruses and does not create chlorinated byproducts, but it has no residual disinfecting effect in the distribution system.

Fluoridation of Drinking Water

Exposure to fluoride at low concentrations in drinking water is well known to prevent tooth decay, a substantial public health benefit. Community **fluoridation** programs aim to achieve fluoride concentrations in drinking water of 0.7 to 1.2 mg/liter in locations with low natural fluoride levels.[38] However, fluoride sometimes occurs naturally in water at concentrations high enough to cause a disfiguring mottling of the teeth called **fluorosis**.

In 1986, the EPA set the enforceable standard (the Maximum Contaminant Level, or MCL) for fluoride in drinking water at 4 mg/liter, and the secondary, nonenforceable limit (the Secondary Maximum Contaminant Level, or SMCL) at 2 mg/liter. The secondary standard reflects concern about the cosmetic effects of fluorosis.

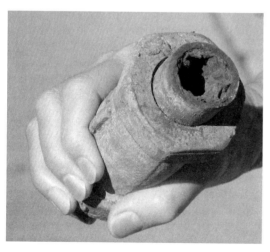

Figure 8.12 This 10-year-old water supply pipe has accumulated mineral deposits that make its internal surface rough.

Courtesy of Keith J. Maxwell

A 2006 assessment of the fluoride standard by the National Research Council recommended that the MCL of 4 mg/liter should be lowered for two reasons[39]: First, the 4 mg/liter standard does not protect against severe fluorosis, which is not just cosmetic but contributes to decay and infection; and second, long-term exposure to fluoride at 4 mg/liter may contribute to the risk of bone fracture. The National Research Council (NRC) also noted that the secondary standard of 2 mg/liter may not fully protect against the cosmetic effects of fluorosis.[39] As of 2020, the drinking water standards for fluoride remain as originally established.

Household-Level Water Supply or Treatment

Although the great majority of Americans now get their water from public supplies, some rely on private wells, mostly in rural areas. And whatever the source of their water, increasing numbers of Americans have installed water treatment devices in their homes in recent years. Finally, bottled water, once a rarity in the United States, has become an everyday consumer item. These alternatives (or supplements) to public water supplies are described here.

Private Wells

Water from private wells is not subject to federal drinking water standards, although some state and local governments set requirements for these sources.[40] In some geologic settings, naturally occurring radon or arsenic is a common contaminant in groundwater. Well water is vulnerable to contamination by activities on land located upgradient of the well, as well as by surface runoff. Because most private wells are located in rural or semirural areas, upgradient land uses often include private septic systems or agriculture. As a result, private wells may be at particular risk of contamination by human fecal waste, animal waste, pesticides, or nitrates from the use of fertilizers. Infants who consume water contaminated with nitrates may suffer methemoglobinemia. Chemical contamination of groundwater supplies may also occur if underground storage tanks located upgradient leak their contents, a common scenario associated with current or former gas stations. Although most groundwater supplies tend to be cleaner than surface supplies, once contamination occurs, it can be impossible to restore groundwater to safe drinking levels.

Devices for Home Water Treatment

Some people choose to install a device to treat drinking water at home. They may do so because their water supply is untreated, or because they are concerned about the quality of their water despite municipal treatment, or simply to improve the taste of their water. Most of these devices are known as **point-of-use treatment systems**; that is, they are installed at a single tap, such as the faucet at the kitchen sink. Many of these devices use carbon filters to remove contaminants; other more complex systems use reverse osmosis or distillation.

Bottled Water

Some consumers prefer the taste of bottled water. During the 1990s and early 2000s, the consumption of commercially bottled water increased dramatically.[41] If the bottled water is labelled as *spring water*, it likely came from a groundwater source, is unlikely to be fluoridated,[42] and is not regulated by the EPA as drinking water, but rather by the U.S. Food and Drug Administration (FDA) as a packaged food. Taste is, of course, a matter of personal preference, but it is not surprising that there should be differences in taste with spring water, given that the taste of any water is affected by its mineral content and by the method of disinfection used to purify the water. The mineral content of bottled water varies with its source, and groundwater is likely to start with higher mineral content than surface waters.[42] Producers of some bottled waters also add minerals for the specific purpose of flavoring the water. Bottled water is also more often disinfected using ozonation or ultraviolet light,[42] compared with chlorination, given that no residual disinfection effect is needed after bottling.

However, more than 60% of bottled water actually comes from municipal drinking water supplies (and, therefore, does meet federal drinking water standards).[43] Whether consumers prefer spring water or just the convenience of regular water, either type is much more expensive per gallon than the price paid for getting water straight from the tap. Sales of water bottled in plastic increased dramatically in the 1990s, but sales have declined since 2010 partially due to concerns with Bisphenyl A exposure and also as awareness grows about the planetary impact of plastic pollution (refer to the Case Study later in this chapter).

Regulation of Drinking Water in the United States

The Safe Drinking Water Act (SDWA) was originally passed in 1974 and substantially amended in 1986 and 1996. It requires the EPA to promulgate national standards (the National Primary Drinking Water Regulations, or NPDWR) for contaminants in public drinking water that are likely to pose a health risk and to be present in waters used to supply drinking water. The EPA is also required to identify, on a regular basis, contaminants that are candidates for future regulation, as discussed in an earlier chapter in the context of emerging concerns with perfluorinated chemicals.

The EPA sets two standards: a Maximum Contaminant Level Goal (MCLG), an unenforceable goal that marks a level where no health effects are anticipated; and a **Maximum Contaminant Level (MCL)**, a standard that must be met. The EPA is to set the MCL as close to the MCLG as is feasible given technological options and costs. The EPA is required to conduct a health risk assessment (using approaches like those described earlier in the context of the science and methods of environmental health) in support of a new MCL and also to estimate its benefits and costs. The EPA can impose fines on public water systems failing to comply with the standards.

Federal MCLs have been set for three types of disinfectants, four types of disinfection byproducts, four categories of radionuclides, eight microorganisms, turbidity, sixteen inorganic chemicals, and more than 50 organic chemical contaminants. The EPA may also set a nonenforceable secondary MCL (SMCL); this is a recommended guideline that individual states may choose to adopt as a standard. An SMCL addresses a contaminant's effect on the taste or odor of water, or its cosmetic effects in those who drink the water (such as discoloration of the teeth from excessive naturally occurring fluoride).

The EPA has set enforceable standards for a small number of specific pathogens, including *Cryptosporidium*, *G. lamblia*, and coliform bacteria.[44] In each case, the MCLG is zero, and the MCL is a requirement for a specific testing regimen and test results. The MCL for coliform bacteria, for example, requires regular sampling for total coliforms; if a threshold for positive results is exceeded, the standard calls for testing for fecal coliform bacteria or for *Escherichia coli* specifically. However, most fecal coliform bacteria are not pathogenic. Nonetheless, any substantial presence of fecal coliforms in drinking water indicates recent sewage contamination and hence the potential presence of fecal pathogens. It is impractical to monitor most fecal pathogens directly, because there are many different ones (including protozoa and viruses as well as noncoliform bacteria), and individually most of them are uncommon. However, because none of these pathogens occurs in the absence of fecal contamination, fecal coliform bacteria serve as *indicator organisms* for sewage contamination and thus for the potential presence of pathogens.

The scope of the Safe Drinking Water Act is much broader than standards for contaminants in water. As amended, it includes provisions for watershed protection at the source of the water and bans the installation of lead pipe and the use of lead solder in public water distribution systems. The law calls for regular monitoring of public drinking water for contaminants, including some not regulated under the law, and requires that information on drinking water quality be provided to the public on a regular basis.

8.4 Solid Waste and Its Management

The amount of ordinary trash generated each year in the United States has increased steadily for decades; in 2017, it stood at 268 million tons, more than double what it was in 1970 (121 million tons).[45] On the other hand, per capita generation appears to be leveling off, hovering between four and five pounds per person per day since 1990.[45] These quantities include trash from businesses—from restaurants to insurance companies—to which everyone contributes indirectly. Including these indirect contributions, the average adult generates his or her weight in trash about every six to eight weeks.

The most common materials in the municipal solid waste stream are paper and plastic products, which together make up approximately 40% of what we throw away (see **Figure 8.13**). Organic wastes (food, yard trimmings, and wood

products) make up roughly another one-third of the total. Looked at another way (not shown in figure), about one-third by weight was made up of containers and other packaging.[46] Perhaps the most dramatic evidence of the scale of global trash production is the very large quantities of floating trash in the world's oceans. For example, an enormous mass, largely made up of plastic items, drifts in the center of the North Pacific, corralled by the circular surface current of the region (described earlier in the context of the global fate and transport of environmental contaminants).

Trash, for all of its homely familiarity, is not easy to manage at the municipal level. For one thing, trash is generated by many individual households across every city and town, so that simply designing routes and schedules for trash trucks is a logistical challenge. In addition, the content of trash is varied; it contains everything from pencils to refrigerators and may sometimes contain hazardous items such as drain cleaners or mothballs. But trash always includes food waste, and this means that it must be removed on a strict schedule: when trash cans overflow, odor quickly becomes a problem, as do rats and other pests. Strikes by trash collectors—for example, in New York in 1981 and in Naples in 2008—provided vivid images of city life without this service. In the bigger picture, most trash is now disposed of in large regional facilities rather than local dumps. However, most towns are not enthusiastic about hosting such a large facility. As a result of such "not-in-my-back-yard" opposition,* it is increasingly difficult to find a final resting place for trash.

There are four basic approaches to managing trash:

- Not generating it in the first place (known as source reduction or waste prevention)
- Recycling, including the composting of organic wastes
- Incineration
- Placement in a landfill

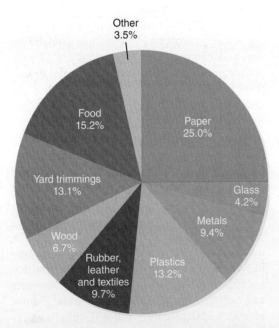

Figure 8.13 Makeup of municipal solid waste by material, 2017.

U.S. Environmental Protection Agency. Advancing Sustainable Materials Management: 2017 Fact Sheet Assessing Trends in Material Generation, Recycling, Composting, Combustion with Energy Recovery and Landfilling in the United States November 2019 pdf Available at: https://www.epa.gov/sites/production/files/2019-11/documents/2017_facts_and_figures_fact_sheet_final.pdf

*There is now another variation on the "not-in-my-back-yard" or NIMBY attitude toward landfills or any type of waste disposal facility; "build-absolutely-nothing-anywhere-near-anyone" or BANANA.

Clearly, it is desirable to reduce the amount of waste we produce and to recycle as much as possible of the waste that we do produce. Unfortunately, only about 25% of the U.S. municipal solid waste stream in 2017 was recycled, with 65% of these recycled materials consisting of paper products.[45] Another 10% was composted, a variation on recycling, with 90% of the composted material consisting of yard trimmings. Almost 13% of municipal solid waste in the United States in 2017 was burned in waste-to-energy incinerators and about slightly more than half was disposed of in landfills.[45]

This section first takes up the four major options for managing municipal solid waste: waste prevention; recycling and composting; incineration, usually with the production of usable energy and referred to as **waste-to-energy (WTE) incineration**; and landfilling. Next, the section briefly describes the handling of two special types of community wastes: hazardous items in household trash, including electronics; and medical wastes, which may include infectious items. The section concludes with a brief description of the U.S. regulatory framework for managing municipal solid waste.

Preventing Waste

Waste prevention (also called source reduction) is difficult to quantify, and is the result of many corporate and individual decisions. Products can be designed to contain less material, to have a longer useful life, or to be repairable rather than disposable, countering a decades-long trend toward more disposable items. Packaging, the major contributor to plastic waste, can be reduced, and reusable glass bottles can be substituted for plastic containers.

At the consumer level, the EPA encourages such practices as double-sided copying, buying in bulk to avoid using single-use containers, and the use of washable plates, silverware, and towels rather than disposable ones. The agency also notes the tradition of reusing both durable and nondurable goods (such as appliances, furniture, or clothing), whether by passing them on informally to friends and family or through donations to charity, as a practice that reduces waste.[6] Thus, much of what is now called consumer-level source reduction has a common-sense ring to it, and in fact was common practice 50 or 75 years ago.

Recycling

Recycling of municipal solid waste removes from the waste stream items made of recyclable materials, such as glass, metal, plastic, and paper, before the wastes are disposed of. A 2015-2016 assessment of over 2,500 communities determined that 94% provided access to recycling.[47] Seventy-three percent of households had access to curb-side recycling, although one-fifth of these homes had to subscribe and opt-in for an additional fee for the curb-side service. Curb-side recycling either requires that households sort into separate recycling containers, called multi-stream recycling, or with single-stream recycling, all household recyclable materials go into the same container to be processed at **materials recovery facilities**, where items are sorted using varying degrees of automation. For example, a series of tumblers perforated with larger and larger holes can be used to sort objects by size; a water bath can separate materials that float (such as wood or plastic) from those that sink (such as metals); and magnets can be used to separate out ferrous metals.

Regional differences in the availability of curb-side recycling are striking and show urban compared to rural variation. Curbside recycling reached a substantially higher percentage of people in the more populous Northeast and West (79% and 67%, respectively) than in the Midwest (43%) or South (23%).[6] This pattern probably partly reflects greater urbanization in the Northeast and West: Although recycling can be challenging in locations of extremely high population density, it is very costly where population density is low. Households without curbside use drop-off recycling programs that either allow for one-stop recycling, typically also affiliated with trash disposal, or must travel to various recycling venues for different types of materials.

Plastic Pollution

The science may still be unclear regarding the true extent of human health risks associated with our reliance on plastic, but the impacts on our environment have become very obvious. The majority of waste found in giant marine garbage patches and along our litter-lined coasts and roadways is composed of plastics. And plastic waste comes in various sizes, from microbeads that pose digestive risks to fish, to six-pack rings and grocery store bags posing entanglement risks to larger marine species, to the *mega-sized* plastic debris associated primarily with fishing and packaging wastes that makes up more than half of those ocean garbage patches.[1] And, unfortunately, there will be plenty of time to research the extent of human health hazards associated with plastic pollution exposure since it will take decades (for toiletry sachets and plastic bags) or centuries (for six-pack rings and plastic bottles) to decompose in our environment.

Although there are some types of plastic that cannot be easily recycled, such as polystyrene food takeout containers and polyvinyl chloride (PVC) pipes, much of the plastic generated yearly by Americans can be recycled and repurposed. However, it must be clean and the lid and other packaging material needs to be removed, even if it is also made from a different type of plastic. Americans are not very good at preparing their plastic waste properly.[2] Among those households that dutifully sort their recyclables curbside, less than 20% of the plastic arrives at the recycling center uncontaminated and in any condition to be recycled. Eighty percent of plastic collected at municipal recycling centers ends up actually being landfilled or incinerated. Much of the plastic recycling collected in the United States was shipped to China until 2016 when they banned U.S. plastics because it was still too contaminated to be economically profitable for China to recycle. Considering some of the dubious disposal practices in China and other Asian nations, it came as quite a shock that American plastic was just not worth it.[2]

Now the future of plastic recycling in the United States needs to be addressed more domestically. Manufacturers need to reduce the total amounts of plastic generated, particularly in packaging materials. Research is underway to discover plastic alternatives or at least more biodegradable plastic materials. Federal and state governments need to subsidize the development of homegrown recycling business infrastructure, including the promotion of green repurposing industries.[3] Finally, Americans need to be educated regarding their cavalier attitude toward all waste disposal, particularly plastics. And remarkably for those who diligently recycle, it is actually better to throw something in the regular trash when in doubt, rather than risk contaminating an entire batch destined to (*hopefully*) be recycled. Developing "pay as you throw away" systems with incentives to reduce and recycle, and fines for polluting, along with public education about the fate of their trash will help ensure a reduced pollution, more sustainable and healthier future.[4]

1. Lebreton, L., Slat, B., Ferrari, F., Sainte-Rose, B., Aitken, J., Marthouse, R., Hajbane, S., Cunsolo, S., Schwarz, A., Levivier, A., Noble, K., Debeljak, P., Maral1, H., Schoeneich-Argent, R., Brambini, R. & Reisser, J. (2018). Evidence that the Great Pacific garbage patch is rapidly accumulating plastic. *Scientific Reports*, 8 (4666), 1-15. https://www.nature.com/articles/s41598-018-22939-w

2. Cho, R. (2020, March 13). Recycling in the U.S. Is broken. How do we fix it? *State of the Planet: Earth Institute*, Columbia University. Retrieved July 25, 2020 from: https://blogs.ei.columbia.edu/2020/03/13/fix-recycling-america/

3. Ritchie, H., (2018, September 2). FAQs on Plastics. *Our World in Data*. Retrieved August 3, 2020 from https://ourworldindata.org/faq-on-plastics#how-long-does-it-take-plastics-to-break-down

4. Rysavy, T.F. (n.d.). Americans are really bad at recycling. But only because we're not trying very hard *Green American Magazine*. Retrieved August 3, 2020 from https://www.greenamerica.org/rethinking-recycling/americans-are-really-bad-recycling-only-because-were-not-trying-very-hard

Composting

A range of organic materials can also be removed from the solid waste stream for **composting**. In many communities, municipal composting is limited to yard trimmings, separated by the consumer before placing trash at the curb.[6] However, as municipalities have seen their costs to dispose of trash soar and encountered resistance to landfilling and incineration, support for community composting has increased from negligible levels thirty years ago.[45] Several major municipalities, such as those in the San Francisco Bay Area, Los Angeles, and Seattle, have incorporated composting into their municipal waste management systems with the stated goal of achieving *zero waste*.[48] Households and businesses sort outgoing trash into food (or organic) wastes, recyclables, and landfill containers. Several strategies, such as tiered waste removal fees and public education, are used to support the composting (and recycling) efforts.

From the municipal point of view, backyard composting by individuals is considered waste prevention rather than recycling, because it prevents waste from entering the municipal waste stream. People with enough yard space can use a composting bin or start a composting pile outdoors. By mixing fresh materials (such as grass clippings and fruit or vegetable scraps) with dry materials (such as dead leaves or twigs) and keeping the mixture damp, the home composter creates conditions in which organic materials slowly decay into compost that can be used as fertilizer and soil conditioner. Even indoors, composting of plant-based food scraps can be done on a small scale using worms. This approach, called **vermicomposting**, uses worms (specifically, redworms) housed in a bin. The worms consume the food scraps and produce castings (worm excrement) that can be used as potting soil.[49]

Waste-to-Energy Incineration

Waste-to-energy (WTE) incineration serves the dual purpose of disposing of municipal solid waste and generating energy, either in the form of electricity or as steam to be used in an industrial process. Energy produced by a municipal solid waste incinerator reduces the demand for energy from traditional sources, such as fossil or nuclear fuels. In addition, when trash is reduced to ash by burning, its volume is decreased by 80% to 90%. This fact makes trash incinerators attractive in principle—but incineration is not a benign technology.

Certain components of trash produce hazardous emissions when burned. This means that either some materials must be removed from the waste stream before burning or the incinerator must be designed to manage the hazards. Metals, mostly as particulates (but in the case of mercury, vapors), must be captured by devices in the smokestack. And burning plastics causes the emission of dioxins and furans unless a very high temperature is maintained in the incinerator. The incineration of trash also poses practical challenges. A trash incinerator is expensive to start up or shut down and; therefore, it requires a steady flow of trash as well as a steady market for the energy it produces.

Incinerators produce two kinds of ash: **fly ash**, captured by pollution control equipment in the smokestack, and **bottom ash**, which remains on the floor of the furnace. Fly ash is produced in smaller quantities but is more toxic. Under federal law, both types of ash must be tested and then either disposed of as hazardous waste or landfilled as municipal solid waste. According to the EPA, between 1990 and 2005, incinerator emissions of dioxins were reduced by more than 99%, emissions of mercury by 93%, and emissions of lead by 95%.[50]

As regulatory controls on incinerator emissions have been tightened, many have shut down, and the majority of today's incinerators are large operations. Of the 66 large WTE facilities still in operation in the United States, almost half (32) are in the Northeast Corridor (from Washington, D.C., through New York and New England), half a dozen are in Florida, and a few are clustered in the Upper Midwest.[50] In 2017, slightly less than 13% of all U.S. waste was incinerated, equal to 34 million tons.[45] The locations where incinerators do exist within municipalities have also raised alarm from environmental justice advocates since many are located in more disadvantaged communities.

Disposal in Landfills

Up through the 1970s, most municipal solid waste in the United States was put in a town dump. As the name suggests, this was simply a location where any type of trash could be dumped on the ground. Some dumps were located in gullies, so that trash could be dumped from above, or in wet locations, which were undesirable for building. Not surprisingly, dumps were food sources that attracted various wild animals, from rats to bears, as well as insect pests. Sometimes, the trash at town dumps was burned to reduce its volume and make it less attractive to pests. Many town dumps were located near a town boundary so as to offend as few local voters as possible.

However, one important environmental impact of the dump—its contamination of groundwater—is largely invisible. As described elsewhere, rainwater seeping through waste leaches out (that is, extracts) some constituents from the wastes. The water carrying these dissolved or suspended substances, now called leachate, trickles downward below the surface of the soil until it reaches the water table and then slowly spreads into the groundwater. Over time,

as domestic trash came to include more chemical products, the problem of groundwater contamination took on a new importance.

Today's **municipal solid waste landfill** is very different from the town dump. It is a licensed facility, usually operated by a corporation. It holds a very large volume of waste and is engineered specifically to prevent rainwater from leaching contaminants into groundwater. About the only feature it has in common with the town dump is that it accepts unsorted municipal solid waste.

A solid waste landfill (see **Figure 8.14**) begins as a depression dug into the ground surface, and as the landfill fills up, it rises above the surface around it. Basic design features guard against groundwater contamination. The pit is double-lined, usually with plastic and clay liners, to prevent leachate from reaching the ground beneath the facility. Next to the liner is a network of pipes that collect leachate, which is pumped

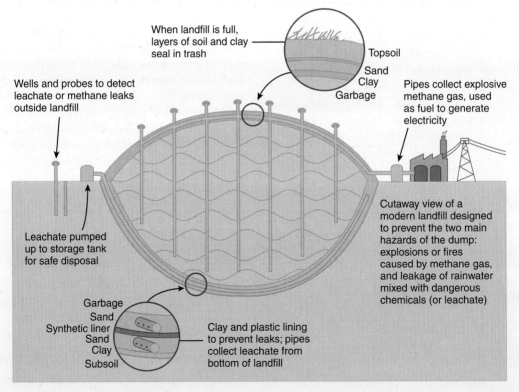

When landfill is full, layers of soil and clay seal in trash

Topsoil
Sand
Clay
Garbage

Wells and probes to detect leachate or methane leaks outside landfill

Pipes collect explosive methane gas, used as fuel to generate electricity

Leachate pumped up to storage tank for safe disposal

Cutaway view of a modern landfill designed to prevent the two main hazards of the dump: explosions or fires caused by methane gas, and leakage of rainwater mixed with dangerous chemicals (or leachate)

Garbage
Sand
Synthetic liner
Sand
Clay
Subsoil

Clay and plastic lining to prevent leaks; pipes collect leachate from bottom of landfill

Figure 8.14 A schematic cross-section of a modern municipal solid waste landfill.

U.S. Environmental Protection Agency, Resource Conservation and Recovery Act (RCRA). Available at: www.epa.gov/superfund/students/clas_act/haz-ed/ff_06.htm. Accessed December 13, 2007 to the surface, where it may be reintroduced into the landfill or removed for disposal elsewhere. As trash arrives at the operating landfill, heavy machinery is used to compact the waste in layers several feet deep, with a layer of soil between layers of waste. The finished landfill is capped with clay, to prevent rainwater from entering. After a landfill is closed and capped, it must be monitored and maintained. However, the surface area can be used for purposes that do not involve construction, such as a public park.

The modern landfill creates one new hazard. Open dumping allowed aerobic decomposition of waste, whereas the environment within a modern landfill is largely anaerobic (or becomes anaerobic over time). Bacteria able to decompose organic wastes in an anaerobic setting produce methane, an explosive gas. To keep methane from building up inside a landfill, pipes inserted throughout the landfill collect the gas, which can either be safely vented into the environment or collected and used as fuel in industry.

As described elsewhere in the context of global climate change, methane is a potent greenhouse gas. On a global scale, it has proved difficult to establish the relative importance of various sources of this gas, given wide regional variation. Landfill emissions accounted for an estimated 15% of U.S. methane emissions in 2017.[51]

Modern landfills meeting federal specifications are expensive to build, and because they are large they can be difficult to site in densely populated areas. However, trash is so bulky that it is not usually economical to transport it over long distances. Like waste incinerators, landfills are becoming fewer and larger—there were 6,326 municipal solid waste landfills in 1990, but only 1,654 in 2005.[52] In contrast to waste incinerators, these landfills are underrepresented in the most densely populated northeastern section of the country, which hosts only 133 such facilities.

With the advent of brominated flame retardants and perfluorinated compounds in consumer products, these hazardous chemicals will increasingly make their way into municipal landfills as products are discarded. Given the persistence of these chemicals, there is some concern that they will outlast the integrity of engineered landfills, resulting in releases to the broader environment over the long term as landfill liners degrade.[53]

Handling of Household Hazardous Wastes

As described earlier in the context of manufacturing pollution, industrial wastes are classified as hazardous under federal law if they are corrosive, toxic, ignitable, or reactive. Using the same criteria, some ingredients of household products are hazardous, and products containing such ingredients are classified as **household hazardous wastes**. Most are common products, such as oven cleaners, drain cleaners, and toilet cleaners; antifreeze and transmission fluid; weed killers, cockroach sprays, mothballs, and rat poison; propane tanks and lighter fluid; paint strippers and photographic chemicals; mercury thermometers and compact fluorescent light bulbs; and ordinary batteries.[54]

Discarded computers pose a special problem. Ideally, they would be reused or recycled, but the U.S. market for outdated computers is very limited, and because computers have many parts, some of which contain toxic materials, they cannot simply be recycled like glass or plastic items. Many end up in landfills. Some communities have special programs to collect computers for recycling, but the actual work of recycling often takes place in a less-developed country, as described elsewhere in the context of disparities in hazards to workers. When the contribution from other electronics is included, eWaste represents the fastest growing domestic waste stream in the United States.[55]

Federal law does not restrict the disposal of household hazardous wastes in municipal trash—consumers are not required to separate hazardous items, and municipalities are not required to provide special handling. However, many communities do maintain sites where household hazardous wastes can be turned in, or hold special collection days for these wastes, and such opportunities make it easier for people to dispose of hazardous items properly (see **Figure 8.15**).

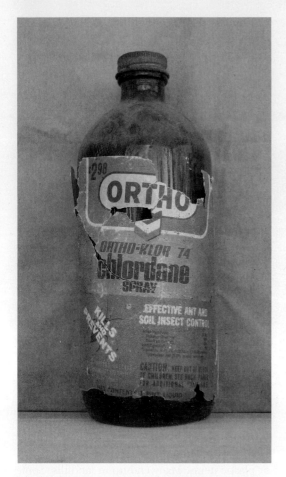

Figure 8.15 This bottle of liquid chlordane, which sat in a garage for 20 years after the sale of the pesticide was prohibited in the United States, was turned in at a municipal collection day for household hazardous wastes.

In the United States, 1.6 million tons of household hazardous waste are generated each year.[54] Like trash more generally, this is a waste stream that can be reduced substantially through individual decisions and actions as more people become aware of these hazards (refer to **Table 8.2**).

Medical Waste

Medical waste, produced by healthcare facilities, includes ordinary trash as well as items that are infectious, hazardous, or radioactive. This waste stream typically contains surgically removed organs or limbs, bandages, gloves, and discarded "sharps," among other items. Under federal law, healthcare facilities are defined broadly to include veterinary hospitals, blood banks, and research laboratories; in some locations, there is also state or local regulation. One particularly influential federal action was to set emissions requirements for all medical waste incinerators built after 1996; these requirements create pressure to develop new approaches to medical waste disposal. Currently, less than 10% of all medical waste is incinerated.[45]

Regulation of Municipal Solid Waste in the United States

The major law governing the handling of municipal solid waste is the Resource Conservation and Recovery Act (RCRA), discussed in Chapter 3. As its name suggests, its goals not only include ensuring that disposal facilities are adequate but also encourages source reduction, recycling, and recovering energy from wastes. Open trash dumping is no longer legal; regulations under RCRA set requirements for municipal landfill features inclusion of liners, leachate collection, and ground-water monitoring. Emissions from trash incinerators must meet emissions limits under the Clean Air Act.

The leading drawback is that RCRA does not directly apply to household waste generation (*the source*), but rather only indirectly as far as affecting how municipalities may manage these waste streams from their residents. Regional governments influence disposal behaviors by how they structure and charge for trash pick-up services. In addition, the use of incentives, such as nickel deposits on aluminum cans, or the leveling of fines for improper disposal or preparation of trash for pick-up, have also been shown to be effective (refer to **Figure 8.16** regarding U.S. recycling rates). Also, municipalities typically have strong educational campaigns to enlist public support and advocacy to "not trash" their own community.

Table 8.2 Alternatives to Using Hazardous Household Products

Instead of	Substitute
Drain Cleaner	Use a plunger or plumber's snake
Glass Cleaner	Mix one tablespoon of vinegar or lemon juice in one quart of water; spray on and use newspaper to dry.
Furniture Polish	Mix one teaspoon of lemon juice in a pint of mineral or vegetable oil and wipe furniture.
Rug Deodorizer	Use baking soda instead
Silver Polish	Boil two to three inches of water in shallow pan with one teaspoon salt, one teaspoon baking soda, and a sheet of aluminum foil. Submerge silver completely and boil for a few minutes. Wipe away tarnish when cooled.
Mothballs	Use cedar chips, lavender flowers, rosemary, or white peppercorns.

Data from U.S. Environmental Protection Agency. *Hazardous Waste Source Reduction Around the Home.* Retrieved July 30, 2020 from: https://www.epa.gov/hw/household-hazardous-waste-hhw.

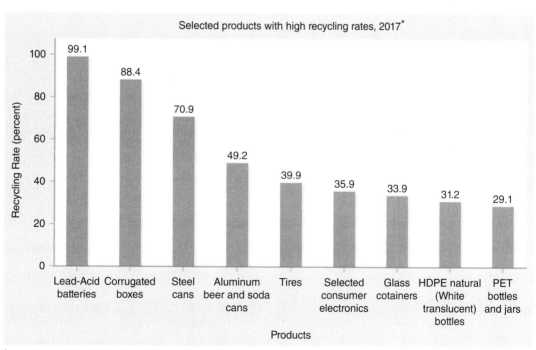

Selected products with high recycling rates, 2017[*]

*Does not include combustion with energy recovery

Figure 8.16 U.S. Recycling rates

Advancing Sustainable Materials Management: 2017 Fact Sheet Assessing Trends in Material Generation, Recycling, Composting, Combustion with Energy Recovery and Landfilling in the United States, November 2019 produced by USEPA

8.5 Urban Settings in Less-Developed Countries

The world's population of almost 7.5 billion people became more than half urban in 2010, and two-thirds of the global population is expected to live in urban settings by 2050.[56] Thus the challenges of managing the urban metabolism—the disposal of toilet waste and trash, and the provision of safe drinking water—are of critical importance worldwide and are especially urgent in less-developed countries. These challenges are amplified by the fact that the world's cities are becoming ever larger; in 2018, some 33 of the world's cities were designated as **megacities**, having at least 10 million inhabitants. **Table 8.3** presents the top 20 largest

Table 8.3 Top 20 Largest Cities in 2000 and 2020

Rank in 2000	Name	Population (millions)	Rank in 2020	Name	Population (millions)
1	Mexico City, Mexico	26.3	1	Tokyo, Japan	37.28
2	Sao Paulo, Brazil	24	2	Mumbai (Bombay), India	25.97
3	Tokyo, Japan	17.1	3	Delhi, India	25.83
4	Calcutta, India	16.6	4	Dhaka, Bangladesh	22.04
5	Mumbai (Bombay), India	16	5	Mexico City, Mexico	21.81
6	New York City, USA	15.5	6	São Paulo, Brazil	21.57
7	Seoul, Republic of Korea	13.5	7	Lagos, Nigeria	21.51
8	Shanghai, China	13.5	8	Jakarta, Indonesia	20.77
9	Rio de Janeiro, Brazil	13.3	9	New York City, USA	20.43
10	Delhi, India	13.3	10	Karachi, Pakistan	18.94
11	Buenos Aires, Argentina	13.2	11	Calcutta, India	18.54
12	Cairo, Egypt	13.2	12	Buenos Aires, Argentina	15.48
13	Jakarta, Indonesia	12.8	13	Cairo, Egypt	14.02
14	Bagdad, Iraq	12.8	14	Manila, Philippines	13.4
15	Teheran, Iran	12.7	15	Los Angeles, USA	13.25
16	Karachi, Pakistan	12.2	16	Rio de Janeiro, Brazil	13.23
17	Istanbul, Turkey	11.9	17	Istanbul, Turkey	12.76
18	Los Angeles, USA	11.2	18	Shanghai, China	12.63
19	Dacca, Bangladesh	11.2	19	Moscow, Russia	11.73
20	Manila, Philippines	11.1	20	Osaka, Japan	11.53

Data from United Nations Department of International and Social Affairs, Estimates and Projections of Urban, Rural and City Populations. 1950-2025: The 1982 Assessment, (New York: United Nations, 1985). p.147 Defense Mapping Agency Hydrographic Topographic Center, World Per Index (10th Edition), 1986 Publication No. 150 Website: https://meteor.geol.iastate.edu/gccourse/issues/pop/cities.html For 2020: Retrieved from 8/4/2020 from https://www.macrotrends.net/cities/largest-cities-by-population

cities in 2000 compared with 2020, and indicates that much of the increase in urbanization is occurring in less-developed countries. As a general rule, urban areas are characterized by sharp socioeconomic disparities within their boundaries, including access to fundamental basic resources.

Rapid urbanization has overwhelmed the capacities of many of these urban governments in low to middle income countries. The World Health Organization (WHO) estimates that about a billion people worldwide live in urban slums.[57] Life in the urban slums of less-developed countries is characterized by extremes of poverty, overcrowding, and lack of sanitation and clean water (see **Figure 8.17**).[57] Ambient air pollution, lead exposure from industry and the relatively recent use of leaded gasoline, toxic wastes, traffic accidents, violence, and fires are also common hazards of these settings.[57]

Many who live in these urban slums are cut off from opportunities for employment, health services, or education,[58] as well as basic municipal services. In Jakarta, for example, less than 60% of the population has access to piped water at communal taps, and water from this source must be boiled before it can be drunk safely.[59] In many cities in less developed countries, street vendors sell water or other drinks, and often expect their consumers to return the container (see **Figure 8.18**). Because sewage and trash are largely uncontrolled,[59] many people live surrounded by wastes. Many families, and often the children, try to earn money from scavenging among these trash piles

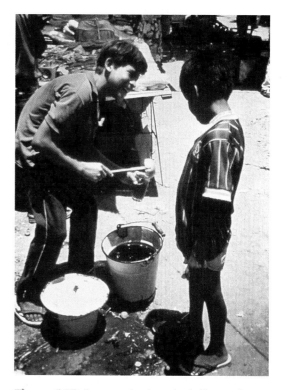

Figure 8.18 A young street vendor in Peru sells a homemade corn drink, using a dipper and a single glass.

Courtesy of CDC Public Health Image Library. ID# 5319. Content provider: CDC. Available at: http://phil.cdc .gov/phil/home.asp. Accessed October 30, 2012.

for anything still of value—a risky activity mentioned previously in the context of eWaste. All of the conditions of these urban slums—crowding, trash, the lack of clean drinking water, and standing water resulting from a lack of wastewater management—are conducive to the transmission of infectious diseases, including diseases of closeness or contact, diseases of fecal origin, and vectorborne illnesses.

8.6 The Built Environment

The cities and suburbs of the more-developed countries today, although not without infrastructure problems, have generally adequate systems for maintaining the "urban metabolism"—provision of drinking water, removal and treatment

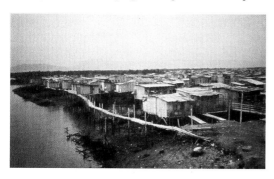

Figure 8.17 Slum dwellings in an Ecuadoran city perch over sewage-contaminated water.

Courtesy of CDC Public Health Image Library. ID# 5323. Content provider: CDC. Available at: http://phil.cdc .gov/phil/home.asp. Accessed October 30, 2012

Suburban Sprawl

Other public health concerns of the built environment stem from the expansive suburban and exurban development that has come to be known simply as **sprawl**. Suburban sprawl in the United States is marked by low-intensity construction (compared with urban settings) and by the separation of land uses in distinct locations compared with the now old-fashioned idea of a multipurpose town square. In these planned communities, housing (in subdivisions, as in **Figure 8.19**), stores (in malls), offices or industry (in office parks or industrial parks), and civic institutions such as high schools (on campuses) are built on large tracts of land designated for one use through zoning laws.[1]

Another hallmark of sprawl is the necessity for a car in daily life—simply to navigate among life's basic functions—and the resulting extensive road systems and heavy traffic.[1] All this driving, of course, contributes to air pollution on a regional scale and, along with the preponderance of single-family housing, increases per capita energy consumption in the suburbs. In contrast, traditional urban neighborhoods were not planned, but rather grew incrementally. In this setting, different land uses are interspersed, and many basic needs can be met by walking or using public transportation. A city is fundamentally a collection of such neighborhoods.

Part of the allure of the suburbs has been that they seem to offer an escape from an unhealthful urban setting characterized by crowding and pollution. But suburban life brings its own risks. Many suburban roadways carry a high volume of traffic, moving at high speed, yet with cars constantly entering traffic or turning off the road; miles driven per capita are also high. In fact, traffic fatality rates are higher in sprawled areas than in denser urban development—for pedestrians specifically, and also for all traffic

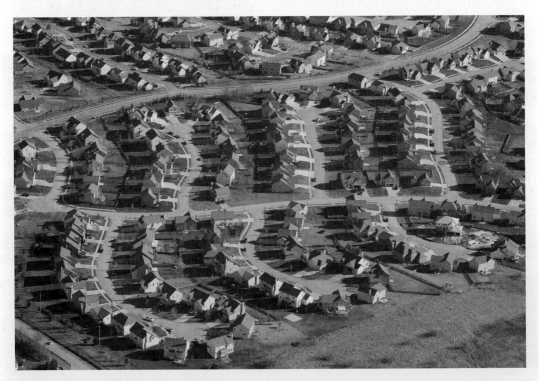

Figure 8.19 Suburban residential developments like this one, with its curving cul-de-sacs and large homes, all similar in design, are found all across the United States.

Courtesy of Craig L. Patterson

fatalities (i.e., involving private vehicles, buses, trains, taxis, bicycles, or pedestrians).[2] The response time for emergency medical services to reach accident scenes is longer in sprawled settings, and the arrival of an ambulance is more likely to be delayed.[3] Research also suggests that some features of urban driving that are in fact hazards (e.g., narrow streets, trees close to the curb) may also signal to drivers that speeding would be hazardous, thereby encouraging slower driving.[4]

Finally, the inconvenience and hazards of walking in sprawled development discourage travel on foot; and such a sedentary lifestyle may be associated with obesity.[5] Obesity has become a serious national problem and one that is rapidly becoming worse. In 1990, the prevalence of obesity was less than 20% in every state, but by 2018, the prevalence was at least 25% in all but three states and more than half of all states have a prevalence of 30% or higher.[6,7]

1. Duany A, Plater-Zyberk E, Speck J. *Suburban Nation: The Rise of Sprawl and the Decline of the American Dream*. North Point Press. 2000.
2. Ewing R, Schieber R, Zegeer CV. Urban sprawl as a risk factor in motor vehicle occupant and pedestrian fatalities. *Am J Public Health*. 2003;93:1541-1545.
3. Trowbridge MJ, Gurka MJ, O'Connor RE. Urban sprawl and delayed ambulance arrival in the U.S. *Am J Prevent Med*. 2009;37(5):428-432.
4. Ewing R, Dumbaugh E. The built environment and traffic safety: a review of empirical evidence. *J Plan Lit*. 2009;23(4):347-367.
5. Frumkin H. Urban sprawl and public health. *Pub Health Rep*. 2002;117:201-212.
6. U.S. Centers for Disease Control and Prevention. (2012). Overweight and Obesity: Adult Obesity Facts. Obesity Trends Among U.S. Adults Between 1985 and 2011 [PowerPoint presentation]. Retrieved December 7, 2012 from: www.cdc.gov/obesity/data/adult.html
7. U.S. Centers for Disease Control and Prevention. Prevalence of self-reported obesity among U.S. adults by state and territory, BRFSS, 2018. Retrieved August 3, 2020 from: https://www.cdc.gov/obesity/data/prevalence-maps.html#states

of wastewater, and removal and disposal of trash. The setting that shapes daily life in urban or suburban settings is often referred to as the *built environment*, and it not only includes buildings but also any transportation systems and public spaces. Recent concern with increasing obesity among Americans has encouraged the development of more *green space* within cities for exercising. Interestingly, these efforts are often combined with the redevelopment of older industrial regions within the city, called *brownfields*.

Indoor Environmental Health Hazards

In 2001, a national survey of activity patterns documented that Americans spent approximately 87% of their time indoors and about 69% of their time in their homes.[60] Among adults, those in the lowest income and education brackets spent the most hours indoors at home.[61] Working adults spend substantial time in their work environments, and similarly, children spend a lot of time in school. Interestingly, although most people tend to assume that indoor air is less polluted than outdoor air, the opposite is often true as the indoor setting is a confined space. Indoor air may not only contain local or naturally occurring ambient air pollutants but also pollutants originating indoors, including some related to construction practices, and others associated with individual lifestyle choices.

Tobacco Smoke

The increasing use of indoor woodstoves in the United States in recent decades has increased the presence of particulates, irritant gases, and other air pollutants in the indoor air of some homes.[62] Other activities (e.g., grilling food) also contribute particulates and other pollutants to indoor air. However, these hazards are dwarfed by those associated with exposure to tobacco smoke.

Exposure to **environmental tobacco smoke**, sometimes called **secondhand smoke**, is hazardous to the health of those who live or work with smokers. Like smokers, adults exposed to secondhand smoke are at increased risk of heart disease, heart attack, and lung cancer; children exposed to secondhand smoke are at increased risk of Sudden Infect Death Syndrome (SIDS) and respiratory effects, including asthma.[63] Young children typically cannot control their exposures while home, if their caregivers smoke. Exposure to secondhand smoke is also a risk factor for hearing loss.[64,65] Adolescents' exposures to secondhand smoke are of concern, given that many are also exposed to noise at high volumes in night clubs or through headphones or earbuds.

Environmental Noise

As detailed elsewhere in the occupational context, noise can damage hearing (causing *threshold shift*, an upward shift in the volume threshold at which sounds can be heard) and has broader health impacts as well. The National Institute for Occupational Safety and Health (NIOSH) has set a Recommended Exposure Limit for noise in the workplace (i.e., for an average exposure over an 8-hour workday) at 85 decibels (dbAs). But not all exposures to excessive noise are work-related. Many recreational activities, such as indoor sporting events, rock concerts, motorcycle or speedboat races, and target shooting, can generate sound at a decibel level high enough to cause noise-induced hearing loss or tinnitus, a continuous ringing or other sound in the ears. There is concern that a whole generation of youngsters who listen regularly to music at high volume through headphones or earbuds may suffer hearing loss.[1,2] **Figure 8.20** presents the decibel levels of some common sounds of outdoor and indoor environments.

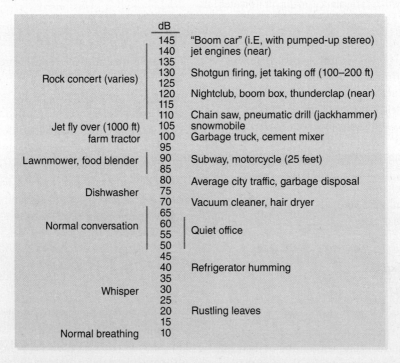

Figure 8.20 Decibel levels of some common sounds.

National Institute on Deafness and Other Communication Disorders. Common Sounds. Available at: www.nidcd.nih.gov/staticresources/health/education/teachers/CommonSounds.pdf. Accessed February 7, 2008.

The National Health and Nutrition Examination Survey (NHANES) dataset has been a rich source of information on hearing loss in the general U.S. population. In the 1999-2004 datasets (NHANES IV), either a unilateral or bilateral threshold shift was documented in almost 13% of adults age 20-69 (unilateral, 9.4%; bilateral, 3.4%).[3] Prevalence of hearing loss was higher in those aged 30 and older, in men, in those with lower educational attainment, and in those with a history of smoking. The hearing of a national sample of U.S. children ages 6 through 19 was also documented. The prevalence of hearing loss was higher in boys (14.8%) than in girls (10.1%), and higher in children ages 12 through 19 (15.5%) than in children ages 6 through 11 (8.5%).[4] Another NHANES analysis showed that the prevalence of hearing loss in adolescents rose from 15% in 1988-1994 to 20% in 2005–2006 (NHANES V).[5]

The most-studied types of environmental noise are traffic noise and airport noise, and this research indicates that the health impacts of noise are not limited to hearing loss. The sounds of airports and traffic clearly cause annoyance in both adults and children, and exposure to airport noise may have cardiovascular effects, although the evidence to date is limited.[6] The best-documented non-hearing impacts of noise to date are its effects on children's cognitive performance: Exposure to airport noise at school has been associated with impairments of both reading comprehension and long-term memory.[6] Other effects of environmental noise have also been suggested. However, the physiological links among noise exposure, sleep disturbance, annoyance, perceived stress, cortisol levels, gender, immune function, cognitive functioning, and mental health are far from clear.[7]

1. Serra MR, Biassoni EC, Richter U, et al. Recreational noise exposure and its effects on the hearing of adolescents. Part I: an interdisciplinary long-term study. *Int J Audiol.* 2005;44(2):65-73.

2. Biassoni EC, Serra MR, Richter U, et al.(Recreational noise exposure and its effects on the hearing of adolescents. Part II: development of hearing disorders. *Int J Audiol.* 2005;44(2):74-85.

3. Mahboudi H, Zardouz S, Oliaei S, Pan D, Bazargan M, Djalilian HR. Noise-induced hearing threshold shift among US adults and implications for noise-induced hearing loss: national Health and Nutrition Examination Surveys. *Eur Arch Otorhinolaryng.* 2013;270:461-467.

4. Niskar AS, Kieszak SM, Holmes AE, Esteban E, Rubin C, Brody DJ. Estimated prevalence of noise-induced hearing threshold shifts among children 6 to 19 years of age: the Third National Health and Nutrition Examination Survey, 1988–1994, United States. *Pediatrics.* 2001;108(1):40-43.

5. Shargorodsky J, Curham SG, Curham GC, Eavey R. Change in prevalence of hearing loss in US adolescents. *JAMA.* 2010;304(7):772-778.

6. Stansfeld SA, Matheson MP. Noise pollution: non-auditory effects on health. *Brit Med Bull.* 2003;68(1):243-257.

7. Smith, A.P. Noise and health: Why we need more research [conference presentation]. InterNoise 2010: Noise and Sustainability, Lisbon, Portugal. 2010, June 13-16. Retrieved September 22, 2012 from: http://psych.cf.ac.uk/home2/smith/ASmith_IN2010.pdf

Radon

As noted elsewhere in the context of exposures to naturally occurring radiation, the global average annual exposure to radon is about 1.15 mSv per capita, but ranges much higher in some locations.[66] Exposure to radon, a natural hazard, can be enhanced by construction practices. In high-granite regions, indoor exposure to naturally occurring radon gas and radon progeny, which emit ionizing radiation, can be substantial, particularly in a building with a basement. Radon rises from the soil and seeps into the basement air, from where it may circulate throughout the house. An exhaust vent in the basement (e.g.,

for a clothes dryer) can create negative pressure, drawing more radon into the basement. In addition, if a home in a high-radon area is served by local groundwater, radon volatilizes into the air of the home whenever tap water is used. Tight construction, although it is desirable for energy efficiency, allows radon to accumulate at higher concentrations indoors. The potential for radon to accumulate indoors was not appreciated as a public health concern until the mid-1980s, when a worker in Eastern Pennsylvania set off a radiation detector as he *entered* the nuclear power plant where he worked; an investigation revealed high radon concentrations in his home.

Because radon has no odor and is not a respiratory irritant, people can be completely unaware of a radon hazard in their homes. Yet, in a high-radon location, radon may be the dominant source of exposure to ionizing radiation from natural sources. Because radon is a gas, and because radon and some radon progeny are alpha emitters, lung cancer is the health risk of greatest concern. Fortunately, inexpensive radon detectors are available, and relatively simple steps, such as sealing cracks in the foundation and installing an appropriate system of vents and fans, can often greatly reduce radon concentrations in indoor air.

Another source of exposure to ionizing radiation is medical X-rays, whose use varies widely with the overall intensity of medical care. For the period 1997–2007, the U.N. Scientific Committee on the Effects of Atomic Radiation (UNSCEAR) estimates that in countries with one or more physicians for every 1,000 population, the average annual exposure to radiation from diagnostic medical X-rays was 1.92 mSv per capita; and in countries with one physician per 1,000–2,999 people, 0.32 mSv per capita.[67] Exposures in other countries are lower on average, but difficult to estimate. This means that in countries with the highest intensity of health care, including the United States, the actual balance between radiation exposure from diagnostic X-rays and inhalation of radon may vary depending upon local geology, construction techniques, and health care.

Sources of Nonionizing Radiation

The household setting also provides exposures to nonionizing radiation from microwaves, appliances and electronics. The rapid adoption of cell phones by a broad segment of the population has outpaced research to assess any associated health risks. Cellular phones emit electromagnetic radiation in the microwave range. The potential for such **microwave radiation** to cause cancer in parts of the brain near the ear, where exposure is highest, is an active area of research. Several large multicountry, case-control studies have suggested that a slight risk exists for brain tumors associated with the heat from a cell phone,[68,69] but have

shown that cell phone radiation does not cause direct DNA carcinogenic mutations. It may still be too early to see results in adults who were exposed as children, who are a vulnerable subgroup for certain brain tumors, and whose brains absorb more radiofrequency radiation than an adult brain.[70] In 2011, about 87% of U.S. 14 to 17 year olds, and 57% of 12 to 13 year olds had a cell phone, and although they are texting more and calling less, 4 of 10 still report that they talk on the phone with friends every day.[71] Although IARC has classified radiofrequency electromagnetic fields (a range that includes cellular phones as well as heating pads and electric blankets) in Group 2B, possibly carcinogenic to humans, cell phones are now a proven risk factor for motor vehicle fatalities associated with distracted driving.

Artificial tanning beds also provide exposure to another type of indoor nonionizing radiation. These devices, found in special tanning salons or associated with nail and hair salons, emit mainly UV-A radiation, along with much smaller quantities of UV-B radiation. More recently, tanning booths, in which the user stands up, have been introduced.

Until the early 1990s, UV-A radiation was generally not considered to cause skin cancer. However, current scientific evidence makes clear that UV-A, like UV-B and UV-C, is carcinogenic. Epidemiologic study has clearly linked the use of tanning beds to risk of malignant melanoma, especially with exposure before age 35, and probably also to risk of squamous cell carcinoma.[72] Despite new understanding on the health effects of UV-A radiation, many tanning salons continue to claim that they offer a "safe" way to tan. IARC classifies solar radiation, ultraviolet radiation (encompassing the UV-A, UV-B, and UV-C wavelengths), and UV-emitting tanning devices in Group 1 (known human carcinogen).[72]

Other Indoor Respiratory Hazards

Asbestos, although not used in new construction in the United States, is present as insulation in many older homes and office buildings, not only in walls and ceilings but also around furnaces and pipes. It was also installed in many schools across the country. People who worked with asbestos on the job are at risk of asbestosis (a fibrotic lung disease), lung cancer, and mesothelioma. The general population continues to be exposed to asbestos fibers released from crumbling insulation in walls or around pipes or boilers in homes, schools, and workplaces. Indeed, in the more developed countries, nearly everyone has asbestos fibers in his or her lungs.[73] People who live with asbestos building materials have exposures much lower than those experienced by workers and are very unlikely to develop asbestosis, because fibrotic disease develops in response to a heavy burden of particles or fibers in the lungs. On the other hand, exposure to asbestos insulation at home or work does carry some risk of lung cancer or mesothelioma, albeit a much lower risk than that borne by workers with substantially higher exposures.

Formaldehyde is widely used in the production of pressed wood products, such as particle-board and plywood (as well as crease-proof and flame-proof fabrics for curtains and furniture).[74] Formaldehyde, a gas at room temperature, is slowly released from products into indoor air. In the 1970s, formaldehyde was used in the manufacture of urea-formaldehyde foam insulation, which resulted in substantial formaldehyde exposure; however, this product is rarely installed today, and insulation from the 1970s is no longer a significant source of exposure. Formaldehyde is a respiratory irritant and can trigger asthma attacks[75,76]; The IARC classification for formaldehyde is as a known carcinogen to humans (Group 1) on the basis of epidemiologic evidence on nasopharyngeal cancer.[77]

Mold and other biological contaminants, such as bacteria and pollen, may grow or accumulate in buildings, usually where water or dampness is present. Many homes that survive the initial damage associated with flooding must subsequently deal with an increased prevalence of these biological pollutants that may cause respiratory or allergic responses in people who live or work in the building (refer **Figure 8.21**).

Personal Care Products

One of the hallmarks of the consumer lifestyle is the very large number of products that people deliberately bring into their homes and apply to their bodies. Unlike cigarettes, these products are not generally seen as unhealthful. Rather, they meet a need to maintain some combination of health, comfort, and physical appearance.

Sometimes called **personal care products**, this group includes soap, shampoo, toothpaste, moisturizers, sunblock, and feminine hygiene products, all of which are important for health or comfort, although they are often marketed (and to some extent formulated) for their cosmetic benefits. These core products are outnumbered by products that are fundamentally cosmetic: deodorants and antiperspirants; products to condition, color, curl, or straighten hair; depilatories to remove hair; nail polish and polish remover; special cleansers, moisturizers, and anti-aging products for the face; creams to lighten the skin or darken it, to screen out some of the sun's rays or enhance their tanning effect; and an array of facial makeup products. Although women use more of these products than men do, cosmetic products are increasingly marketed to men.

It is challenging to assess the health risks of personal care products because both exposure and toxicity are hard to document. For example, a woman may use a rather long list of products, and the list changes over time. Similarly, a single product may have many ingredients, and its composition may change often in a competitive marketplace. And, although a listing of ingredients must appear on the label of a cosmetic product, listed in order of predominance (by weight), **inert ingredients** need not be listed. Inert ingredients are those that do not serve the primary function of a particular product but have some supporting function—as solvents or spreading agents, for example. This designation does not mean either that the ingredient is harmless or that it is chemically inert. Similarly, ingredients that are trade secrets need not be named.

The toxicity of many ingredients has not been well characterized. Phthalates, for example, have been used as plasticizers in nail polish, hair spray,

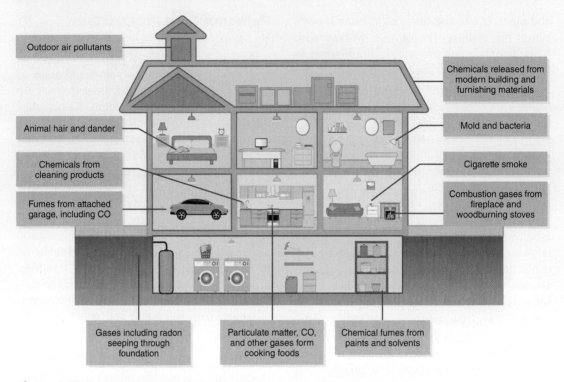

Outdoor air pollutants

Chemicals released from modern building and furnishing materials

Animal hair and dander

Mold and bacteria

Chemicals from cleaning products

Cigarette smoke

Fumes from attached garage, including CO

Combustion gases from fireplace and woodburning stoves

Gases including radon seeping through foundation

Particulate matter, CO, and other gases form cooking foods

Chemical fumes from paints and solvents

Figure 8.21 Sources of Indoor Air Pollution.

U.S. Environmental Protection Agency. Sources of Indoor Air Pollution. Available at: https://www.epa.gov/expobox/exposure-assessment-tools-media-air

and fragrances for some years, but have only, rather recently, come under scrutiny as endocrine disruptors. When, in 2001, the Centers for Disease Control and Prevention (CDC) did its first survey of body burdens of chemicals in the U.S. population, which included measurements of phthalate metabolites in urine, the results were a surprise.[78] The most prominent phthalates were not breakdown products of the phthalates produced in the largest quantities and used to make plastic products (diethylhexyl and diisononyl phthalate). Rather, they were breakdown products of the phthalates used in personal care products (dibutyl phthalate and diethyl phthalate). Some chemicals long used in personal care products— toluene in nail polish and polish remover, acetone in polish remover, and chemicals known as meth(acrylates) in artificial nails—are known to have neurotoxic effects.[79]

Antibacterial soaps and hand sanitizers are increasingly popular. Even in 2000, researchers found that among national brand products at national chain stores, 26% of bar soaps and 78% of liquid soaps contained an antibacterial agent.[80] This very widespread use of antimicrobial products is mostly unnecessary and contributes to the emerging problem of antibiotic resistance among bacteria.

History shows clearly that some ingredients named as selling points, in past marketing of personal care products, were poor choices. For example, during the 1950s, magazine advertisements touted estrogenic hormones in skin creams and foundation makeup, and hormones made a comeback in the advertising of hair and scalp products in the late 1970s and 1980s.[81] Yet today, there is great concern about hormonally active environmental chemicals. Similarly, during the 1950s and 1960s, hexachlorophene was advertised regularly in magazines as the active ingredient in underarm deodorant, as was ammoniated mercury as the active ingredient in skin bleaching creams marketed to African American women.[81] Both of these chemicals are neurotoxic. In the early

1970s, the FDA prohibited the use of mercury in most cosmetics and restricted hexachlorophene to bacteriostatic skin cleansers, with appropriate labeling.[82]

Products for Housekeeping

Recent decades have also seen a proliferation of chemical products for housekeeping—detergents, fabric softeners, and stain removers for the laundry; and many products offering protection against germs or odors, such as toilet bowl cleaners and air fresheners. Many disinfectants and other household cleaning products contain respiratory irritants, and asthma is an occupational hazard for those who work as indoor cleaners.[83] Yet, it is difficult for many people to see these mundane products as potentially harmful.

Air fresheners range from solid blocks (from which chemicals volatilize) to aerosol sprays to programmable electronic mist dispensers. Many air fresheners contain formaldehyde—the same chemical present in pressed wood products—or paradichlorobenzene.[73] Both are respiratory irritants; as described previously, formaldehyde can also trigger asthma attacks and is carcinogenic.[73,74] Moreover, solid air fresheners are often fatal if eaten by children or pets.[73] Paradichlorobenzene is also a key ingredient of mothballs, along with naphthalene, which can cause damage to red blood cells.[84]

Household Pesticides

Application of pesticides in the home also creates conditions for substantial exposure because pesticide residues may cling to certain items (including furniture, carpet, or plush toys) for some time. Young children risk being highly exposed because of their hand-to-mouth behaviors and their tendency to mouth or chew toys. People living in urban areas, and especially those in substandard housing, are likely to have more problems with some insect pests, such as cockroaches, and may resort more often to pesticide use.

Also of concern is the accidental ingestion, mostly by children, of illegal household pesticides. A series of accidental poisonings in the city

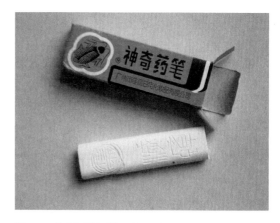

Figure 8.22 This illegal pesticide, known as Chinese chalk, resembles ordinary blackboard chalk.
Courtesy of Dion Lerman, Pennsylvania Integrated Pest Management Program/Pennsylvania State University

of New York in the 1990s revealed that an illegal rat poison known as Tres Pasitos ("three little steps," taken by a rat before dying) contained the carbamate insecticide aldicarb, not licensed for use as a rodenticide. Tres Pasitos continues to be sold illegally.[85,86] Similarly, an insecticide known as "Chinese chalk" (cockroaches are said to die if they cross a line drawn on the floor) contains deltamethrin, a potent pyrethroid pesticide.[87] Mostly illegally imported from China, it resembles ordinary blackboard chalk, and as a result, children are likely to see it as harmless (see **Figure 8.22**).

Sick Building Syndrome

A so-called **sick building** is one whose occupants report a range of acute symptoms when they are in the building and usually feel better shortly after they leave the building but cannot pinpoint what is causing their symptoms. Occupants report such nonspecific symptoms as headache; irritation of the eyes, nose, or throat; dry cough; itchy skin; dizziness; nausea; difficulty in concentrating; and fatigue, which together are referred to as **sick building syndrome**.[88] The causes, which are usually not clearly established, may include organic chemicals in the air of the building originating from construction materials; biological agents such as mold spores, bacterial toxins, or insect feces; airborne particulates from many sources; or chemicals originating from activities in the building—all of which may be compounded by shoddy maintenance or poor ventilation. Industry standards for required ventilation rates in buildings, which were reduced in the 1970s to conserve energy, are now at least 15 cubic feet of outside air per minute per person and are higher in many specific settings.[88] In contrast to sick building syndrome, a specific diagnosable illness that has been clearly linked to a specific feature of a building is referred to as building-related illness.

Regulation Related to Hazards of Indoor, Modern Life

In addition to the EPA, both the FDA and the Consumer Product Safety Commission (CPSC) have roles in the regulation of consumer products and indoor air. As described elsewhere in the context of the pervasive production and use of synthetic organic chemicals, the Consumer Product Safety Improvement Act of 2008 banned the use of a specific class of chemicals—phthalates—in children's toys and certain other products for children. However, the CPSC's regulation of the physical safety of various consumer products, such as lawn mowers, is outside of the scope of this discussion.

With an addition to the Toxic Substances Control Act, named the Residential Lead-Based Paint Hazard Reduction Act of 1992, the federal government directed the EPA to provide technical information about managing lead hazards, as well as public education and outreach activities. The EPA authorizes state programs for the surveillance and abatement of lead hazards, but it is the states that train and certify inspectors and contractors.

Similarly, the federal government provides financial support and technical assistance to states for radon programs, although states are required to neither monitor nor control radon. The Consumer Product Safety Commission regulates the safety of household products containing chemicals, including products such as cleaning

chemicals and air fresheners, but mainly with regard to packaging and labeling.

For the most part, restrictions on smoking in specific locations are set at the state and local levels; an exception is the prohibition of smoking on domestic airline flights.[89] The major federal actions have been to require warnings on cigarette packages and to prohibit cigarette advertising on television and radio; however, agencies have passed up opportunities to regulate cigarettes as a hazardous substance, as a chemical substance, and as a consumer product.[89]

Under the Federal Food, Drug, and Cosmetic Act (FFDCA), the FDA has only limited authority to regulate cosmetics. Cosmetic products and ingredients are not subject to premarket approval by the FDA (except for color additives), and recall of a cosmetic product from the market is a voluntary action by the manufacturer.[90] The safety of cosmetics ingredients is reviewed by a panel of scientists, the Cosmetic Ingredient Review, established in 1976 by the Cosmetic, Toiletry, and Fragrance Association, a trade group. The FDA has a nonvoting liaison member on the panel. The FDA does have authority to initiate the removal of adulterated or misbranded cosmetics from the market. As of December of 2006, the FDA had prohibited a total of 10 ingredients for use in cosmetics, including mercury and two ingredients whose regulation originates outside the realm of cosmetics (chlorofluorocarbon propellants and prohibited cattle material). A manufacturer can ask the FDA to grant trade secret status for an individual ingredient with special properties that is not well known; in this case, the label need not list the ingredient but must add the words "and other ingredients."

8.7 Sharing Global Impacts and Resources

As described throughout this text, modern Western-style development, although it brings many benefits in health and comfort, has often been long on hubris and short on foresight.

We have developed classes of synthetic organic chemicals that are both toxic and persistent—pesticides, PCBs, brominated and perfluorinated compounds—and dispersed them into the environment. We are using nanotechnology in many applications without a clear understanding of the health effects of these tiny engineered particles. We have allowed the overuse of antibiotics to shape resistant bacterial populations, and we have released engineered plants to take part in nature's genetic reshuffling. We have pumped up carbon dioxide in the troposphere and depleted ozone in the stratosphere. We subsidize our agriculture with chemicals made from fossil fuels and tractors powered by fossil fuels. Ecologically speaking, we eat meat to excess, and we have been relentless in taking fish from the oceans and in converting undeveloped land into developed land.

As consumers in a consumer society, we live surrounded by our *stuff* and its wastes—both the byproducts of production and the discards of daily life. These wastes may collect in heaps on land or as floating masses in the ocean; they may be buried; they may disperse in water or air; and they may even change form. But they do not simply go away. The products and byproducts of modern life, and their various environmental health impacts, have been the focus through most of this text, but we conclude by stepping back to take a broader view of the ecological impact of Western-style development and its implications for the future.

Quantifying the Impacts of Development

The impact of development on an ecosystem or on the global environment is often conceptualized this way:

Impact = Population × Consumption per capita

or

$$I = P \times C$$

a formulation known simply as the impact equation. Alternatively, with the C expanded into the component factors of Affluence and Technology, the equation can be written as:

$$I = P \times A \times T$$

a formulation commonly referred to as the IPAT equation. This expanded version incorporates both sides of a historical difference of opinion between two leading environmentalists,[91,92] both biologists by training: Paul Ehrlich, who emphasized the importance of affluence as a driving force in environmental pollution; and Barry Commoner, who emphasized technology as the key factor.

Ecosystems cannot support and sustain unlimited impacts. Rather, as described earlier, any ecosystem (or the Earth as a whole) has an inherent **carrying capacity**: the maximum impact that it can support for an extended period. This means that if the combination of population and per capita consumption pushes impact above the carrying capacity, this condition cannot be sustained without permanent, or long-term, damage to the ecosystem. In contrast, **sustainable development** is defined as development that can be maintained over many generations, within the constraints of a regional ecosystem or the global ecosphere.

The Global Footprint Network[93] has developed a useful website to calculate an impact of development, the **ecological footprint**: the area on the Earth's surface that is required to provide resources for, and absorb the wastes of, an individual or a population with a given standard of living. The ecological footprint is conceptualized as the sum of five inputs[94]: the built-up land area occupied by human settlement, the areas required to produce food on land (comprising croplands and pastures) and at sea (fisheries), the forested area required to produce wood products, and the forested area needed to absorb the carbon dioxide produced by burning fossil fuels (called the **carbon footprint** or energy footprint).

The global ecological footprint in 2018 was 1.6 planet Earths, meaning that global ecological resources were being used up 1.6 times faster than they could be replenished.[93] This projected deficit is referred to as **ecological overshoot** and it has doubled from one Earth to almost two in the past 50 years.[93] In high-income countries (using the World Bank's classification of countries into high-, upper-middle-, lower-middle-, and low-income groups), the carbon footprint dominates, usually making up one-half to three-quarters of the total footprint. In contrast, in most countries in the low-income category, the food and forest footprints dominate, making up at least three-quarters of the total footprint. The high-income countries represent 15% of the world's population and account for 35% of the global ecological impact; the low-income countries represent 20% of the population and account for 9% of the impact.[93] At present, the per capita ecological footprint in the United States demands four times the resources and waste mitigation than our planet can absorb annually.[93]

Moreover, we are depleting two gifts of nature in ways not captured by the ecological footprint. Over the span of a few generations, we are now using up fossil fuel resources that were laid down over geologic time scales. Similarly, shortages of potable water are now looming in locations around the world as water becomes polluted by sewage, industrial wastes, or the extraction of fuels; or is lost to evaporation through the irrigation of crops; or is withdrawn from freshwater aquifers but ultimately is conveyed out to sea; or worse, is wasted by consumers. The United Nations estimates that about a quarter of the world's population lives with water scarcity.[95]

Facing a Challenging Future

From the vantage point of the early 21st century, three realities stand out starkly. First, as just described, modern Western-style development patterns are simply not sustainable at the global scale: It would take three to four Earths to sustain the world's population living at the per capita impact of the United States or Western European countries.

Second, enormous disparities persist between the world's richer and poorer countries. The benefits of modern development have accrued mainly to the wealthier countries; the negative impacts, however, are more broadly shared. And finally, despite the high per capita ecological footprints of the United States and other more developed countries, the strain on the Earth's total carrying capacity in the future is likely to be driven mostly by increasing footprints in regions with much larger populations. In particular, China and India, with populations of about 1.4 billion and 1.35 billion, respectively—more than one-third of the world's people—are rapidly embracing many aspects of Western-style development. Indeed, China has been referred to as "the factory of the world" and India as "the office of the world."[96]

In light of these ecological and demographic realities, the world faces a daunting challenge in devising a global future that is both more sustainable and more equitable than the present one. The IPAT equation, although it frames the limits of environmental sustainability, also offers some hope of a more positive role for technology. As the framework was originally conceived, technological development was seen as a contributor to environmental impact. But to the extent that technology is reoriented toward the "green"—reflecting a broader social shift toward environmentally conscious decision making—it may become a part of the solution.[90]

For those living in the more developed countries, and especially in the United States, with its generous natural endowments, the Earth's physical limits have not always been apparent. They were not of concern when we elected to use clean water to carry sewage, or began to draw down the Ogallala Aquifer, or embraced the automobile, or subsidized meat with grain subsidized in turn by oil. But today, common sense calls for a more sustainable way of living in a world that is burdened by ecological debt, linked by the global transport of pollutants and pathogens, and framed by a climate whose intricate balance we have only begun to appreciate.

Study Questions

1. Explain how the major objectives of sewage treatment are met through the major processes of sewage treatment.
2. Do you know where your drinking water comes from? Locate a current Consumer Confidence Report to assess your drinking water's quality.
3. Do you know what happens to your solid waste once you throw something away?
4. Using an online calculator, estimate your ecological footprint and test out the effects of some variations. Are there changes you could readily make that would reduce your footprint?
5. What environmental health issue do you feel so strongly about that you would advocate for protective risk policies at the regional or national or global level?

References

1. Tarr J. *The Search for the Ultimate Sink: Urban Pollution in Historical Perspective.* University of Akron Press; 1996.
2. Strasser S. *Waste and Want.* Henry Holt & Company; 1999.
3. U.S. Environmental Protection Agency. *How We Use Water.* Retrieved July 25, 2020 from: www.epa.gov/watersense/how-we-use-water
4. Onsite Installer. *New Study Shows Decline in Residential Water Use.* 2017. Retrieved August 4, 2020 from: https://www.onsiteinstaller.com/online_exclusives/2017/08/new_study_shows_decline_in_residential_water_use
5. Dieter CA, Maupin MA, Caldwell RR, et al. Estimated use of water in the United States in 2015. *US Geological Survey Circular.* 2018;1441, 65.
6. US Environmental Protection Agency. Municipal solid waste generation, recycling and disposal in the United States: Facts and Figures for 2010. Retrieved July 25, 2020 from: www.epa.gov/msw/pubs/mswchar10.pdf
7. U.S. Environmental Protection Agency. Combined Sewer Overflows/Demographics. Retrieved July 25, 2020 from: https://www.epa.gov/npdes/combined-sewer-overflows-csos
8. Massachusetts Water Resources Authority. About MWRA: Massachusetts Water Resources Authority. Retrieved April 25, 2012 from: www.mwra.state.ma.us/02org/html/whatis.htm
9. Massachusetts Water Resources Authority. Combined Sewer Overflows. 2007. Retrieved March 31, 2012 from: www.mwra.state.ma.us/03sewer/html/sewcso.htm
10. Hale RC, La Guardia MJ. Have risks associated with the presence of synthetic organic contaminants in land-applied sewage sludge been adequately assessed? *New Solut.* 2002;12(4):371-386.
11. Gale P. Land application of treated sewage sludge: quantifying pathogen risks from consumption of crops. *J Appl Microbiol.* 2005;98(2):380-396.
12. Sahlström L, de Jong B, Aspan A. *Salmonella* isolated in sewage sludge tracked back to human cases of salmonellosis. *Letters Appl Microbiol.* 2006;43(1):46-52.
13. Rideout K, Teschke K. Potential for increased human foodborne exposure to PCDD/F when recycling sewage sludge on agricultural land. *Environ Health Perspect.* 2004;112(9):959-969.
14. Hale RC, La Guardia MJ, Harvey EP, Gaylor, MO, Matteson Mainor T, Duff WH. Persistent pollutants in land-applied sludges. *Nature.* 2001;412:140–141.
15. Golet E, Strehler A, Alder A, Giger W. Determination of fluoroquinolone antibacterial agents in sewage sludge and sludge-treated soil using accelerated solvent extraction followed by solid-phase extraction. *Analyt Chem.* 2002; 74(21):5455-5462.
16. Clarke BO, Smith SR. Review of 'emerging' organic contaminants in biosolids and assessment of international research priorities for the agricultural use of biosolids. *Environ Int.* 2011;37(1):226-247.
17. U.S. Environmental Protection Agency. Basic information about biosolids. Retrieved August 4, 2020 from: https://www.epa.gov/biosolids/basic-information-about-biosolids
18. Minnesota Pollution Control Agency. Sewage treatment in a soil system. Waste/Wastewater-ISTS #1.11. 2001. Retrieved December 7, 2012 from: http://attfile.konetic.or.kr/konetic/xml/use/31A1B0245005.pdf
19. U.S. Environmental Protection Agency and U.S. Department of Agriculture. A Handbook of Constructed Wetlands. 2012.
20. Zezima, K. Vermont blends "green" flush toilets and a greenhouse. 2005. *New York Times.*
21. Rockefeller A, Goodland R. What is environmental sustainability in sanitation? In Goodland R, Orlando L, Anhang J, eds. *Toward Sustainable Sanitation (pp. 7-16).* The International Association of Impact Assessment. 2001:7-16.
22. U.S. Environmental Protection Agency. Sewage Sludge (Biosolids)/Frequently Asked Questions. Retrieved April 25, 2012 from: http://water.epa.gov/polwaste/wastewater/treatment/biosolids/genqa.cfm
23. U.S. Environmental Protection Agency. Biosolids/Final Action Not to Regulate Dioxins in Land-Applied Sewage Sludge. Retrieved April 25, 2012 from: http://water.epa.gov/scitech/wastetech/biosolids/dioxinfs.cfm
24. U.S. Environmental Protection Agency. Public drinking water systems: facts and figures. 2006. Retrieved

December 27, 2007 from: www.epa.gov/ogwdw/pws/index.html

25. VanDerslice J. Drinking water infrastructure and environmental disparities: evidence and methodological considerations. *Am J Pub Health.* 2011;101, S109-S116.

26. U.S. Geological Survey. Probing the Los Angeles basin—insights into ground-water resources and earthquake hazards. Fact Sheet 086-02. 2002. Retrieved April 29, 2008 from: http://geopubs.wr.usgs.gov/fact-sheet/fs086-02/

27. Troesken W, Beeson PE. The significance of lead water mains in American cities: Some historical evidence. In Costa DL, ed. *Health and Labor Force Participation Over the Life Cycle: Evidence from the Past.* University of Chicago Press; 2003.

28. U.S. Environmental Protection Agency. National primary drinking water regulations: proposed lead and copper rule revisions. *Fed Regist.* 2019. Retrieved August 5, 2020 from https://www.federalregister.gov/documents/2019/11/13/2019-22705/national-primary-drinking-water-regulations-proposed-lead-and-copper-rule-revisions

29. US Environmental Protection Agency. Lead and copper rule: a quick reference guide. 2004. Retrieved June 20, 2012 from https://www.epa.gov/dwreginfo/lead-and-copper-rule#rule-history

30. Villanueva CM, Cantor KP, Grimalt JO, et al. Bladder cancer and exposure to water disinfection by-products through ingestion, bathing, showering, and swimming in pools. *Am J Epidemiol.* 2007;165(2):148-156.

31. Chang CC, Ho SC, Wang LY, Yang CY. Bladder cancer in Taiwan: relationship to trihalomethane concentrations present in drinking-water supplies. *J Toxicol Environ Health Part A.* 2007;70(20):1752-1757.

32. Nieuwenhuijsen MJ, Toledano MB, Eaton NE, Fawell J, Elliott P. Chlorination disinfection byproducts in water and their association with adverse reproductive outcomes: a review. *Occupat Environ Med.* 2000;57(2):73-85.

33. Wright JM, Schwartz J. Dockery DW. Effect of trihalomethane exposure on fetal development. *Occupat Environ Med.* 2003;60(3):173-180.

34. Howards PP, Hertz-Picciotto I. Invited commentary: disinfection by-products and pregnancy loss—lessons. *Am J Epidemiol.* 2006;164(11):1052-1055.

35. Savitz DA, Singer PC, Herring AH, Hartmann KE, Weinberg HS, Makarushka C. Exposure to drinking water disinfection by-products and pregnancy loss. *Am J Epidemiol.* 2006;164(11):1043-1051.

36. Villanueva CM, Gracia-Lavedán E, Ibarluzea J, et al. Exposure to trihalomethanes through different water uses and birth weight, small for gestational age, and preterm delivery in Spain. *Environ Health Perspect.* 2011;119(12):1824-1830.

37. U.S. Environmental Protection Agency. Chloramines in drinking water. 2007. Retrieved December 27, 2007 from https://www.epa.gov/dwreginfo/chloramines-drinking-water

38. U.S. Centers for Disease Control and Prevention. Community water fluoridation. 2007. Retrieved December 27, 2007 from www.cdc.gov/fluoridation/

39. National Academy of Sciences. Fluoride in drinking water: a scientific review of EPA's standards (report in brief). 2006. Retrieved April 29, 2008 from https://www.actionpa.org/fluoride/nrc/NRC-2006.pd

40. U.S. Environmental Protection Agency. Private drinking water wells. 2006. Retrieved December 27, 2012 from www.epa.gov/safewater/privatewells/index2.html

41. US Food and Drug Administration, Center for Food Safety and Applied Nutrition. Bottled Water Regulation and the FDA. *Food Safety Magazine.* 2002. Retrieved December 27, 2012 from https://www.foodsafetymagazine.com/magazine-archive1/augustseptember-2002/bottled-water-regulation-and-the-fda/

42. U.S. Environmental Protection Agency. Bottled water basics. 2005. Retrieved December 7, 2012 from https://www.epa.gov/sites/production/files/2015-11/documents/2005_09_14_faq_fs_healthseries_bottledwater.pdf

43. Conley, J. *Report: 64% of Bottled Water Is Tap Water, Costs 2000x More.* Common Dreams, EcoWatch. 2018. Retrieved August 4, 2020 from https://www.ecowatch.com/bottled-water-sources-tap-2537510642.html

44. US Environmental Protection Agency. Drinking water contaminant candidate list 3-draft. 2008. Retrieved April 30, 2008 from https://www.federalregister.gov/documents/2008/02/21/E8-3114/drinking-water-contaminant-candidate-list-3-draft

45. U.S. Environmental Protection Agency. *Advancing sustainable materials management: 2017 Fact Sheet - Assessing trends in material generation, recycling, composting, combustion with energy recovery and landfilling in the United States.* 530-F-19-007. 2019. Retrieved August 4, 2020 from https://www.epa.gov/sites/production/files/2019-11/documents/2017_facts_and_figures_fact_sheet_final.pdf

46. U.S. Environmental Protection Agency. Packaging. Retrieved April 26, 2012 from https://www.epa.gov/facts-and-figures-about-materials-waste-and-recycling/containers-and-packaging-product-specific-data#main-content

47. Sustainable Packaging Coalition. Study examines recycling availability. *Recycling Today.* 2017. Retrieved August 5, 2020 from: https://www.recyclingtoday.com/article/recycling-availability-study-spc/

48. Rysavy TF. Americans are really bad at recycling. But only because we're not trying very hard. *Green American Magazine.* Retrieved August 3, 2020 from https://www.greenamerica.org/rethinking-recycling/americans-are-really-bad-recycling-only-because-were-not-trying-very-hard

49. U.S. Environmental Protection Agency. *Vermicomposting.* 2007. Retrieved December 12, 2007 from www.epa.gov/compost/vermi.htm

50. Wayland R. *Clean Air Act Section 129: waste to energy overview.* Presentation for the Waste-to-Energy: An

Integrated Waste Management Option Conference. 2007.

51. U.S. Environmental Protection Agency. *Basic information about landfill gas.* Landfill Methane Outreach Program. Retrieved August 5, 2020 from: https://www.epa.gov/lmop/basic-information-about-landfill-gas#:~:text=Landfill%20gas%20(LFG)%20is%20a,of%20non%2Dmethane%20organic%20compounds

52. U.S. Environmental Protection Agency. Municipal solid waste generation, recycling, and disposal in the United States: facts and figures for 2010. 530-F-11-005. 2011. Retrieved April 25, 2012 from: www.epa.gov/waste/nonhaz/municipal/pubs/msw_2010_factsheet.pdf

53. Weber R, Watson A, Forter M, Oliaei F. Persistent organic pollutants and landfills—a review of past experiences and future challenges. *Waste Manag Res.* 2011;29(1):107-121.

54. US Environmental Protection Agency. Household hazardous waste (HHW). 2006. Retrieved March 30, 2007 from https://www.epa.gov/hw/household-hazardous-waste-hhw

55. U.S. Environmental Protection Agency. *At a glance: improved information could better enable EPA to manage electronic waste and enforce regulations,* 13-P-0298. 2013. Retrieved August 4, 2020 from: https://www.epa.gov/sites/production/files/2015-09/documents/20130621-13-p-0298.pdf

56. United Nations, Department of Economic and Social Affairs, Population Division *World Urbanization Prospects: The 2018 Revision* (ST/ESA/SER.A/420). United Nations. 2019.

57. World Health Organization. *A Billion voices: listening and responding to the health needs of slum dwellers and informal settlers in new urban settings.* 2005. Retrieved October 30, 2012 from www.who.int/social_determinants/resources/urban_settings.pdf

58. Vlahov D, Galea S, Gibble E, Freudenberg N. Perspectives on urban conditions and population health. *Cad Saude Publica.* 2005;21(3)949-957.

59. Marshall J. Megacity, mega mess... *Nature.* 2005;437:312-314.

60. Klepeis N, Nelson WC, Ott WR, et al. The National Human Activity Pattern Survey (NHAPS): a resource for assessing exposure to environmental pollutants. *J Expos Analyt Environ Epidemiol.* 2001;11:231-252.

61. Echols SL, Macintosh DL, Hammerstrom KA, Ryan B. Temporal variability of microenvironmental time budgets in Maryland. *J Expos Analyt Environ Epidemiol.* 1999;9:502-512.

62. Naeher LP, Brauer M, Lipsett M., et al. Woodsmoke health effects: a review. *Inhal Toxicol.* 2007;19(1):67-106.

63. U.S. Centers for Disease Control and Prevention. *Smoking & Tobacco Use: Secondhand Smoke (SHS) Facts.* Retrieved December 7, 2012 from: www.cdc.gov/tobacco/data_statistics/fact_sheets/secondhand_smoke/general_facts/index.htm

64. Mahboudi H, Zardouz S, Oliaei S, Pan D, Bazargan M, Djalilian H. Noise-induced hearing threshold shift among US adults and implications for noise-induced hearing loss: National Health and Nutrition Examination Surveys. *Eur Arch Otorhinolaryngol..* 2012;270:461-467.

65. Niskar AS, Kieszak SM, Holmes AE, Esteban E, Rubin C, Brody DJ. Estimated prevalence of noise-induced hearing threshold shifts among children 6 to 19 years of age: the Third National Health and Nutrition Examination Survey, 1988–1994, United States. *Pediatrics.* 2001;108(1):40-43.

66. United Nations Scientific Committee on the Effects of Atomic Radiation (UNSCEAR). *UNSCEAR 2006 Report Vol. I: Effects of Ionizing Radiation, Annex A.* 2008. Retrieved June 20, 2012 from https://www.epa.gov/hw/household-hazardous-waste-hhw

67. United Nations Scientific Committee on the Effects of Atomic Radiation (UNSCEAR). *Sources and Effects of Ionizing Radiation: UNSCEAR 2008.* Report to the General Assembly with Scientific Annexes. 2010. Retrieved June 20, 2012 from: www.unscear.org/unscear/en/publications/2008_1.html

68. Saracci R, Samet J. Commentary: call me on my mobile phone . . . or better not?—a look at the INTERPHONE study results. *Int J Epidemiol.* 2010;39(10):695-698.

69. INTERPHONE Study Group. Brain tumour risk in relation to mobile telephone use: results of the INTERPHONE international case–control study. *Int J Epidemiol.* 2010;39(3):675-694.

70. Mead MN. Cancer: strong signal for cell phone effects. *Environ Health Perspect.* 2008;116(10), A422.

71. Lenhart, A. *Teens, Smartphones & Texting: overview.* Washington, DC: Pew Research Center. 2012. Retrieved June 20, 2012 from https://www.pewresearch.org/internet/2012/03/19/teens-smartphones-texting/

72. International Agency for Research on Cancer Working Group on artificial ultraviolet (UV) light and skin cancer. The association of use of sunbeds with cutaneous malignant melanoma and other skin cancers: a systematic review. *Int J Cancer.* 2006;120(5):1116-1122.

73. Robinso BS, Musk AW, Lake RA. Malignant mesothelioma. *Lancet.* 2005;366(9483):397-408.

74. Miller, E.W. & Miller, R.M. *Indoor Pollution.* Santa Barbara, CA: ABC-CLIO. 1998.

75. U.S. Environmental Protection Agency. *Learn about Chemicals Around Your House: Air Fresheners.* Retrieved April 4, 2007 from: www.epa.gov/kidshometour/products/airf.htm

76. U.S. Environmental Protection Agency. *An Introduction to Indoor Air Quality: Formaldehyde.* Retrieved October 30, 2012 from: www.epa.gov/iaq/formaldehyde.html

77. International Agency for Research on Cancer. *Agents Classified by the IARC Monographs, Volumes 1–104.* 2012. Retrieved April 7, 2012 from http://monographs.iarc.fr/ENG/Classification/ClassificationsAlphaOrder.pdf

78. U.S. Centers for Disease Control and Prevention. *National Report on Human Exposure to Environmental Chemicals.* 2001. Retrieved January 20, 2002 from www.cdc.gov/exposurereport/

79. LoSasso GL, Rapport LJ, Axelrod BN, Whitman RD. Neurocognitive sequelae of exposure to organic solvents and (meth)acrylates among nail studio technicians. *Neuropsychiatr Neuropsychol Behav Neurol.* 2002;15(1):44-55.

80. Perencevich EN, Wong MT, Harris AD. National and regional assessment of the antibacterial soap market: a step toward determining the impact of prevalent antibacterial soaps. *Am J Infect Control.* 2001;29(5): 281-283.

81. Maxwell NI. Social differences in women's use of personal care products: a study of magazine advertisements, 1950–1994. 2000. Silent Spring Institute.

82. U.S. Food and Drug Administration. *Prohibited & Restricted Ingredients in Cosmetics.* 2006. Retrieved October 30, 2012 from: https://www.fda.gov/cosmetics /cosmetics-laws-regulations/prohibited-restricted -ingredients-cosmetics

83. Zock JP, Kogevinas M, Sunyer J, et al Asthma risk, cleaning activities and use of specific cleaning products among Spanish indoor cleaners. *Scand J Work Environ Health.* 2001;27(1):76-81.

84. U.S. Agency for Toxic Substances and Disease Registry. *ToxFAQs for Naphthalene.* 2005. Retrieved December 7, 2012 from www.atsdr.cdc.gov/toxfaqs/index.asp

85. Centers for Disease Control and Prevention (CDC). Poisonings associated with illegal use of aldicarb as a rodenticide—New York City, 1994–1997. *Mortality and Morbidity Weekly Report.* 1997;46(41):961-963.

86. City of New York, Department of Health and Mental Hygiene. *Poisonings Associated with the Use of an Illegal Pesticide.* 2006.

87. US Environmental Protection Agency. *Avoid Illegal Household Pesticide Products.* Retrieved April 5, 2007 from https://www.epa.gov/safepestcontrol/avoid-illegal -household-pesticide-products#main-content

88. U.S. Environmental Protection Agency. *Indoor Air Facts no. 4 (revised): Sick Building* Syndrome. 1991. Retrieved October 30, 2012 from https://www.epa.gov/sites /production/files/2014-08/documents/sick_building _factsheet.pdf

89. U.S. Centers for Disease Control and Prevention. *Smoking and Tobacco Use.* 2007.

90. U.S. Food and Drug Administration. *FDA Authority Over Cosmetics.* Retrieved October 30, 2012 from www.fda.gov /Cosmetics/GuidanceComplianceRegulatoryInformation /ucm074162.htm

91. Chertow, M. The IPAT equation and its variants: changing views of technology and environmental impact. *J Indust Ecol.* 2001;4(4):13-29.

92. Chertow, M. IPAT equation. In *Encyclopedia of Earth.* Environmental Information Coalition, National Council for Science and the Environment. Retrieved October 30, 2012 from www.eoearth.org/article/IPAT_equation

93. Global Footprint Network. *Ecological Footprint.* Retrieved August 5, 2020 from https://www.footprintnetwork.org /our-work/ecological-footprint/

94. Global Footprint Network. *Footprint basics—Overview.* Retrieved May 1, 2012 from: www.footprintnetwork.org /en/index.php/GFN/page/footprint_basics_overview/

95. United Nations Department of Economic and Social Affairs. *Water Scarcity.* Retrieved August 3, 2020 from https:www.un.org/waterforlifedecade/scarcity.shtml

96. Ghosh J. *Poverty Reduction in China and India: Policy Implications of Recent Trends* (DESA Working Paper No. 92; ST/ESA/2010/DWP/92). United Nations, Department of Economic and Social Affairs. 2010. Retrieved June 21, 2012 from: www.un.org/esa/desa /papers/2010/wp92_2010.pdf

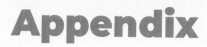

Appendix

Table A.1 Overview of U.S. Regulatory Framework for Environmental Health

Environmental Health Domain	Major Laws and Key Provisions for the Control of Environmental Health Hazards
Overall	National Environmental Policy Act—established creation of the Environmental Protection Agency (EPA); created mandate for Environmental Impact Assessments (EIA)
Food supply	Federal Insecticide, Fungicide, and Rodenticide Act—requirements to register new pesticides
	Federal Food, Drug, and Cosmetic Act—setting pesticide tolerances in food; BSE surveillance and controls on feed for ruminants; requirements for HACCP systems for food safety; setting food defect action levels; approval of food additives including potential chemical byproducts of irradiation
Industrial wastes	Comprehensive Environmental Response, Compensation and Liability Act ("Superfund") (CERCLA)—identify, assess health risks of, and remediate abandoned hazardous waste sites
	Clean Water Act (CWA)—ambient standards (Ambient Water Quality Criteria) for about 125 pollutants; technology requirements and permitting system for industrial discharges to ambient water
	Resource Conservation and Recovery Act (RCRA)—"cradle-to-grave" manifest system for hazardous wastes; standards and permits for hazardous waste storage or disposal facilities; provisions to promote hazardous waste minimization (source reduction) and recycling of hazardous wastes
Workplace hazards	Occupational Safety and Health Act—ambient standards (permissible exposure limits) for workplace air; modifications to work environment take priority over use of personal protective equipment; employers must provide Materials Safety Data Sheets (MSDSs) to workers
Toxic chemicals	Toxic Substances Control Act—premanufacture notice for new chemicals; EPA can restrict manufacture, distribution, or use if new chemical poses unreasonable risk
	Consumer Product Safety Improvement Act of 2008—ban on six phthalates in toys and children's products
	Emergency Planning and Community Right-to-Know Act—local and state emergency response commissions; yearly chemical reporting requirements for manufacturing facilities; data available as Toxics Release Inventory; facilities must provide Materials Safety Data Sheets (MSDSs) to local commissions

(continues)

Table A.1 Overview of U.S. Regulatory Framework for Environmental Health   *(continued)*

Environmental Health Domain	Major Laws and Key Provisions for the Control of Environmental Health Hazards
Air pollution	Clean Air Act—ambient standards (NAAQS) for criteria air pollutants; emissions standards for hazardous air pollutants, including mercury; emission allowances for SO_2 (to control acid deposition); banning of leaded gasoline; requirement to sell reformulated gasoline in high-smog areas; regulation of CO_2 as a greenhouse gas
Nuclear fuel cycle	Nuclear Waste Policy Act—requirements to build and regulate a repository for radioactive wastes, including spent reactor fuel Uranium Mill Tailings Radiation Control Act—standards for cleanup and management of mill tailings at abandoned sites Low-Level Radioactive Waste Policy Act—requires states to take responsibility for low-level radioactive wastes generated within their boundaries; states may form groups ("compacts") for this purpose
Alternative energy sources	Energy Policy Act—modest supports for alternative energy sources
Municipal wastewater	Clean Water Act—ambient standards and water supply permitting system for discharges to ambient water from municipal wastewater treatment plants; requirement for both primary and secondary sewage treatment; procedures for land application of treated sewage sludge
Community water supply	Safe Drinking Water Act—standards for drinking water: Maximum Contaminant Level Goal (MCLG) and Maximum Contaminant Level (MCL), which is the standard Federal Food, Drug, and Cosmetic Act—regulation of bottled water as packaged food
Municipal solid waste	Resource Conservation and Recovery Act—requirements for municipal solid waste landfills and waste-to-energy incinerators

Table A.2 Location of Environmental Health Topics within the Text

Familiar Topics	Chapter 2 Science of Environmental Health	Chapter 3 Managing Environmental Health Risks	Chapter 4 Living with Nature	Chapter 5 Producing Food	Chapter 6 Producing Manufactured Goods	Chapter 7 Producing Energy	Chapter 8 Living in the World We've Made
Air pollution, including climate change						✓	✓
Built environment							✓
Drinking water							✓
Environmental health policy and principles		✓					
Environmental risk assessment	✓						
Epidemiology	✓						
Food safety				✓			
Infectious disease			✓				
Municipal solid waste			✓				✓
Natural disasters			✓				
Noise					✓		✓
Occupational hazards					✓		
Organic chemicals					✓		
Pesticides			✓	✓			
Radiation						✓	
Sewage					✓		✓
Toxic metals							✓
Toxicology	✓						

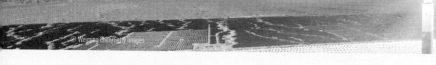

Glossary

A

absorbed dose the quantity of a toxicant that passes through the human envelope, thereby entering the body

acid deposition (or *acid rain*) precipitation made acidic by the atmospheric conversion of nitric oxide and nitrogen dioxide to nitrates and nitric acid and of sulfur dioxide to sulfates and sulfuric acid

acid mine drainage water, originating as rainwater, that has been made acidic by passing through mine shafts or the waste rock from a coal mine

acid rain see *acid deposition*

active immunity the immunity, usually permanent, that results after the immune system has mounted a counterattack against a foreign substance

active ingredient in a pesticide, the chemical ingredient that is intended to kill the pest

acute exposure a brief exposure

aerosol very fine airborne solid or liquid particles

aflatoxin a mycotoxin produced by a mold, *Aspergillus flavus*, that grows most commonly on peanuts and corn in storage; a potent liver carcinogen

Air Quality Index the Environmental Protection Agency's (EPA's) daily rating of local air quality, and associated health concern, for five major air pollutants

airborne transmission (of pathogens) transmission of pathogens in very fine liquid droplets or solid particles (aerosols) remaining suspended in the air for some time

allergen a type of antigen that produces an abnormally vigorous immune response in which the immune system fights off a perceived threat that would otherwise be harmless to the body

allergic rhinitis (hay fever) an allergic reaction in the upper airway, with symptoms of sneezing, runny nose, and watery eyes

allergy a disease in which the immune system mounts an unnecessary response to a foreign, but harmless, substance

alpha particle a particle consisting of two protons plus two neutrons that is ejected from the nucleus of an atom during radioactive decay

alveolar ducts the smallest airways of the lungs, whose walls have many clusters of tiny sacs

alveoli tiny sacs, occurring in clusters as outpocketings of the alveolar ducts, where gas exchange occurs in the lungs

analytic epidemiology epidemiology using a study design intended to test a hypothesized association between risk factor and health outcome

antagonism the occurrence of a joint effect of two exposures that is less than the sum of their individual effects

anthropogenic originating from human activities as opposed to natural sources; manmade

antibiotic resistance bacterial resistance to an antibiotic

antibiotics pharmaceuticals that kill or inhibit bacteria

antibodies special proteins produced as part of the immune system's response to an antigen

antigen a foreign substance, such as a bacteria or virus, that elicits a response from the body's immune system

aquaculture the farming of fish, crustaceans, mollusks, aquatic plants, algae, and other organisms

aqueous solubility the tendency of a chemical to dissolve in water

aquifer geologic material that is porous enough to hold and transmit water

arbovirus (arthropod-borne virus) a virus transmitted by an arthropod

artesian well a well drilled into a confined aquifer in which water under pressure rises without pumping to a level above the top of the aquifer or sometimes above ground level

arthropod any of a group of animals that includes insects (e.g., mosquitoes, flies, lice, and fleas) and arachnids (e.g., ticks, mites, and spiders)

asbestos a durable and noncombustible mineral fiber used as insulation in many products and settings

asbestosis a debilitating fibrotic lung disease

asthma an immune illness in which the bronchi are chronically inflamed and prone to bronchoconstriction

asthma attack a condition in which a person's airways become inflamed, narrow, and swell, and produce extra mucus, making it difficult to breathe

autoimmune disease a condition in which your immune system mistakenly attacks your body

B

bacteria single-celled microorganisms, smaller than protozoa and containing DNA but no true nucleus; some are pathogenic; some are spore-forming

bacterial spore dormant bacterial cell with a hard coating, able to survive inhospitable conditions

bar screen parallel bars that screen out relatively large objects, such as children's toys and dead rats

basal cell carcinoma a type of skin cancer originating in the deeper cells of the epidermis

Becquerel (Bq) unit of radioactivity of a source of radiation (disintegrations per second); replaces Curie's of earlier terminology

beta particle an electron ejected from the nucleus of an atom during radioactive decay

bias in epidemiology, a systematic error in the way subjects were selected or information was gathered

bioaccumulation the building up of a chemical in an individual organism's tissues over its lifetime, as the organism continually takes in more than it excretes

bioassay toxicity test in rodents or other laboratory animals

biochemical oxygen demand (BOD) the demand for oxygen created by the biochemical process of decomposition of organic matter in surface waters receiving sewage wastes

bioconcentration the movement of a chemical from water into the fatty tissues of animals; a biological consequence of a chemical's lipophilic tendency

biohazards see *biological hazards*

biological hazards (or *biohazards*) hazards stemming from living things, most prominently agents of infectious disease

biological vector an organism that is a host species of an infectious disease and which also transmits the disease to one or more other host species (e.g., a mosquito that transmits malaria to humans by biting)

biologically effective dose the quantity of a toxicant (or toxin) or its breakdown product that is available to interact with some vulnerable tissue in the body (not the quantity of a toxicant or its breakdown product that is required to induce a biological effect); measured as a concentration in a specific vulnerable tissue

biomagnification the process by which a chemical becomes more concentrated in the tissues of organisms at each higher level of the food chain within an ecosystem

biomarker a measured change in tissue structure or function within the body, indicating the biological effect of a toxicant

biomass any plant material or animal dung

biomass energy energy stored in plant material or animal dung

biomass fuel any fuel that either consists of biomass or is derived from biomass

biosolids a term coined to refer to treated sewage sludge

biotech gene see *transgene*

biotechnology often used synonymously with genetic engineering but may refer more broadly to applied biological science

bioterrorism the use of pathogens as weapons

bioweapons pathogens that are deliberately transmitted by human action as weapons; or, the means for such transmission

bisphenol A (BPA) a synthetic organic chemical widely used in the production of plastics

black lung pneumoconiosis associated with exposure to coal dust

blood lead action level the blood's lead level at which action should be taken to reduce a child's exposure to lead

blood lead level (BLL) the concentration of lead in blood measured in micrograms of lead per deciliter of blood (μg/dL) and used as a biomarker of children's exposure to lead

blue baby syndrome see *methemoglobinemia*

body burden the total quantity of a chemical present in the body at a given point in time

bottom ash ash produced by a waste-to-energy incinerator which settles to the floor of the furnace

bovine growth hormone (or *bovine somatotropin*) a natural hormone in cows that, among other things, regulates milk production

bovine spongiform encephalopathy (BSE) (or *mad cow disease*) a prion disease of cattle

broiler a chicken raised for its meat

bronchi (singular bronchus) the two cartilaginous airways, one serving each lung, into which the trachea divides

bronchioles small airways formed by the branching of the bronchi

bronchoconstriction a reduction in the diameter of the bronchi caused by muscle constriction

brown lung see *byssinosis*

brownfields contaminated industrial sites

built environment the manmade structures which shape life in urban and suburban settings, including buildings, transportation systems, and public spaces

byssinosis (or *brown lung*) fibrotic lung disease caused by exposure to cotton dust

C

***Campylobacter* species** common bacterial contaminants of raw poultry

cancer a disease of cells in which cells divide without restraint, operating outside of the body's normal controls

cancer latency the period between the exposure that initiates a malignant tumor and the recognition of the cancer

cancer slope factor (CSF) the slope of the dose–response curve for the carcinogenicity of a chemical in humans; specifically, the slope in the low-dose range where human exposures may actually occur; the cancer slope factor has units of incremental risk per unit increase in dose

carbamate insecticides a class of synthetic organic insecticides

carbon footprint the forested area of the Earth's surface required to absorb the carbon dioxide produced through the burning of fossil fuels by an individual or a population with a given lifestyle

carcinogen a substance that increases the risk of cancer

carcinogenesis the process by which cancer occurs in the body

carrying capacity the maximum impact that an ecosystem, or the global environment as a whole, can support for an extended period

case-control study an observational epidemiologic study in which subjects are selected according to their disease status (e.g., lung cancer [cases], no lung cancer [controls]), and then compared on their past exposures to some factor of interest (e.g., cigarette smoking)

case study a research method involving an up-close, in-depth, and detailed examination of a particular case

chelation a treatment for lead poisoning that increases the excretion of circulating lead

chemical hazards environmental hazards that are chemical in nature; many, but not all, are synthetic (manmade) organic chemicals

chloracne a painful and disfiguring skin condition caused by acute exposure to PCBs or dioxins, which can last for months or years

chlorinated hydrocarbon insecticides see *organochlorine insecticides*

chlorofluorocarbons (CFCs) a subgroup of halocarbons containing chlorine, fluorine, and carbon in different combinations; the major cause of stratospheric ozone depletion

chronic exposure a long-term exposure, typically at a low level

chronic obstructive pulmonary disease (COPD) a condition in which breathing is impaired by changes to the airways or alveoli, as in emphysema or chronic bronchitis

chronic rodent bioassay a rodent bioassay lasting about 2 years, approximately the lifetime of the test animals, which provides information on both cancer and noncancer effects

ciguatera poisoning an illness with a range of symptoms caused by eating food, usually warm-water reef fish, contaminated with toxins produced by marine algae

cilia tiny finger-like protrusions of the cells that line the trachea and bronchi

circadian referring to the cycles of roughly 24 hours that occur in various physiological processes

Clostridium botulinum a foodborne pathogen that produces a neurotoxin that can be denatured by heat but is potentially fatal

coagulation and flocculation a step in the treatment of municipal drinking water in which the negative charge of very fine suspended particles is neutralized, allowing the particles to form flocs that settle out

cohort study an observational epidemiologic study in which subjects are selected according to exposure status (e.g., smoker, nonsmoker) and then compared on disease status (e.g., lung cancer, no lung cancer)

combined sewer overflow (CSO) an overflow valve in a combined sewer system that releases some wastewater untreated when the combined flow of municipal wastewater and storm runoff exceeds the capacity of the wastewater treatment plant

comminutor a grinder through which municipal wastewater flows after passing through a bar screen

composting a type of recycling in which organic materials slowly decay into compost that can be used as fertilizer

composting toilet a toilet that stabilizes human waste in a composter that is part of the unit, avoiding the use of water to carry sewage

concentrated animal feeding operation (CAFO) open feedlot (for cattle) or building (for swine and poultry) in which animals are held while being brought to market weight

confined aquifer an aquifer that is sandwiched between layers of impermeable or nearly impermeable rock

confounds factors that fluctuate with the independent variable and whose affects on the dependent variable are subsequently hard to distinguish through empirical observation from the influence of the independent variable

confounding in epidemiology, the mixing of effects that occurs when a third factor is associated both with the risk for the disease and the exposure under investigation

constructed wetland a manmade marsh designed to act as a wastewater treatment system

control rods in the core of a nuclear reactor, rods of a neutron-absorbing material used to slow down the nuclear chain reaction

cosmic radiation the shortest-wavelength electromagnetic radiation, originating in outer space; a type of ionizing radiation

Creutzfeldt-Jakob disease (CJD) a transmissible spongiform encephalopathy that occurs sporadically in humans

criteria air pollutants six widespread air pollutants regulated under the Clean Air Act: carbon monoxide, nitrogen dioxide, sulfur dioxide, particulate matter, lead, and ground-level ozone

critical control point a point in the production of food at which food safety hazards can be controlled or eliminated in the context of a Hazard Analysis and Critical Control Point (HACCP) system

cross-contamination in food safety, the contamination of food after cooking by an implement or a surface previously in contact with the raw food

cross-sectional study an observational epidemiologic study in which the subjects are cross-classified on exposure and health outcome; in this type of prevalence survey design, it may not be clear that exposure preceded outcome

crude incidence rate calculated as the number of new cases that arise in a given population divided by the person-years of observation

Curie see *Becquerel*

D

danger zone in food safety, the temperature range from 40°F to 140°F at which human pathogens can survive and multiply

DDT (dichloro-diphenyl-trichloroethane) an early organochlorine pesticide, still in use in some parts of the world

decibel (dB) unit of intensity (wave amplitude) of sound; a logarithmic, composite, weighted scale

deoxyribonucleic acid (DNA) the hereditary material in the cells of human beings and other organisms

depleted uranium the excess uranium-238 removed from yellowcake through enrichment

dermal contact a major route of exposure to environmental contaminants, through the skin

descriptive epidemiology epidemiologic activities that describe patterns of disease and help formulate hypotheses associating a potential exposure with a specific disease of interest

deterministic effect a (non-cancer) health effect that increases in severity with increasing dose

developmental toxicity the occurrence of an adverse effect on the developing organism in utero, during infancy, or during childhood (i.e., before puberty)

dioxins and furans a large group of structurally related chlorinated compounds that often co-occur; never manufactured, but rather created as byproducts of various chemical processes

direct discharge a discharge of industrial waste to some body of water, separate from the municipal wastewater system

DALY disability adjusted life years; a measure of morbidity or mortality that accounts for the quality of life as affected by disability or disease severity

disease of fecal origin see *infectious diarrheal disease*

disinfection a treatment with the specific objective of killing pathogens

disinfection byproducts (DBPs) organic compounds formed when residual chlorine from the disinfection of drinking water combines with organic matter present in the water

distribution movement of a toxicant (or toxin) around the body via the bloodstream or lymph system

dose the quantification of an exposure

dose–response the magnitude of the response of an organism, as a function of exposure (or doses) to a stimulus or stressor (usually a chemical) after a certain exposure time

dose–response curve the graphical representation of a dose–response relationship, plotting dose on the *x*-axis and response on the *y*-axis, and typically having the shape of a flattened S

dose–response relationship the quantitative relationship between a dose and a toxic effect ("response"), often summarized in a graph

downgradient in the direction of groundwater flow within an aquifer; analogous to downstream in surface water

drainage basin the area drained by a river and the streams that feed it (see also *watershed*)

E

ecologic study an observational epidemiologic study in which all information on health outcomes, exposures, or other characteristics is at the level of the community rather than at the level of the individual

ecological fallacy a limitation of ecologic studies where something observed at the group level fails to be true when assessed with individual-level data

ecological footprint the area on Earth's surface that is required to provide resources for, and absorb the wastes of, an individual or a population with a given lifestyle

ecological overshoot the belief that the human population, or its resource-consumption patterns, has or in the future may rise above the sustainable use of resources

ecosystem a local or regional community of living things (including animals, plants, and microorganisms) and the physical setting in which they live

effect modification in epidemiology, a joint effect of two risk factors that is either greater than or less than the sum of their individual effects

electricity a form of energy resulting from the existence of charged particles (such as electrons or protons), either statically as an accumulation of charge or dynamically as a current.

electricity generation the process of generating electric power from sources of primary energy

electromagnetic radiation energy traveling through space in the form of waves that have electric and magnetic components

electromagnetic spectrum the set of distinct types of electromagnetic radiation, arranged in order of wavelength

electronic waste discarded electrical or electronic devices. Used electronics, which are destined for refurbishment, reuse, resale, salvage recycling through material recovery, or disposal are also considered e-waste.

emerging (or reemerging) infectious diseases infectious diseases that have only recently been identified or are making an unexpected comeback

endemic (adjective, referring to a disease) normally present at a low to moderate level in a given population or location

endocrine-disrupting compound see *endocrine disruptor*

endocrine disruptor (or *endocrine-disrupting compound*) a chemical that interferes in some way with the body's endocrine system (hormone system)

energy conservation reducing the amount of energy consumed

energy efficiency getting more out of energy that is consumed

enrichment (of yellowcake) a process that increases the ratio of uranium-235 to uranium-238 in yellowcake, achieved by removing uranium-238

environment the complex natural system comprising all living things on the earth as well as the elements of the physical setting (air, water, soil, rock) in which they live

environmental epidemiology the use of epidemiologic methods to study environmental hazards to human health

environmental half-life the period of time after which one-half of the original quantity of a chemical in a given environmental medium is expected to have been chemically or biologically transformed

environmental hormone an endocrine disruptor in the environment

environmental impact statement (EIS) a report, required of federal agencies in the executive branch of government under the National

Environmental Policy Act, that discloses and evaluates the environmental impacts of a proposed action

environmental justice narrowly defined, equal protection from environmental health hazards and equal access to governmental decision-making processes for people of all incomes and racial or ethnic groups; more broadly, includes redress of social inequities in the burden of environmental pollution and industrial facilities, especially unjust burdens on people of color

Environmental Kuznets Curve (EKC) a Kuznets curve graphs the hypothesis that as an economy develops, market forces first increase and then decrease economic inequality

environmental modeling mathematical estimation of the concentration of a toxicant at or near the location of exposure, using information from farther back along the exposure pathway

environmental monitoring measurement of the concentration of a toxicant in air, water, or soil

environmental risk management environmental risk management seeks to determine what environmental risks exist and then determine how to manage those risks in a way best suited to protect human health and the environment.

environmental sustainability environmental sustainability is the rate of renewable resource harvest, pollution creation, and nonrenewable resource depletion that can be continued indefinitely. If they cannot be continued indefinitely then they are not sustainable

environmental tobacco smoke (or *second-hand smoke*) cigarette smoke, mostly in indoor air, from smoking by other people

epidemic the occurrence of a disease at an unusually high rate in a population; now sometimes used for chronic as well as infectious diseases; also used as an adjective

epidemiology a quantitative research method for the study of the distribution and determinants of health outcomes in human populations

epigenetics the study of heritable changes in gene expression (active versus inactive genes) that do not involve changes to the underlying DNA

sequence—a change in phenotype without a change in genotype—which in turn affects how cells read the genes

ergotism poisoning caused by eating a toxin produced by the mold ergot

***Escherichia coli* O157:H7** a serotype of the bacteria species *Escherichia coli* and is one of the Shiga-like toxin–producing types of *E. coli*. It is a cause of disease, typically foodborne illness, through consumption of contaminated and raw food, including raw milk and undercooked ground beef

eutrophication an overgrowth of algae and other plant life in surface water, caused by overloading of the nutrients phosphorus and nitrogen

eWaste hazardous waste generated from discarding electronics

excretion removal of a toxicant (or toxin) or its metabolites outside the human envelope by way of exhaled air, urine, feces, or other routes

experimental study a type of epidemiologic study, used to evaluate associations between risk factors and health outcomes, in which the researcher assigns study subjects to different exposure or treatment groups and then gathers information on health outcomes

exposure contact of an environmental toxicant with the human envelope

exposure assessment an applied science comprising methods to measure or estimate human contact with environmental contaminants; in a risk assessment for a chemical or site, an estimation of the exposure of the population(s) of concern to the chemical(s) of concern

exposure modeling the mathematical estimation of exposure, using information or assumptions about contact by ingestion, by inhalation, or through the skin

exposure pathway the pathway linking the environmental source of a contaminant to the point of exposure

externality a cost or impact associated with the use of an environmental resource that is not reflected in the price paid by users benefiting from its usage

extremely low-frequency radiation a type of nonionizing electromagnetic radiation emitted by electric power lines and electrical appliances

F

fate and transport the behavior of contaminants in the environment, including their chemical or physical transformations (fate) and their movements within or between environmental media (transport)

fecal–oral pathway any exposure pathway by which pathogens that cause infectious diarrheal disease are transmitted from feces to the mouth

fibrosis excessive fibrous tissue (scar tissue) in the lungs, causing a loss of flexibility that impairs breathing; fibrotic lung disease

fine particulates generally, particulates 2.5 microns or less in diameter

floc a loose mass of fine particles

fluoridation the addition of fluoride to community drinking water at low concentrations to prevent tooth decay

fluorosis a disfiguring mottling of the teeth caused by an excess of fluoride in drinking water

fly ash ash that is produced by a waste-to-energy incinerator and is captured by pollution control equipment in the smokestack

fomite an inanimate object that passively transmits pathogens in the environment

food additive the U.S. regulatory term for a substance deliberately added to a food during processing to achieve a specific purpose (e.g., a preservative or a sweetener)

food defect the U.S. regulatory term for a foreign substance in food (e.g., insect fragments or rodent hairs)

foodborne illness any infectious illness transmitted in food

foodborne transmission (of pathogens) transmission in food of pathogens from fecal or other sources

formaldehyde a chemical used in many applications and products; a gas at room temperature and a respiratory irritant

fossil fuels (or *hydrocarbon fuels*) fuels formed from decayed plants and animals laid down millions of years ago and then subjected to heat and pressure underground (e.g., coal, petroleum, and natural gas); also refers to fuels derived from fossil fuels (e.g., gasoline)

fracking see *hydraulic fracturing*

fuel a substance that releases energy when it is changed, mostly through burning or nuclear fission

fuel fabrication the production of fuel rods (metal tubes containing pellets of enriched uranium) to be used in nuclear reactors

fungi a simple organism, or living thing, that is neither a plant nor an animal

fungicide a pesticide used against fungi

furans see *dioxins and furans*

G

gamma radiation a high-frequency, ionizing type of electromagnetic radiation emitted from the nucleus of an atom undergoing radioactive decay

genetic engineering the use of technology to create genetically modified organisms

genetic traits inherited characteristics, encoded in an individual's DNA

genetically engineered see *transgenic*

genetically modified (GM) see *transgenic*

geographic information system (GIS) a computerized system combining a database of spatially linked information with application software for spatial analyses and mapping

geothermal energy the Earth's internal heat energy

global carbon cycle the set of natural processes by which carbon moves from the physical environment through living things and back into the physical environment

global climate change the enhancement of the natural greenhouse effect by the production of anthropogenic greenhouse gases, resulting in overall warming and other impacts on climate

global warming the enhancement of the natural greenhouse effect by the production of anthropogenic greenhouse gases; this term has been supplanted in the scientific literature by *global climate change*

Gray (Gy) unit of dose of ionizing radiation (energy delivered per gram of tissue); replaces rads of earlier terminology

green chemistry a preventive approach to reducing chemical hazards, which seeks to eliminate the worst actors altogether; to reduce the overall quantity and toxicity of chemicals produced and used, and wastes generated; and to make products safer

Greenhouse effect The trapping of the sun's warmth in a planet's lower atmosphere, due to the greater transparency of the atmosphere to visible radiation from the sun than to infrared radiation emitted from the planet's surface.

greenhouse gases gases in the troposphere that absorb some of the heat energy radiated outward from the Earth and then reradiate this energy back toward the Earth's surface

grit chamber a step in primary wastewater treatment in which heavier particles such as sand settle out

groundwater water in the saturated zone of an aquifer

gyre large system of circulating ocean currents

H

half-life the time it takes for half the atoms in a sample of a radioactive element to undergo radioactive decay

halogens a group of highly reactive chemicals including chlorine, fluorine, bromine, and iodine

hand-to-mouth exposure exposure to a contaminant in soil or dust that is carried to the lips by the hands (e.g., in eating or smoking)

hand-to-mouth transmission (of pathogens, especially fecal pathogens) transmission of pathogens from feces or soil to the mouth via the hands while eating, smoking, or gesturing

Hazard Analysis and Critical Control Point (HACCP) a systematic approach to food safety that rests on identifying critical control points in the production of food, and then establishing preventive, monitoring, and corrective procedures around these control points

hazard identification in a risk assessment for a chemical, a qualitative evaluation of the toxic effect(s) of a chemical, focused separately on carcinogenicity or on noncancer effects; in a risk assessment for a site, identification of the chemicals contaminating the various environmental media on the site, and characterization of the degree of contamination

hazard index where people are exposed to multiple substances, the sum of the hazard quotients for a set of individual substances affecting the same organ or organ system, ideally through the same toxicological mechanism

hazard quotient the ratio of an actual or estimated dose to a reference dose for an individual substance

hazardous waste under U.S. law, any waste that is corrosive, toxic, ignitable, or reactive; the definition also lists specific commercial chemical products (e.g., pesticides) when they are discarded and some specific wastes from named industries or industrial processes

hazardous waste landfill under current U.S. regulations, a landfill designed and managed specifically to hold hazardous wastes safely; formerly, any landfill in which hazardous wastes had been placed

heavy metal a metal with a high atomic weight; lead, mercury, arsenic, cadmium, and chromium are heavy metals

herbicide a pesticide used against plant pests

herd immunity the practical protection from an infectious disease experienced by a community when enough of its members have immunity against a disease that it becomes difficult to maintain a chain of infection

host (in infectious disease) an organism in which a pathogen becomes established

household hazardous waste any item in household waste that meets the legal definition of hazardous waste

human envelope the envelope that separates the interior of the human body from the exterior environment; in environmental health, refers mostly to the skin, the lining of the gastrointestinal tract, and the lining of the respiratory tract

hybrid car a car that uses both a gasoline-powered combustion engine and electric power

hydraulic fracturing (or *fracking*) a technique for extracting natural gas from shale formations by injecting a mixture of water, sand, and chemicals into a well at high pressures, thus creating many small cracks in the rock so that gas can flow from the well

hydrocarbon fuels see *fossil fuels*

hydrocarbons organic compounds composed of only hydrogen and carbon; methane, propane, and benzene are hydrocarbons

hydrogen fuel cell a device in which a simple chemical reaction converts hydrogen fuel and oxygen into electricity, producing water as a byproduct

hydrologic cycle the complex web of processes through which the Earth's water moves through the environment

hydropower the energy of moving water, captured by a turbine or a water wheel

I

in situ leaching the use of an acidic or alkaline solution to dissolve uranium from the ore in which it is embedded; an alternative to mining

incidence the occurrence of new (incident) cases of a disease in a given population during a given period of time

incidental ingestion inadvertent swallowing of small amounts of water or dust

incremental lifetime cancer risk the additional cancer risk, over a 70-year lifetime, that would result from a particular exposure

indirect discharge a discharge of industrial wastes into the municipal wastewater treatment system

inert ingredient a regulatory term referring to an ingredient that does not serve the primary function of a particular product but rather has some supporting function

infection (foodborne) foodborne illness in which pathogens cause symptoms in the host simply through infection

infectious diarrheal disease (or *disease of fecal origin*) an infectious disease with diarrhea as a major symptom; most often transmitted by the fecal–oral pathway

infectious disease illness caused by microorganisms or worms that become established in a host organism and that can be transmitted to other hosts by various means

informed consent consent by a subject in a research study to participate in the study, after having been informed of the potential risks and benefits of such participation

ingestion a major route of exposure to environmental contaminants, through eating or drinking

inhalation a major route of exposure to environmental contaminants, through ordinary continuous breathing

insecticide a pesticide used against insect or arachnid pests

integrated pest management (IPM) an approach using multiple tactics (e.g., biological and chemical) to manage multiple pests in a manner consistent with ecological principles

intervention study an experimental epidemiologic study in which subjects are randomly assigned to groups receiving different health interventions, and the effectiveness of the interventions is compared across groups

intoxication (foodborne) foodborne illness in which pathogens produce toxins that cause the symptoms of foodborne illness

ionizing radiation radiation that has enough energy to knock an electron out of orbit, creating an ion

isolation the separation of persons who have an infectious illness

isotope a variant of a chemical element; different isotopes of an element have the same number of protons but different numbers of neutrons in their nuclei

K

kuru a transmissible spongiform encephalopathy of humans documented in New Guinea and linked to the ritual eating of body parts of corpses of people also afflicted with the disease

L

lag phase in the growth of a population of bacteria, the first few hours in a new environment, during which time the bacteria multiply only slowly

LD$_{50}$ the dose of a test chemical that is acutely lethal to 50% of test animals exposed to it

leach field (or *drainage field*) as part of a septic system, the area over which wastewater is distributed through a system of perforated pipes

leachate the liquid substance, containing dissolved or suspended materials, that results from leaching

leaching the dissolving or suspension of some components of a substance (e.g., soil or wastes) in water as the water percolates through it

lead a neurotoxic heavy metal

lead paint paint containing the pigment known as white lead, which contains an inorganic lead compound

limiting factor characteristic factors in an environment that regulate the growth and distribution of a species

lipophilic fat-soluble; tending to move from water to an oily medium

liquefied natural gas (LNG) natural gas that has been cooled to a very low temperature, transforming it into liquid form

Listeria monocytogenes a highly fatal foodborne pathogen common in mammals, birds, and soil

log phase a period of logarithmic growth in a population of bacteria, following the lag phase

low-level radioactive wastes radioactive wastes originating from nuclear power production or from other sources (e.g., research, medicine), and which have much lower levels of radioactivity than spent reactor fuel

lowest observed adverse effect level (LOAEL) the lowest dose at which an effect is observed in a chronic rodent bioassay

M

mad cow disease see *bovine spongiform encephalopathy*

malignant melanoma a cancer of melanocytes, cells in the skin that produce pigment (melanin)

mammalian feed ban a ban on feeding any mammalian protein (i.e., meat and bone meal from rendered mammals) to ruminants

materials recovery facility (MRF) a facility where recyclable materials are separated from municipal solid waste (if not separated at curbside) and are sorted by type (e.g., glass, metal, plastic, paper)

Materials Safety Data Sheet (MSDS) a summary of an individual chemical's health effects, which employers must provide to workers under U.S. law; also available to the public

Maximum Contaminant Level (MCL) under U.S. law, the maximum allowable concentration of a specific contaminant in drinking water

mechanical vector an organism that is not a host species of an infectious disease but transmits the disease in mechanical fashion (e.g., a housefly that transfers fecal pathogens that cling to its feet)

meat and bone meal fed to farm animals as a high-protein dietary supplement, shortening the time needed to bring the animals to market. It is also an ingredient in many pet foods.

medical waste waste produced by healthcare facilities; includes some ordinary trash but also items that are infectious, hazardous, or radioactive

megacity an urban conglomeration with at least 10 million inhabitants

mercury a neurotoxic heavy metal that is liquid at room temperature

mesothelioma a cancer of the pleura (the membranes that coat the outsides of the chest organs and the inside of the chest cavity) or the peritoneum (a similar membrane in the abdominal cavity)

metabolism chemical transformation of a toxicant (or toxin) by enzymes in the body

metabolite a product of the body's metabolism of a chemical; a breakdown product

metal an element that is shiny, is solid at room temperature (mercury is an exception), can be melted or formed using heat, and conducts electricity and heat

methemoglobinemia (or *blue baby syndrome* when it occurs in infants) a medical condition in which hemoglobin in the bloodstream is converted into a form that cannot carry oxygen; most common in infants and young children

methicillin-resistant *Staphylococcus aureus* (MRSA) a virulent strain of *Staphylococcus aureus*, widespread in hospitals, that is resistant not only to methicillin but also to related antibiotics including penicillin and amoxicillin

methylmercury a neurotoxic organic mercury compound formed by the action of bacteria on elemental mercury

miasma in early theories of infectious disease causation, an atmospheric emanation that rose from the earth or from rotting organic matter and that caused disease

microwave radiation a nonionizing type of electromagnetic radiation emitted by devices including cellular phones; also used to heat food in microwave ovens

morbidity a nonfatal diseased (morbid) state

mortality the number of deaths in a given population during a given period of time

mucociliary escalator the slow movement of mucus upward in the trachea and bronchi, propelled by cilia beating in unison

municipal solid waste (or *trash*) a community waste stream consisting mainly of paper, plastics, metals, glass, and organic wastes

municipal solid waste landfill under current U.S. regulations, a waste disposal facility in which waste is buried, usually in layers, and with features intended to isolate the wastes from the surrounding environment; formerly, any site where waste was buried

municipal wastewater (see also *sewage*) a community waste stream consisting mainly of urine and feces but including everything that goes down the drain in homes or offices

mutagen an agent that binds chemically to DNA, causing a change in its structure

mutation a change to the DNA of a cell

mycotoxins toxins produced by molds or other fungi

N

nanomaterials see *nanoparticles*

nanoparticles (or *nanomaterials*) engineered particles fewer than 100 nanometers (0.1 microns) in diameter

nanotechnology technology for designing and producing nanoparticles

National Ambient Air Quality Standards (NAAQS) maximum allowable concentrations for the six criteria air pollutants as regulated under the Clean Air Act

National Priorities List a national register of abandoned hazardous waste sites, created under the Comprehensive Environmental Response, Compensation, and Liability Act (Superfund)

no observed adverse effect level (NOAEL) the highest nonzero dose at which no effect is observed in a chronic rodent bioassay

noise unwanted sound; sound that can damage hearing or otherwise harm health

nonionizing radiation radiation that does not have enough energy to knock an electron out of orbit

nonpoint source a U.S. regulatory term referring to a source of water pollution that releases contaminants over a large area

nonrenewable or finite energy resources energy resources that cannot be renewed (produced in nature) on the human time scale

nonselective herbicide an herbicide that kills all types of plants

nuclear fission the splitting of the nucleus of an atom, with the release of energy

nuclear fuel cycle the full sequence of activities related to the production of nuclear power

nuclear power the production of energy through the use of controlled nuclear fission

obesogen foreign chemical compounds that disrupt normal development and balance of lipid metabolism, which, in some cases, can lead to obesity

observational study a type of epidemiologic study, used to evaluate associations between risk factors and health outcomes in which the researcher does not manipulate exposures but rather observes and documents exposures and outcomes

occupational asthma asthma caused by an exposure at work

odds ratio an epidemiologic measure of association appropriate for quantifying the relationship between exposure and disease in case-control study designs

organic chemical any of a large group of chemicals that includes most carbon-containing chemicals

organic farming agriculture employing sustainable practices and does not use synthetic pesticides or commercial fertilizers

organic solvent (or *solvent*) an organic chemical that dissolves other substances

organochlorine insecticides (or *chlorinated hydrocarbon insecticides*) the first generation of synthetic organic insecticides; includes DDT

organophosphate insecticides a class of synthetic organic insecticides

ozone the triatomic form of oxygen (O_3)

ozone layer a layer in the earth's stratosphere at an altitude of about 6.2 miles (10 km) containing a high concentration of ozone, which absorbs most of the ultraviolet radiation reaching the earth from the sun

pandemic an infectious disease epidemic of global proportions; also used as an adjective

paralytic shellfish poisoning an illness with neurologic symptoms caused by eating food, usually mollusks, contaminated with toxins produced by marine algae

parasite an organism that must spend a part of its lifecycle inside an animal host on which it depends for certain benefits, but to which it gives no benefit

particulate matter (PM) or particulates a complex mixture that may consist of both small solid particles and fine liquid droplets, and may include soil particles (dust), sulfates, metals, and organic chemicals; long, narrow fibers, such as asbestos fibers, are considered elongated mineral particles

passive immunity the temporary immunity gained from a vaccine that contains antibodies or from antibodies transported across the placenta to an infant in utero

pathogen an agent that causes a specific infectious disease in a host

perfluorinated compounds (PFCs) see *perfluorochemicals*

perfluorochemicals (or *perfluorinated compounds [PFCs]*) a group of synthetic fluorine-containing chemicals, used in producing nonstick coatings

Permissible Exposure Limit (PEL) under U.S. regulations, the allowable concentration of a specific chemical in workplace air; as an 8-hour time-weighted average, a 15-minute time-weighted average, and a ceiling

persistence the tendency of a chemical to remain in the environment without being transformed into another chemical or chemicals

persistent toxic substances chemicals that are persistent in the environment and known to be toxic to human beings (see text for a discussion of related terms: persistent organic pollutants; persistent, bioaccumulative, and toxic chemicals; and ubiquitous bioaccumulative toxins)

personal care product a product that people apply to their bodies for the sake of physical comfort and/or physical appearance

personal monitoring measurement of the concentration of a toxicant in an individual's personal environment

personal protective equipment equipment worn by a worker to reduce exposure to workplace hazards; for example, goggles, ear protectors, and respirators

pest any animal or plant judged to interfere with people's well-being or interests (not a biological category)

pesticide any chemical used to kill pests

pesticide resistance the capacity of a pest to survive exposure to a pesticide as a result of its genetic makeup

pesticide tolerance in the U.S. regulatory framework, the maximum pesticide residue allowed in human food

photochemical smog smog created through a complex series of chemical reactions among nitrogen oxides, volatile organic compounds, and other chemicals in the presence of sunlight

photovoltaic cell (or *solar cell*) a device that converts sunlight directly into electrical energy

phthalates a group of semivolatile synthetic organic chemicals used as plasticizers

physical hazards hazards that stem from contact with some form of energy; for example, radiation and noise

plasticizers chemicals used in manufacturing plastics to make them flexible (i.e., plastic)

plastics a large group of materials made with high-molecular-weight synthetic organic chemicals, which have at least some flexibility (plasticity) and can be formed into items of almost any shape (e.g., three-dimensional objects, thin sheets, filaments)

plume a trail of smoke in air, or of a chemical in groundwater, which becomes broader and less concentrated with increasing distance from the source

PM$_{10}$ particulate matter 10 microns or fewer in diameter

PM$_{2.5}$ particulate matter 2.5 microns or fewer in diameter

pneumoconiosis fibrosis formed as a reaction to a physical irritant such as particulates and thus associated with exposure to dust or other particulate matter

point-of-use treatment system a treatment device for drinking water (e.g., a carbon filter) installed at a single tap, such as the faucet at the kitchen sink

point source a U.S. regulatory term referring to a source of water pollution that releases contaminants at a specific location

polluter-pays principle the idea that the party responsible for pollution should pay the costs of remediation

pollution any output of human activity that is considered harmful or unpleasant; historically referred mostly to chemical wastes, smoke, and dust, but by extension used to refer to, for example, radiation, unwanted sights or sounds, or genetically modified plant species

polybrominated diphenyl ethers (PBDEs) a large group of structurally related synthetic brominated compounds, used mainly as flame retardants

polychlorinated biphenyls (PCBs) a group of high-molecular-weight synthetic organic chemicals, used mainly to insulate electrical devices

polycyclic aromatic hydrocarbons (PAHs) a group of related organic compounds that are products of incomplete combustion and are ubiquitous in the environment

potable water water deemed suitable for drinking

precautionary principle the concept that early indications that a substance or activity causes serious harm should trigger precautionary measures before harm is proven

pretreatment (of industrial wastes) treatment of industrial wastes before they enter a municipal wastewater system

prevalence the proportion of a population that has a disease at a given point in time

primary clarifier a step in primary wastewater treatment in which suspended solids containing organic matter settle out

primary prevention in public health, steps taken to prevent a health outcome from occurring (e.g., through the elimination of an exposure)

primary sewage treatment a mechanical process during which ever-finer materials are removed from municipal wastewater through a sequence of steps

prion a type of protein found on the surface of normal nerve cells of some mammalian species; abnormal prions cause a set of degenerative brain diseases called transmissible spongiform encephalopathies

protozoa single-celled microorganisms with a true nucleus containing DNA; some are pathogenic and parasitic

pufferfish a fish in which some organs may contain potentially fatal neurotoxins

pyrethroid insecticides a class of synthetic organic insecticides

pyrethrum a pesticide extracted from chrysanthemums

Q

quarantine the separation of persons who have been exposed to an infectious agent and may become ill

R

rad see *Gray*

radiation energy that is radiated from a source as particles or as waves

radiation sickness the set of symptoms caused by high-level exposure to radiation, characterized by effects on the central nervous system, the gastrointestinal tract, and the bone marrow

radioactive exhibiting radioactive decay

radioactive decay the spontaneous ejection of a part of the nucleus of an atom

radiolytic chemical a chemical created by the action of radiation

radionuclide a radioactive isotope

radon a gaseous radioactive element in the decay chain of uranium-238

radura the symbol used to signify that food has been irradiated

recharge the replenishing of water in an aquifer by water trickling downward through the zone of aeration

recharge area the area on the ground surface through which rainfall feeds an aquifer

recombinant bovine growth hormone (rBGH) a genetically engineered version of bovine growth hormone

recycling separating and processing of waste materials so that they can be used again

reference dose (RfD) a dose expected to have no adverse effects in people who are particularly sensitive to the chemical's effects and who are exposed over a 70-year lifetime; the reference dose has units mg/(kg × day)

regulatory toxicology toxicity testing done in support of regulatory decision making

relative biological effectiveness (RBE) a factor used in radiation dosimetry to adjust for the fact that some types of radiation do more damage to tissue than others, per unit of energy delivered

relative risk (RR) relative risk is used in the statistical analysis of the data of experimental, cohort, and cross-sectional studies, to estimate the strength of the association between treatments or risk factors, and outcomes

rem see *Sievert*

rendering the heating of animal remains in batches for the purpose of separating fat from other material

renewable energy source an energy source that is either continually renewed in nature or can readily be renewed through human effort

reprocessing (of spent nuclear fuel) extracting remaining uranium-238 from nuclear power plant wastes and fabricating it again into fuel pellets to be used in a reactor

reproductive toxicity the occurrence of an adverse effect on the reproductive system or reproductive capacity of an organism

reservoir a natural or artificial place where water is collected and stored for use, especially water for supplying a community, irrigating land, furnishing power, etc. A receptacle or chamber for holding a liquid or fluid

respirable particulates generally, particulates 10 microns or fewer in diameter

respiratory bronchioles very small conducting airways formed by the branching of the bronchioles

ricin a potent toxin produced by the castor bean plant

risk assessment an applied science consisting of formal procedures for evaluating and integrating scientific information on exposure and toxicity to estimate the real-world public health risk of a hazard

risk communication the provision or exchange of information about environmental health hazards; more broadly, public participation in research or policymaking

risk factor a factor that has been shown to pose a risk of a specific harm

risk management actions taken to prevent or mitigate environmental health hazards; the process balances risks, benefits, and costs, and also considers social context

rodenticide a pesticide used against rodents

routes of exposure routes by which people contact and absorb environmental contaminants (mainly inhalation, ingestion, and dermal contact)

ruminant an animal that has a multichambered stomach and regurgitates and rechews previously swallowed food

ruminant feed ban a ban on feeding ruminant protein (i.e., meat and bone meal from rendered ruminants) to ruminants

S

Salmonella (nontyphoid species) common bacterial contaminants of raw poultry

sand filter a filter in which water trickles gently through a bed of sand, driven by gravity; used in drinking water treatment

sanitation the control of environmental factors, especially human waste and food waste, to prevent disease and promote health

saturated zone the underground zone below the zone of aeration in which all pore spaces are filled with water and in which water can move in any direction

scombroid poisoning foodborne poisoning by a toxin produced by certain types of bacteria, usually associated with the spoilage of tuna and related fish

scrapie a transmissible spongiform encephalopathy that affects sheep

secondary pest outbreak a rapid increase in the population of a pest that was the prey of a target pest following the application of a pesticide to kill the target pest

secondary pollutant a pollutant formed in the environment through the chemical transformation of the original pollutant

secondary prevention in public health, steps taken to prevent a health problem from progressing (e.g., through early detection of disease)

secondary sewage treatment a biological process in which bacteria digest organic wastes in an aerobic environment

secondhand smoke see *environmental tobacco smoke*

sedimentation a step in the treatment of municipal drinking water in which flocs are allowed to settle out by gravity

selective herbicide an herbicide either kills broad-leaved plant species but not plants in the grass family or the reverse

sensitization an immune response on first exposure to a specific allergen, after which any future exposure to this allergen will produce an allergic response

sentinel illness an illness caused solely (or almost solely) by exposure to a single substance and which is, therefore, considered a marker of exposure to that substance

septic system a system, consisting of a septic tank and a leach field, used for the on-site treatment of household wastewater

septic tank a buried steel or concrete holding tank that receives wastewater from a building or buildings

sewage urine and fecal waste; but often used interchangeably with *municipal wastewater*

sewage sludge material that originates as sludge and scum removed from the municipal wastewater stream during primary and sometimes secondary treatment

shipbreaking the dismantling of oceangoing vessels to obtain scrap metal

sick building a building whose occupants report a range of nonspecific symptoms when they are in the building

sick building syndrome the set of nonspecific symptoms reported by occupants of a so-called sick building

Sievert (Sv) unit of dose of ionizing radiation (energy delivered per gram of tissue), weighted by the relative biological effectiveness of the radiation; replaces rems of earlier terminology

silicosis pneumoconiosis associated with exposure to silica

slope (of a dose–response curve) the increase in toxic response for a given increase in dose

sludge digester a large tank, used in sewage sludge treatment, in which thickened sludge is digested by anaerobic organisms in a warm, well-circulated environment

smog (a contraction of smoke and fog) visible air pollution; or photochemical smog specifically

social or behavioral hazards hazards that originate in a person's social circumstances or from the person's own behaviors

solar cell see *photovoltaic cell*

solar power the energy in sunlight, captured using various technologies

solvent see *organic solvent*

source reduction (or *waste prevention*) an approach to managing pollution by reducing the amount of waste produced

sprawl the style of development typical of modern U.S. suburbs, which is of relatively low density overall and in which major land uses are generally separated rather than intermixed

squamous cell carcinoma type of skin cancer that originates in the most superficial cells of the epidermis

stabilization (of sewage sludge) the second step in the treatment of sewage sludge; digestion of sludge by anaerobic organisms in a warm, well-circulated environment

standardized rate (SR) the rate of disease (or death) that would occur in a given location if it had the age distribution of some reference population but its age-specific rates were unchanged

standardized rate ratio (SRR) the ratio of two standardized rates, both of which are standardized to the same reference population

stakeholders a person or group with an interest or concern associated with an environmental risk management decision

Staphylococcus aureus a common foodborne pathogen that is a normal inhabitant of human skin

statistically significant of a statistical association; unlikely to be due to chance alone (according to an agreed upon criterion)

stochastic effect a health effect whose probability of occurring increases with increasing dose; typically refers to cancer risks

stratosphere the layer of the Earth's atmosphere above the troposphere, reaching to an altitude of about 30 miles (48 kilometers)

strip mining see *surface mining*

subchronic rodent bioassay a 90-day rodent bioassay, conducted as a preliminary to a chronic bioassay

Superfund colloquial name for the Comprehensive Environmental Response, Compensation, and Liability Act; also refers to the fund for the cleanup of abandoned hazardous waste sites created by this law

surface mining (or *strip mining*) a coal-mining technique in which the earth overlying a seam of coal is removed

surface water water located on top of the Earth's surface such as in lakes, rivers, creeks, and wetlands

surveillance the tracking of disease or injury rates and the comparison of rates over time or across places or diseases; a type of descriptive epidemiology

surveillance biomonitoring biomonitoring undertaken at the population level as a means of surveillance

sustainable development development capable of being maintained indefinitely within the constraints of an ecosystem or the global environment

synergism the occurrence of a joint effect of two exposures that is greater than the sum of their individual effects

synthetic organic chemical any manufactured organic chemical

T

tallow the animal fat product of the rendering process

target organ in toxicity testing, the organ that is affected first as the dose of a test chemical is increased from zero (not an organ that a toxic chemical seeks out in the body)

target pest the specific pest that is the target of a pesticide application

target pest resurgence the rebounding of the target pest population after the population of a natural predator is reduced through the use of a pesticide

temperature inversion a local weather condition in which a mass of cooler, heavier air becomes trapped at ground level beneath a layer of warmer, less dense air

teratogenic agent or teratogen an agent that may cause embryonic or fetal malformations

teratogenesis the occurrence of a structural defect in the developing organism as a result of an exposure that occurs between conception and birth

tertiary sewage treatment specialized treatment technologies, used after primary and secondary sewage treatment, and tailored to local needs

thermohaline circulation the global circulation of deep ocean waters along predictable paths, driven mainly by differences in the density of the

water related to temperature (thermo) and salinity (haline)

thickening (of sewage sludge) the first step in the treatment of sewage sludge, usually accomplished by centrifuging or adding coagulants

threshold (of a dose–response curve) the highest dose at which no toxic effect occurs

Threshold Limit Value (TLV) concentration of a specific chemical in workplace air that is expected to be without material adverse health effect; published by ACGIH

threshold shift in an individual person, an upward shift in the threshold at which sound of a certain frequency can be perceived; a marker of hearing loss

tinnitus a continuous ringing, roaring, or other sound in the ears that occurs after exposure to loud noise

toxicant a toxic substance that results from human activities; also, naturally occurring agents that are not produced by a plant or animal

toxicity poisonous effect; harm to the body

toxicity testing the practical work of assessing chemicals' toxicity to living things

toxicodynamics the processes that constitute the effects of a toxicant in the body; changes in tissue structure or function, and the resulting adverse effects on health

toxicokinetic modeling estimation of the ultimate disposition of a chemical from what is known about its absorption, distribution, metabolism, storage, and excretion

toxicokinetics the combined processes of absorption, distribution, metabolism, storage, and excretion

toxicology the study of the adverse effects of toxic agents (both chemicals, including natural toxins, and physical hazards, such as fibers or radiation) on the normal structure and function of biological systems

Toxics Release Inventory (TRI) a publicly available online database of the quantities of chemicals released to air or water, placed on land, or transferred offsite by industrial facilities

toxics use reduction a preventive approach that calls for both the use of less toxic chemicals and the use of smaller quantities of toxic chemicals

toxin a naturally produced toxic substance, especially one produced by a plant or animal

trachea the cartilaginous windpipe below the larynx, considered a part of the lower respiratory system

transgene (or *biotech gene*) a gene that codes for a desired characteristic and that is transferred from the DNA of one species into the DNA of the species being modified (e.g., corn)

transgenic (or *genetically engineered* or *genetically modified*) modified by the insertion of a transgene

transpiration a process through which water taken up by the roots of plants is released to the atmosphere through their leaves

trash see *municipal solid waste*

trickling filter in secondary sewage treatment, a bed of rocks coated with bacteria-containing slime over which municipal wastewater is sprayed and allowed to trickle downward to facilitate bacterial digestion of organic wastes

trihalomethanes (THMs) a family of chemicals that are common disinfection byproducts

troposphere the innermost layer of the Earth's atmosphere, extending to an altitude of approximately 8 miles (13 kilometers)

turbidity the cloudiness of water; specifically, a measure of how much the transmission of light through water is impaired

U

ultrafine particulates generally, particulates 0.1 microns or fewer in diameter

ultraviolet radiation a form of electromagnetic radiation that includes both ionizing wavelengths (UV-C radiation) and nonionizing wavelengths (UV-A and UV-B)

uncertainty factor a multiplier, used in deriving a reference dose, to set the reference dose lower (i.e., to make it more protective) to account for a specific limitation in the available toxicity data

unconfined aquifer (or *water table aquifer*) an aquifer in which the recharge area is directly above the aquifer, with no intervening impermeable layer

upgradient in the direction opposite to the direction of groundwater flow within an aquifer; analogous to upstream in surface water

uranium a radioactive metallic element used as fuel in nuclear power reactors

uranium mill tailings depleted uranium ore in the form of sandy sludge, a waste of the production of yellowcake

uranium mine tailings crushed rock wastes of uranium mining

V

vaccine an antigen preparation administered to a person to produce an immune response without causing illness

vaccine-preventable diseases the set of diseases for which a vaccine is presently available

variant Creutzfeldt-Jakob disease (vCJD) a transmissible spongiform encephalopathy of humans, linked to eating beef from cattle afflicted with bovine spongiform encephalopathy

vector (of infectious disease) any living transmitter of pathogens

vectorborne disease an infectious disease that is transmitted by biological vector

vermicomposting indoor composting of plant-based food scraps by worms housed in a bin

virus a parasite consisting of a strand of DNA or RNA with a coat of protein; cannot reproduce without a host organism

volatile organic compound (VOC) a naturally occurring or manmade organic compound that volatilizes significantly at ordinary environmental temperatures

volatility the tendency of a liquid chemical to change into gaseous form (i.e., to volatilize)

volume threshold the lowest volume at which sound at a given frequency can be heard

W

waste prevention see *source reduction*

waste-to-energy (WTE) incineration burning of municipal solid waste in an incinerator that also generates energy

waterborne illness caused by recreational or drinking water contaminated by disease-causing microbes or pathogens

waterborne transmission a highly effective means for spreading infectious agents to a large portion of the population through various bodies of water

water table the boundary between the zone of aeration and the saturated zone

waterborne illness any infectious disease transmitted in drinking water; often fecal in origin

waterborne transmission (of infectious disease) the transmission of pathogens, often pathogens of fecal origin, in water used for drinking

watershed in environmental health, the area drained by a river and the streams that feed it (synonymous with drainage basin); in common speech, also refers to the divide between two drainage basins

weed a plant pest

weight-of-the-evidence categories a set of categories describing the likely human carcinogenicity of a chemical, based on the total body of scientific evidence

wind farm a group of wind turbines installed together

wind power the energy of moving air, captured by a wind turbine

worms multicellular (helminthic) organisms ranging widely in size, but all visible to the naked eye; some are parasitic and pathogenic

X

xenobiotics anthropogenic substances found in the environment that mimic the function of human hormones or other metabolic enzymes

xenoestrogen an environmental chemical that mimics the effect of estrogen in the human body

X-rays an ionizing form of electromagnetic radiation, widely used for medical imaging

Y

yellowcake the uranium concentrate that is extracted from uranium ore through milling

Z

zone of aeration a subsurface zone within which the pore spaces are partly filled by water and water moves only downward

zoonosis an infectious disease that can be transmitted to humans from nonhuman animals, either domestic or wild

Index

Note: Page numbers followed by *f* and *t* indicate material in figures and tables respectively.

Turbidity, 240
Type 1 Diabetes (T1D), 81
Typhus, 77

U

Ultrafine particulates, 194, 196
Ultraviolet radiation, 88, 92, 150–152, 192, 266
Uncertainty factors in risk assessment, 40
Unconfined aquifer, 14
UNHCR. *See* U.N.'s High Commissioner for Refugees
United Kingdom, 118, 119
United Nations Environment Programme, 200
United Nations World Commission on Environment and Development, 60
United States
    air pollution in, 139–140, 140*f*
    CAFOs profile in, 111–112
    community water systems in, 247
    ecological footprint of, 271
    environmental health agencies and organizations, 54–55*t*
    industrial pollution and workplace exposures in, 167–171, 168*f*, 170*f*
    Kyoto Protocol and, 203–204
    leaded gasoline in, 191
    phthalates, 143
    precautionary principle and, 49
    recycling, 253
    regulation of drinking water in, 251
    regulation of municipal solid waste in, 258, 259*f*
Unsaturated zone, 13
U.N. Scientific Committee on the Effects of Atomic Radiation (UNSCEAR), 266
U.N.'s High Commissioner for Refugees (UNHCR), 94
Uranium, 86–87, 208–210, 210–211, 210*f*, 213–217, 221
Uranium-238 decay chain, 88*t*
Uranium Mill Tailings Radiation Control Act, 221
Uranium mine and mill tailings, 210
Urban community garden, 128*f*
Urban metabolism, 236, 261
Urban settings, in less developed countries, 260–261

U.S. Consumer Product Safety Commission, 55*t*
U.S. Department of Agriculture, 55*t*, 223
U.S. Department of Energy, 55*t*
U.S. Department of Health and Human Services, 54*t*
U.S. Department of Labor, 55*t*
U.S. Environmental Protection Agency (EPA), 55*t*, 204
U.S. farming. Survey data from the Department of Agriculture (USDA), 105, 129
    organic seal, 130*f*
U.S. General Accounting Office (GAO), 168
U.S. Geological Survey, 109
U.S. Nuclear Regulatory Commission, 55*t*

V

Vaccine-preventable diseases, 82
Vaccines, 80
Vadose, 13
Variant Creutzfeld-Jakob disease (vCJD), 119, 120
    risk factor for, 119
Varicella, 82
vCJD. *See* Variant Creutzfeld-Jakob disease
Vector, 67
Vectorborne disease, 76, 203
Vectorborne transmission of infectious disease, 76–78
Venereal diseases, 68
Vermicomposting, 255
Vibrio cholerae, 4
Vinyl chloride, 206
Virus, 66, 66*f*
Volatile organic compounds (VOCs), 189–193, 189*t*, 190*f*, 192*t*, 206
Volatility of chemicals, 15
Volume threshold, 164

W

Waste prevention, 173, 253–255
Wastes
    animals, 114
    of slaughterhouse, 118
Waste-to-energy (WTE) incineration, 253, 255
Wastewater management
    industrial wastes and, 239–240

in municipalities, 238, 238*f*, 241
    regulation of, 246–247
    sewage treatment and, 240–244
    storm runoff and, 238–239, 239*f*
Water. *See also* Drinking water supply and treatment
    crop production consumption, 109
    environmental contaminants and, 10–15
    fresh water, 12–15
    global hydrologic cycle, 10–11
    municipal supplies, 236–238
    nonfecal organisms in, 71–72
    ocean waters, 11–12
Waterborne illness, 69
Waterborne transmission of disease, 69
Water-quality violations, 57
Water source in Jakarta, 261
Water table, 13
Water table aquifer, 14
Watson, James, 19
Weeds, 99
Weight-of-the-evidence categories for carcinogenicity, 41*t*
Wells, private, 250
West Nile virus, 76
WHO. *See* World Health Organization
Wholesome Meat Act, 128, 130
Whooping cough, 68, 82, 83
Wild fish stocks, 122
Wind farms, 225
Windmills, 224*f*
Wind patterns, 9
Wind power, 224
Wind turbine, 225*f*
Workers
    CAFO, 115–117
    global disparity in protections for, 169–170, 169*f*, 170*f*
Workers health, 171–172
Workplace
    exposures in United States, 167–169, 168*f*
    hazards in, 159–166
World Health Organization (WHO), 54, 79, 92, 94
    on DDT, 103
    on irrigation and water supply, 109
    on malnutrition, 83
World Meteorological Organization, 200
Worms, 64, 65*f*
    in recycling, 255
WTE incineration. *See* Waste-to-energy incineration